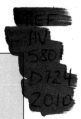

W9-BNH-153

Learning Disabilities Sourcebook, 3rd Edition

Leukemia Sourcebook

Liver Disorders Sourcebook

Lung Disorders Sourcebook

Medical Tests Sourcebook, 3rd Edition

Men's Health Concerns Sourcebook, 2nd Edition

Mental Health Disorders Sourcebook, 4th Edition

Mental Retardation Sourcebook

Movement Disorders Sourcebook, 2nd Edition

Multiple Sclerosis Sourcebook

Muscular Dystrophy Sourcebook

Obesity Sourcebook

Osteoporosis Sourcebook

Pain Sourcebook, 3rd Edition

Pediatric Cancer Sourcebook

Physical & Mental Issues in Aging Sourcebook

Podiatry Sourcebook, 2nd Edition

Pregnancy & Birth Sourcebook, 2nd Edition

Prostate & Urological Disorders Sourcebook

Prostate Cancer Sourcebook

Reconstructive & Cosmetic Surgery Sourcebook

Rehabilitation Sourcebook

Respiratory Disorders Sourcebook, 2nd Edition

Sexually Transmitted Diseases Sourcebook, 3rd Edition

Sleep Disorders Sourcebook, 3rd Edition

Smoking Concerns Sourcebook

Sports Injuries Sourcebook, 3rd Edition

Stress-Related Disorders Sourcebook, 2nd Edition

Stroke Sourcebook, 2nd Edition

Surgery Sourcebook, 2nd Edition

Thyroid Disorders Sourcebook

Transplantation Sourcebook

Traveler's Health Sourcebook

Urinary Tract & Kidney Diseases & Disorders Sourcebook, 2nd Edition

Vegetarian Sourcebook

Women's Health Concerns Sourcebook, 3rd Edition

Workplace Health & Safety Sourcebook

Worldwide Health Sourcebook

Teen Health Series

Abuse & Violence Information for Teens

Accident & Safety Information for Teens

Alcohol Information for Teens, 2nd Edition

Allergy Information for Teens

Asthma Information for Teens, 2nd Edition

Body Information for Teens

Cancer Information for Teens

Complementary & Alternative Medicine Information for Teens

Diabetes Information for Teens

Diet Information for Teens, 2nd Edition

Drug Information for Teens, 3rd Edition

Eating Disorders Information for Teens, 2nd Edition

Fitness Information for Teens, 2nd Edition

Learning Disabilities Information for Teens

Mental Health Information for Teens, 3rd Edition

Pregnancy Information for Teens

Sexual Health Information for Teens, 2nd Edition

Skin Health Information for Teens, 2nd Edition

Sleep Information for Teens

Sports Injuries Information for Teens, 2nd Edition

Stress Information for Teens

Suicide Information for Teens, 2nd Edition

Tobacco Information for Teens, 2nd Edition

Drug Abuse

SOURCEBOOK

Third Edition

Health Reference Series

Third Edition

Drug Abuse
SOURCEBOOK

*Basic Consumer Health Information about the Abuse of
Cocaine, Club Drugs, Hallucinogens, Heroin, Inhalants,
Marijuana, and Other Illicit Substances, Prescription
Medications, and Over-the-Counter Medicines*

*Along with Facts about Addiction and Related
Health Effects, Drug Abuse Treatment and Recovery,
Drug Testing, Prevention Programs, Glossaries of
Drug-Related Terms, and Directories of Resources
for More Information*

Edited by
Joyce Brennfleck Shannon

Omnigraphics

P.O. Box 31-1640, Detroit, MI 48231

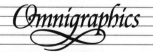

Bibliographic Note

Because this page cannot legibly accommodate all the copyright notices, the Bibliographic Note portion of the Preface constitutes an extension of the copyright notice.

Edited by Joyce Brennfleck Shannon

Health Reference Series

Karen Bellenir, *Managing Editor*
David A. Cooke, MD, FACP, *Medical Consultant*
Elizabeth Collins, *Research and Permissions Coordinator*
Cherry Edwards, *Permissions Assistant*
EdIndex, Services for Publishers, *Indexers*

* * *

Omnigraphics, Inc.

Matthew P. Barbour, *Senior Vice President*
Kevin M. Hayes, *Operations Manager*

* * *

Peter E. Ruffner, *Publisher*

Copyright © 2010 Omnigraphics, Inc.
ISBN 978-0-7808-1079-2

Library of Congress Cataloging-in-Publication Data

Drug abuse sourcebook : basic consumer health information about the abuse of cocaine, club drugs, hallucinogens, heroin, inhalants, marijuana, and other illicit substances, prescription medications, and over-the-counter medicines ... / edited by Joyce Brennfleck Shannon. -- 3rd ed.
    p. cm. -- (Health reference series)
  Includes bibliographical references and index.
  Summary: "Provides basic consumer health information about the abuse of illegal drugs and misuse of prescription and over-the-counter medications, with facts about addiction, treatment, and recovery. Includes index, glossary of related terms and directory of resources"--Provided by publisher.
  ISBN 978-0-7808-1079-2 (hardcover : alk. paper) 1. Drug abuse--Prevention--Handbooks, manuals, etc. 2. Drug abuse--Treatment--Handbooks, manuals, etc. 3. Drug addiction--Treatment--Handbooks, manuals, etc. I. Shannon, Joyce Brennfleck.
  HV5801.D724 2010
  362.29--dc22
                                                                    2010000748

Printed in the United States

Table of Contents

Visit www.healthreferenceseries.com to view *A Contents Guide to the Health Reference Series*, a listing of more than 15,000 topics and the volumes in which they are covered.

Preface xiii

Part I: Facts about Drug Abuse in the United States

Chapter 1—Prevalence of Illicit Drug Use
            and Substance Abuse 3

Chapter 2—Drug Abuse Cost to Society 11

Chapter 3—Deaths from Drug Overdoses 15

Chapter 4—The Controlled Substances Act 21

Chapter 5—Purchasing Controlled Substances 29

            Section 5.1—Prescriptions for
                         Controlled Substances 30

            Section 5.2—Online Dispensing and
                         Purchasing of Controlled
                         Substances 33

            Section 5.3—Facts about Medical
                         Marijuana 36

Chapter 6—Combat Methamphetamine
            Epidemic Act 41

Chapter 7—Initiation of Substance Use 45

Chapter 8—Substance Abuse and Children 53

       Section 8.1—Prenatal Exposure to Illicit
                Drugs and Alcohol 54

       Section 8.2—Drug Endangered Children 59

Chapter 9—Adolescents at Risk for Substance
             Use Disorders 65

Chapter 10—Adolescent Drug Abuse 73

       Section 10.1—Teen Use of Illicit
                Drugs Is Declining 74

       Section 10.2—Prescription and Over-the-
                Counter Drug Abuse 75

       Section 10.3—Impact of Nonmedical
                Stimulant Use 80

       Section 10.4—Teen Marijuana Use
                Worsens Depression 83

Chapter 11—Women, Girls, and Drugs 87

Chapter 12—Minorities and Drugs 93

Chapter 13—Substance Use in the Workplace 97

Chapter 14—Drug Use and Crime 101

Chapter 15—Drugged Driving 107

Part II: Drugs of Abuse

Chapter 16—2C-I 115

Chapter 17—Anabolic Steroids 119

Chapter 18—Blue Mystic 123

Chapter 19—Buprenorphine 127

Chapter 20—BZP 131

Chapter 21—Clenbuterol 135

Chapter 22—Cocaine and Crack Cocaine 139

Chapter 23—Dextromethorphan (DXM) 145

Chapter 24—DMT 149

Chapter 25—Downers 153

Chapter 26—Ecstasy (MDMA) 155

Chapter 27—Fentanyl 161

Chapter 28—Foxy 165

Chapter 29—Gamma Hydroxybutyrate (GHB) 167

Chapter 30—Heroin 171

Chapter 31—Human Growth Hormone 177

Chapter 32—Kava 181

Chapter 33—Ketamine 185

Chapter 34—Khat 189

Chapter 35—Kratom 193

Chapter 36—Lysergic Acid Diethylamide (LSD) 197

Chapter 37—Marijuana, Hashish, and Hash Oil 201

Chapter 38—Methadone 207

Chapter 39—Methamphetamine 213

Chapter 40—Oxycodone 217

Chapter 41—PCP 221

Chapter 42—Ritalin and Other ADHD Medications:
            Methylphenidate and Amphetamines 225

Chapter 43—*Salvia Divinorum* and Salvinorin A 231

Chapter 44—Spirals 235

Chapter 45—Toonies (Nexus) 239

Part III: The Causes and Consequences of Drug Abuse and Addiction

Chapter 46—Understanding Drug Abuse and Addiction 245

Chapter 47—Factors That Impact Drug Abuse
            and Addiction 251

Chapter 48—How Drugs Affect the Brain 259

Chapter 49—Uses and Effects of Drugs That Are Abused 263

Chapter 50—Misuse of Over-the-Counter Cough
and Cold Medications 269

Chapter 51—Nonmedical Use and Abuse of Prescription
Drugs 273

Section 51.1—Scientific Research on
Prescription Drug Abuse 274

Section 51.2—Pain Reliever Abuse 278

Section 51.3—Tranquilizer Abuse 282

Section 51.4—Stimulant Abuse 285

Section 51.5—Sedative Abuse 288

Chapter 52—Mixing Alcohol and Other Drugs 293

Section 52.1—Risk of Substance
Dependence following
Initial Use of Alcohol or
Illicit Drugs 294

Section 52.2—Simultaneous Polydrug Use ... 298

Section 52.3—Alcohol Abuse Makes
Prescription Drug Abuse
More Likely 302

Chapter 53—Am I an Addict? 305

Chapter 54—Medical Consequences of Drug Addiction 309

Chapter 55—Club Drugs' Health Effects 313

Chapter 56—Health Effects of Hallucinogens:
Ecstasy, LSD, Peyote, Psilocybin, and PCP 317

Chapter 57—Impact of Inhalants on the Brain and Health 323

Chapter 58—Adverse Health Effects of Marijuana Use 329

Chapter 59—Drug Abuse and Infectious Disease 333

Section 59.1—Link to Human Immun-
odeficiency Virus (HIV)/
Acquired Immunodeficiency
Syndrome (AIDS) and Other
Infectious Diseases 334

Section 59.2—Syringe Exchange Programs 337

Chapter 60—Comorbidity (Dual Diagnosis):
Addiction and Other Mental Illnesses 341

Chapter 61—Serious Psychological Distress (SPD)
and Substance Use Disorder 347

    Section 61.1—SPD and Substance Use
among Veterans 348

    Section 62.2—Higher Rates of Substance
Use among Young Adult Men
with SPD 351

Chapter 62—Suicide, Severe Depression, and
Substance Use 355

Part IV: Drug Abuse Treatment and Recovery

Chapter 63—Recognizing Drug Use 365

    Section 63.1—Signs and Symptoms
of Drug Use.............................. 366

    Section 63.2—Drug Paraphernalia 372

Chapter 64—Drug Abuse First Aid.. 375

Chapter 65—How People View Addictions and Recovery........ 379

Chapter 66—Brief Guide to Intervention 383

Chapter 67—Treatment Approaches for Drug Addiction 389

Chapter 68—Detoxification: One Part of Substance
Abuse Treatment... 395

Chapter 69—Withdrawal from Drugs 401

Chapter 70—Mutual Support Groups for Alcohol
and Drug Abuse.. 407

Chapter 71—Treatment for Methamphetamine Abusers 415

Chapter 72—Therapy That Reduces Drug Abuse among
Patients with Severe Mental Illness 419

Chapter 73—Drug Abuse Treatment in the Criminal
Justice System... 427

    Section 73.1—Drug Courts 428

    Section 73.2—Treating Drug Abuse
Offenders Benefits Public
Health and Safety 432

Chapter 74—Employee Assistance Programs (EAPs)
for Substance Abuse 437

Section 74.1—Addressing Workplace
Substance Use Problems 438

Section 74.2—Symptoms and Intervention
Techniques When Employees
Abuse Drugs 442

Section 74.3—Employment Status Is
Relevant to Substance
Abuse Treatment
Outcomes 444

Section 74.4—EAPs for Substance Abuse
Benefit Employers and
Employees 447

Chapter 75—Individual Rights When in Recovery from
Substance Abuse Problems 451

Chapter 76—Substance Abuse Treatment Statistics 459

Section 76.1—Treatment Received for
Substance Abuse 460

Section 76.2—Predictors of Substance
Abuse Treatment
Completion 468

Section 76.3—Treatment Outcomes for
Clients Discharged from
Residential Substance
Abuse Treatment 471

Part V: Drug Abuse Prevention

Chapter 77—Effective Responses to Reducing
Drug Abuse 479

Chapter 78—Testing for Drugs of Abuse 485

Section 78.1—How Drug Tests Are Done 486

Section 78.2—Why Drug Tests Are Done 488

Section 78.3—Home Use Test for Drugs
of Abuse 494

Chapter 79—Talking to Your Child about Drugs 497

Chapter 80—Making Your Home Safe 501

Chapter 81—Preventing Adolescent Drug Abuse 505

    Section 81.1—Keeping Your Teens
              Drug-Free 506

    Section 81.2—Youth Prevention-
              Related Measures 510

    Section 81.3—Family Dinners Reduce
              Likelihood That Teens
              Will Abuse Drugs 516

Chapter 82—Drug Abuse Prevention in Schools 521

    Section 82.1—Drug Testing in Schools 522

    Section 82.2—Health Education and
              Services 528

Chapter 83—Keeping the Workplace Drug Free 531

    Section 83.1—Drug-Free Workplace
              Policies 532

    Section 83.2—Drug Testing in the
              Workplace 538

Chapter 84—Religious Involvement Can Be a Protective
           Factor against Substance Use among Adults 543

Part VI: Additional Help and Information

Chapter 85—Glossary of Terms Related to Drug Abuse 551

Chapter 86—Glossary of Street Terms for Drugs of Abuse 557

Chapter 87—Directory of State Substance Abuse Agencies 571

Chapter 88—Directory of Organizations with Information
           about Drug Abuse 581

Index 589

Preface

About This Book

According to the National Institute on Drug Abuse, the costs of substance abuse and addiction in the United States—including health expenses and costs associated with crime—exceed half a trillion dollars annually. The consequences affect people at all ages, beginning even before birth when infants are sometimes exposed to drugs in the womb. Furthermore, substance abuse can play a role in family disintegration, school failure, loss of employment, and other societal concerns. Although treatments for addiction are available, they are used by fewer than 11% of those in need of them, and while some prevention programs have proven successful, nearly 8,000 individuals use an illicit drug for the first time each day in the United States.

Drug Abuse Sourcebook, Third Edition provides updated information about the abuse of illegal substances and the misuse of over-the-counter and prescription medications. It offers facts about the most commonly abused drugs and discusses the causes and consequences of addiction. Drug abuse treatment options are described, and obstacles to recovery are explained. A section on drug abuse prevention discusses some of the strategies that have been successful in helping people avoid drug-related problems. The book concludes with glossaries of drug-related terms and directories of resources for additional help and information.

How to Use This Book

This book is divided into parts and chapters. Parts focus on broad areas of interest. Chapters are devoted to single topics within a part.

Part I: Facts about Drug Abuse in the United States describes the prevalence of substance abuse in the United States, the legal steps that have been taken to address drug-related concerns, and problems among specific populations. It also summarizes statistical information about economic costs associated with drug use and provides facts about the number of lives lost.

Part II: Drugs of Abuse provides facts about more than thirty substances that are often abused. The individual chapters—which include facts about each drug's legal and illicit uses, effects, user populations, distribution channels, and legal status—are arranged alphabetically.

Part III: The Causes and Consequences of Drug Abuse and Addiction describes the physical and mental risk factors associated with substance abuse, including facts about the alterations of brain processes that may occur when drugs are misused. It discusses the health effects of abusing over-the-counter medications and prescription drugs as well as those associated with the use of illegal substances. Information is also presented about the hazards associated with drug and alcohol interactions, drug-related infectious diseases, the co-occurrence of addiction and mental illness, and the role substance use plays in depression and suicide.

Part IV: Drug Abuse Treatment and Recovery discusses various therapies and care approaches used to help people with substance-related concerns. Because recognizing a problem is often the first step, the part begins with information about the signs, symptoms, and paraphernalia that may accompany drug use. The detoxification and withdrawal processes and the roles of support groups, drug courts, and employee assistance programs are also discussed. The part concludes with statistical information about treatment outcomes.

Part V: Drug Abuse Prevention talks about some of the practices found to be most effective in the battle against the misuse of illicit drugs and medications. Facts about drug testing are included, and suggestions are offered for parents, schools, and employers.

Part VI: Additional Help and Information provides glossaries of terms related to drug abuse and street terms for drugs of abuse. Directories of state substance abuse agencies and resources for additional information about drug abuse are also included.

Bibliographic Note

This volume contains documents and excerpts from publications issued by the following U.S. government agencies: Centers for Disease Control and Prevention (CDC); Drug Enforcement Administration (DEA); Federal Bureau of Investigation (FBI); National Institute on Alcohol Abuse and Alcoholism (NIAAA); National Institute on Drug Abuse (NIDA); National Youth Anti-Drug Media Campaign; Office of National Drug Control Policy; Substance Abuse and Mental Health Services Administration (SAMHSA); U.S. Department of Education; U.S. Department of Justice; U.S. Department of Labor; and the U.S. Food and Drug Administration (FDA).

In addition, this volume contains copyrighted documents from the following individuals and organizations: A.D.A.M., Inc.; American Association for Clinical Chemistry; American Psychiatric Association (APA); Steven M. Melemis, MD; Narcotics Anonymous; National Center on Addiction and Substance Abuse (CASA) at Columbia University; Nemours Foundation; and Partnership for a Drug-Free America.

Acknowledgements

In addition to the listed organizations, agencies, and individuals who have contributed to this *Sourcebook*, special thanks go to managing editor Karen Bellenir, research and permissions coordinator Liz Collins, and document engineer Bruce Bellenir for their help and support.

About the Health Reference Series

The *Health Reference Series* is designed to provide basic medical information for patients, families, caregivers, and the general public. Each volume takes a particular topic and provides comprehensive coverage. This is especially important for people who may be dealing with a newly diagnosed disease or a chronic disorder in themselves or in a family member. People looking for preventive guidance, information about disease warning signs, medical statistics, and risk factors for health problems will also find answers to their questions in the *Health Reference Series*. The *Series*, however, is not intended to serve as a tool for diagnosing illness, in prescribing treatments, or as a substitute for the physician/patient relationship. All people concerned about medical symptoms or the possibility of disease are encouraged to seek professional care from an appropriate health care provider.

A Note about Spelling and Style

Health Reference Series editors use *Stedman's Medical Dictionary* as an authority for questions related to the spelling of medical terms and the *Chicago Manual of Style* for questions related to grammatical structures, punctuation, and other editorial concerns. Consistent adherence is not always possible, however, because the individual volumes within the *Series* include many documents from a wide variety of different producers and copyright holders, and the editor's primary goal is to present material from each source as accurately as is possible following the terms specified by each document's producer. This sometimes means that information in different chapters or sections may follow other guidelines and alternate spelling authorities. For example, occasionally a copyright holder may require that eponymous terms be shown in possessive forms (Crohn's disease *vs.* Crohn disease) or that British spelling norms be retained (leukaemia *vs.* leukemia).

Locating Information within the Health Reference Series

The *Health Reference Series* contains a wealth of information about a wide variety of medical topics. Ensuring easy access to all the fact sheets, research reports, in-depth discussions, and other material contained within the individual books of the *Series* remains one of our highest priorities. As the *Series* continues to grow in size and scope, however, locating the precise information needed by a reader may become more challenging.

A Contents Guide to the Health Reference Series was developed to direct readers to the specific volumes that address their concerns. It presents an extensive list of diseases, treatments, and other topics of general interest compiled from the Tables of Contents and major index headings. To access *A Contents Guide to the Health Reference Series*, visit www.healthreferenceseries.com.

Medical Consultant

Medical consultation services are provided to the *Health Reference Series* editors by David A. Cooke, MD, FACP. Dr. Cooke is a graduate of Brandeis University, and he received his MD degree from the University of Michigan. He completed residency training at the University of Wisconsin Hospital and Clinics. He is board-certified in Internal Medicine. Dr. Cooke currently works as part of the University of Michigan Health System and practices in Ann Arbor, MI. In his free time, he enjoys writing, science fiction, and spending time with his family.

Our Advisory Board

We would like to thank the following board members for providing guidance to the development of this *Series*:

- Dr. Lynda Baker, Associate Professor of Library and Information Science, Wayne State University, Detroit, MI

- Nancy Bulgarelli, William Beaumont Hospital Library, Royal Oak, MI

- Karen Imarisio, Bloomfield Township Public Library, Bloomfield Township, MI

- Karen Morgan, Mardigian Library, University of Michigan-Dearborn, Dearborn, MI

- Rosemary Orlando, St. Clair Shores Public Library, St. Clair Shores, MI

Health Reference Series *Update Policy*

The inaugural book in the *Health Reference Series* was the first edition of *Cancer Sourcebook* published in 1989. Since then, the *Series* has been enthusiastically received by librarians and in the medical community. In order to maintain the standard of providing high-quality health information for the layperson the editorial staff at Omnigraphics felt it was necessary to implement a policy of updating volumes when warranted.

Medical researchers have been making tremendous strides, and it is the purpose of the *Health Reference Series* to stay current with the most recent advances. Each decision to update a volume is made on an individual basis. Some of the considerations include how much new information is available and the feedback we receive from people who use the books. If there is a topic you would like to see added to the update list, or an area of medical concern you feel has not been adequately addressed, please write to:

Editor
Health Reference Series
Omnigraphics, Inc.
P.O. Box 31-1640
Detroit, MI 48231-1640
E-mail: editorial@omnigraphics.com

Part One

Facts about Drug Abuse in the United States

Chapter 1

Prevalence of Illicit Drug Use and Substance Abuse

The 2007 National Survey on Drug Use and Health (NSDUH), an annual survey sponsored by the Substance Abuse and Mental Health Services Administration (SAMHSA), is the primary source of information on the use of illicit drugs, alcohol, and tobacco in the civilian, noninstitutionalized population of the United States aged 12 years old or older. The survey interviews approximately 67,500 persons each year.

Illicit Drug Use

The National Survey on Drug Use and Health (NSDUH) obtains information on nine different categories of illicit drug use: use of marijuana, cocaine, heroin, hallucinogens, and inhalants; and the nonmedical use of prescription-type pain relievers, tranquilizers, stimulants, and sedatives. In these categories, hashish is included with marijuana, and crack is considered a form of cocaine. Several drugs are grouped under the hallucinogens category, including lysergic acid diethylamide (LSD), phencyclidine (PCP), peyote, mescaline, psilocybin mushrooms, and Ecstasy (methylenedioxymethamphetamine [MDMA]). Inhalants include a variety of substances, such as nitrous oxide, amyl nitrite,

This chapter includes excerpts from "Results from the 2007 National Survey on Drug Use and Health: National Findings," Substance Abuse and Mental Health Services Administration (SAMHSA), September 2008. The complete report is available online at http://oas.samhsa.gov/nsduh/2k7nsduh/2k7 Results.pdf.

cleaning fluids, gasoline, spray paint, other aerosol sprays, and glue. The four categories of prescription-type drugs (pain relievers, tranquilizers, stimulants, and sedatives) cover numerous medications available by prescription and drugs within these groupings that may be manufactured illegally, such as methamphetamine, which is included under stimulants. Respondents are asked to report only "nonmedical" use of these drugs, defined as use without a prescription of the individual's own or simply for the experience or feeling the drugs caused. Use of over-the-counter drugs and legitimate use of prescription drugs are not included. NSDUH reports combine the four prescription-type drug groups into a category referred to as psychotherapeutics.

Estimates of illicit drug use reported from NSDUH reflect the use of any of the nine drug categories listed. Revised estimates are included of the nonmedical use of prescription psychotherapeutic drugs and prescription stimulants that take into account data on methamphetamine use based on information obtained from survey items added to NSDUH in 2005, 2006, and 2007. The 2006 NSDUH national findings report incorporated revised estimates for methamphetamine use based on these additional items (Office of Applied Studies [OAS], 2007b), and this report extends the revisions to use of stimulants and any prescription psychotherapeutics. In a methodological study, these measures were found to be noticeably higher when the data from the additional methamphetamine use items were taken into account. Estimates for use of illicit drugs overall and use of illicit drugs other than marijuana, however, were affected only minimally by these methamphetamine use items and were not revised.

- In 2007, an estimated 19.9 million Americans aged 12 or older were current (past month) illicit drug users, meaning they had used an illicit drug during the month prior to the survey interview. This estimate represents 8.0% of the population aged 12 years old or older. Illicit drugs include marijuana/hashish, cocaine (including crack), heroin, hallucinogens, inhalants, or prescription-type psychotherapeutics used nonmedically.

- The rate of current illicit drug use among persons aged 12 or older in 2007 (8.0%) was similar to the rate in 2006 (8.3%).

- Marijuana was the most commonly used illicit drug (14.4 million past month users). Among persons aged 12 or older, the rate of past month marijuana use in 2007 (5.8%) was similar to the rate in 2006 (6.0%).

4

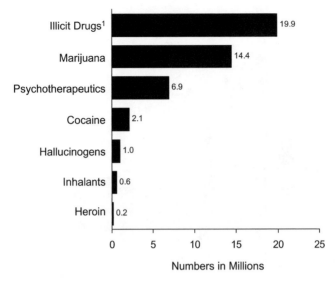

¹Illicit Drugs include marijuana/hashish, cocaine (including crack), heroin, hallucinogens, inhalants, or prescription-type psychotherapeutics used nonmedically.

Figure 1.1. Past Month Illicit Drug Use among Persons Aged 12 or Older: 2007

- In 2007, there were 2.1 million current cocaine users aged 12 or older, comprising 0.8% of the population. These estimates were similar to the number and rate in 2006 (2.4 million or 1.0%).

- Hallucinogens were used in the past month by 1.0 million persons (0.4%) aged 12 or older in 2007, including 503,000 (0.2%) who had used Ecstasy. These estimates were similar to the corresponding estimates for 2006.

- There were 6.9 million (2.8%) persons aged 12 or older who used prescription-type psychotherapeutic drugs nonmedically in the past month. Of these, 5.2 million used pain relievers, the same as the number in 2006.

- In 2007, there were an estimated 529,000 current users of methamphetamine aged 12 or older (0.2% of the population). These estimates were not significantly different from the estimates for 2006 (731,000 or 0.3%).

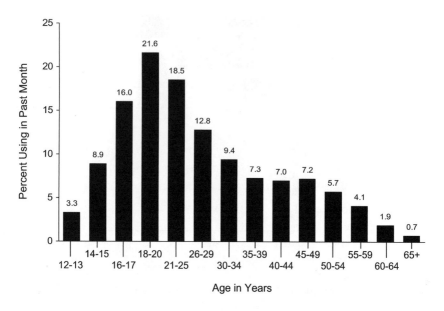

Figure 1.2. *Past Month Illicit Drug Use among Persons Aged 12 or Older, by Age: 2007*

- Among youths aged 12 to 17, the current illicit drug use rate remained stable from 2006 (9.8%) to 2007 (9.5%). Between 2002 and 2007, youth rates declined significantly for illicit drugs in general (from 11.6% to 9.5%) and for marijuana, cocaine, hallucinogens, LSD, Ecstasy, prescription-type drugs used nonmedically, pain relievers, stimulants, methamphetamine, and the use of illicit drugs other than marijuana.

- The rate of current marijuana use among youths aged 12 to 17 declined from 8.2% in 2002 to 6.7% in 2007. The rate decreased for both males (from 9.1% to 7.5%) and females (from 7.2% to 5.8%).

- Among young adults aged 18 to 25, there were decreases from 2006 to 2007 in the rate of current use of several drugs, including cocaine (from 2.2% to 1.7%), Ecstasy (from 1.0% to 0.7%), stimulants (from 1.4% to 1.1%), methamphetamine (from 0.6% to 0.4%), and illicit drugs other than marijuana (from 8.9% to 8.1%).

6

- From 2002 to 2007, there was an increase among young adults aged 18 to 25 in the rate of current use of prescription pain relievers, from 4.1% to 4.6%. There were decreases in the use of hallucinogens (from 1.9% to 1.5%), Ecstasy (from 1.1% to 0.7%), and methamphetamine (from 0.6% to 0.4%).

- Among those aged 50 to 54, the rate of past month illicit drug use increased from 3.4% in 2002 to 5.7% in 2007. Among those aged 55 to 59, current illicit drug use showed an increase from 1.9% in 2002 to 4.1% in 2007. These trends may partially reflect the aging into these age groups of the baby boom cohort, whose lifetime rates of illicit drug use are higher than those of older cohorts.

- Among persons aged 12 or older who used pain relievers nonmedically in the past 12 months, 56.5% reported that the source of the drug the most recent time they used was from a friend or relative for free. Another 18.1% reported they got the drug from just one doctor. Only 4.1% got the pain relievers from a drug dealer or other stranger, and 0.5% reported buying the drug on the internet. Among those who reported getting the pain reliever from a friend or relative for free, 81.0% reported in a followup question that the friend or relative had obtained the drugs from just one doctor.

- Among unemployed adults aged 18 or older in 2007, 18.3% were current illicit drug users, which was higher than the 8.4% of those employed full time and 10.1% of those employed part time. However, most illicit drug users were employed. Of the 17.4 million current illicit drug users aged 18 or older in 2007, 13.1 million (75.3%) were employed either full or part time.

- In 2007, there were 9.9 million persons aged 12 or older who reported driving under the influence of illicit drugs during the past year. This corresponds to 4.0% of the population aged 12 or older, similar to the rate in 2006 (4.2%), but lower than the rate in 2002 (4.7%). In 2007, the rate was highest among young adults aged 18 to 25 (12.5%).

Substance Dependence, Abuse, and Treatment

The National Survey on Drug Use and Health (NSDUH) includes a series of questions to assess the prevalence of substance use disorders (for example, dependence on or abuse of a substance) in the past 12 months. Substances include alcohol and illicit drugs, such as marijuana, cocaine, heroin, hallucinogens, inhalants, and the nonmedical use of prescription-type psychotherapeutic drugs. These questions are used to classify persons as dependent on or abusing specific substances based on criteria specified in the *Diagnostic and Statistical Manual of Mental Disorders, 4th edition* (DSM-IV) (American Psychiatric Association [APA], 1994).

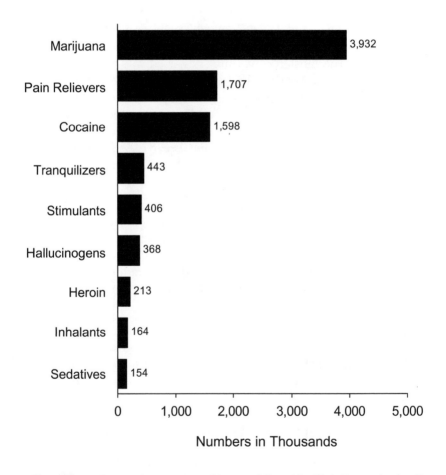

Figure 1.3. Dependence on or Abuse of Specific Illicit Drugs in the Past Year among Persons Aged 12 or Older: 2007.

The questions related to dependence ask about health and emotional problems associated with substance use, unsuccessful attempts to cut down on use, tolerance, withdrawal, reducing other activities to use substances, spending a lot of time engaging in activities related to substance use, or using the substance in greater quantities or for a longer time than intended. The questions on abuse ask about problems at work, home, and school; problems with family or friends; physical danger; and trouble with the law due to substance use. Dependence is considered to be a more severe substance use problem than abuse because it involves the psychological and physiological effects of tolerance and withdrawal. Although individuals may meet the criteria specified here for both dependence and abuse, persons meeting the criteria for both are classified as having dependence, but not abuse. Persons defined with abuse in this report do not meet the criteria for dependence.

- In 2007, an estimated 22.3 million persons (9.0% of the population aged 12 or older) were classified with substance dependence or abuse in the past year based on criteria specified in the *Diagnostic and Statistical Manual of Mental Disorders, 4th edition* (DSM-IV*)*. Of these, 3.2 million were classified with dependence on or abuse of both alcohol and illicit drugs, 3.7 million were dependent on or abused illicit drugs but not alcohol, and 15.5 million were dependent on or abused alcohol but not illicit drugs.

- Between 2002 and 2007, there was no change in the number of persons with substance dependence or abuse (22.0 million in 2002, 22.3 million in 2007).

- The specific illicit drugs that had the highest levels of past year dependence or abuse in 2007 were marijuana (3.9 million), followed by pain relievers (1.7 million) and cocaine (1.6 million).

- The rate of substance dependence or abuse for males aged 12 or older in 2007 was about twice as high as the rate for females (12.5% versus 5.7%). Among youths aged 12 to 17, however, the rate of substance dependence or abuse among males was the same as the rate among females (7.7% for both).

Chapter 2

Drug Abuse Cost to Society

Substance abuse clearly is among the most costly health problems in the United States. Among national estimates of the costs of illness for 33 diseases and conditions, alcohol ranked second, tobacco ranked sixth, and drug disorders ranked seventh (National Institutes of Health [NIH], 2000).

National Drug Threat Assessment

The trafficking and abuse of illicit drugs inflict tremendous harm upon individuals, families, and communities throughout the country. The violence, intimidation, theft, and financial crimes carried out by drug trafficking organizations (DTO), criminal groups, gangs, and drug users in the United States pose a significant threat to our nation. The cost to society from drug production, trafficking, and abuse is difficult to fully measure or convey; however, the most recent data available are helpful in framing the extent of the threat. For example:

- More than 35 million individuals used illicit drugs or abused prescription drugs in 2007.

This chapter begins with an excerpt from "Substance Abuse Prevention Dollars and Cents: A Cost-Benefit Analysis," Center for Substance Abuse Prevention, Substance Abuse and Mental Health Services Administration (SAMHSA), DHHS Pub. No. (SMA) 07-4298, 2009; and continues with text from the "National Drug Threat Assessment 2009," National Drug Intelligence Center, U.S. Department of Justice, December 2008, No. 2008-Q0317-005.

- In 2006, individuals entered public drug treatment facilities more than one million times seeking assistance in ending their addiction to illicit or prescription drugs.

- More than 1,100 children were injured at, killed at, or removed from methamphetamine laboratory sites from 2007 through September 2008.

- For 2009 the federal government has allocated more than $14 billion for drug treatment and prevention, counter-drug law enforcement, drug interdiction, and international counter-drug assistance.

Table 2.1. Estimated Economic Cost of Drug Abuse to Society in 1999 (in billions).

Costs	Drug Abuse
Resource Costs	
Specialty treatment and prevention services	7.6
Treatment of medical consequences	5.4
Goods and services related to crashes, fires, crime, criminal justice	31.1
Total Resource Costs	44.1
Productivity Costs	
Work loss due to premature death	20.9
Work loss due to illness related to substance abuse	26.7
Work loss by crime victims	2.0
Work loss by perpetrators due to incarceration and criminal careers	57.7
Total Productivity Costs	107.3
Total Resource and Productivity Costs	151.4

Source: Harwood and Bouchery (2004). Similar costs are incurred annually.

- In September 2008 there were nearly 100,000 inmates in federal prisons convicted and sentenced for drug offenses, representing more than 52 percent of all federal prisoners.

- In 2007 more than 1.8 million drug-related arrests in the United States were carried out by federal, state, and local law enforcement agencies.

- Mexican and Colombian drug trafficking organizations generate, remove, and launder between $18 billion and $39 billion in wholesale drug proceeds annually.

- Diversion of controlled prescription drugs costs insurance companies up to $72.5 billion annually, nearly two-thirds of which is paid by public insurers.

Drug trafficking organizations (DTOs) rapidly adapt to law enforcement and policy initiatives that disrupt their drug trafficking operations. Law enforcement and intelligence reporting revealed several strategic shifts by DTOs in drug production and trafficking in 2007 and early 2008, attributed in part to the success of counter-drug agencies in disrupting the operations of DTOs. Many of these shifts represent immediate new challenges for policy makers and resource planners.

Chapter 3

Deaths from Drug Overdoses

Unintentional Poisoning Deaths

Unintentional drug poisoning mortality rates increased substantially in the United States during 1999–2004. Previous studies, using multiple cause-of-death data, have indicated that the trend can be attributed primarily to increasing numbers of deaths associated with prescription opioid analgesics (for example, oxycodone) and secondarily to increasing numbers of overdoses of cocaine and prescription psychotherapeutic drugs (for example, sedatives), and cannot be attributed to heroin, methamphetamines, or other illegal drugs.

The mortality increases might be the result of greater use and abuse of potentially lethal prescription drugs in recent years, behaviors that are more common among whites than nonwhites. The substantial increase in deaths among persons aged 15–24 years is consistent with substantial recent increases in recreational prescription drug and cocaine use among adolescents and young adults.

Studies by state health agencies have reported recent increases in prescription drug poisoning mortality in rural communities, despite historically higher rates in urban areas. The South and Midwest regions, which had the largest relative and absolute increases among regions in this study, are the most rural regions of the country.

Text in this chapter is from "Unintentional Poisoning Deaths–United States, 1999–2004," *MMWR Weekly*, February 9, 2007, Centers for Disease Control and Prevention (CDC); and from "Increase in Fatal Poisonings Involving Opioid Analgesics in the United States, 1999–2006," CDC, September 2009.

The findings are subject to at least three limitations. First, mortality coding assigns the underlying cause of death to broad drug categories rather than to specific drugs. Second, death certificates do not reveal the circumstances of drug use. Third, determining the intent of a person who took a drug is often difficult for a coroner or medical examiner and might result in misclassification; some of these deaths might have been suicides, although not classified as such, and some deaths categorized as suicides or of undetermined intent might have been unintentional and therefore not analyzed in this study. The extent of this error is not known.

Increase in Fatal Poisonings Involving Opioid Analgesics in the United States, 1999–2006

Data from the National Vital Statistics System Mortality File indicates the following:

- From 1999 through 2006, the number of fatal poisonings involving opioid analgesics more than tripled from 4,000 to 13,800 deaths.

- Opioid analgesics were involved in almost 40% of all poisoning deaths in 2006.

- In 2006, the rate of poisoning deaths involving opioid analgesics was higher for males, persons aged 35–54 years, and non-Hispanic white persons than for females and those in other age and racial/ethnic groups.

- In about one-half of the deaths involving opioid analgesics, more than one type of drug was specified as contributing to the death, with benzodiazepines specified with opioid analgesics most frequently.

- The age-adjusted death rate for poisoning involving opioid analgesics varied more than eight-fold among the states in 2006.

Poisoning is the second leading cause of injury death overall, and the leading cause of injury death for people aged 35–54 years, surpassing both firearm-related and motor vehicle-related deaths in this age group. Drug poisonings are the largest portion of the poisoning burden and opioid analgesic-related deaths are among the fastest increasing drug poisoning deaths.

From 1999 through 2006, the number of poisoning deaths nearly doubled from almost 20,000 to more than 37,000. In 2006, over 90%

of poisoning deaths involved drugs. Opioid analgesics were involved in almost 40% of all poisoning deaths in 2006, up from about 20% in 1999. The death records for about one-fifth of poisoning deaths each year indicated drug involvement, but did not specify the substance involved; an unknown proportion of these deaths involved opioid analgesics.

From 1999 through 2006, poisoning deaths involving methadone rose more rapidly than those involving other opioid analgesics, cocaine, or heroin. The number of poisoning deaths involving methadone increased nearly sevenfold from almost 790 in 1999 to almost 5,420 in 2006, which is the most rapid increase among opioid analgesics and other narcotics involved in poisoning deaths. Between 2005 and 2006, the number of poisoning deaths involving other synthetic narcotics increased by more than 50%. This increase may be related to the illicit manufacture of non-pharmaceutical fentanyl in 2006.

Throughout the period 1999–2006, people aged 35–54 years had higher poisoning death rates involving opioid analgesics than those in other age groups. From 1999 to 2006, poisoning death rates involving opioid analgesics increased for every age group from 15–24 years through 65 years and older, males and females, and non-Hispanic white and non-Hispanic black persons. Increases among age groups ranged from about twofold (65 years and over) to more than fivefold (15–24 years). Males had higher age-adjusted poisoning death rates involving opioid analgesics than females throughout the period. In 2006, the rate for males was about 75% higher than for females. In 2006, the age-adjusted death rate for poisoning involving opioid analgesics among non-Hispanic white persons was about twice that of non-Hispanic black persons and almost three times that of Hispanic persons.

More than one type of drug was mentioned in the majority of poisoning deaths that involved opioid analgesics in 2006. About one-third of opioid analgesic-related poisoning deaths involved no other drugs and 16% involved nonspecified drug(s). Deaths with a nonspecified drug could potentially involve only opioid analgesics. About one-half of opioid analgesic-related deaths involved at least one other drug that was specified on the death certificate; benzodiazepines were involved in 17% of the deaths, cocaine or heroin in 15%, and benzodiazepines with cocaine or heroin in 3%.

Death rates for poisoning involving opioid analgesics varied more than eight-fold among the states in 2006. In 2006, age-adjusted death rates for poisoning deaths involving opioid analgesics ranged from 1.8 to 15.6 deaths per 100,000 population among the states. In 16 states, the rate was statistically significantly higher than the U.S. rate of 4.6 deaths per 100,000. In 2006, West Virginia, Utah, New

Mexico, Oklahoma, and Nevada had the five highest rates, ranging from 10.5 to 15.6 per 100,000. State-specific comparisons should be interpreted with caution as there is some variation in the reporting of substances on death records.

Summary

Opioid analgesics are drugs that are usually prescribed to treat pain. Poisoning death rates involving opioid analgesics have more than tripled in the United States since 1999. Among opioid analgesic-related deaths, those involving methadone increased the most during the period 1999–2006.

Methadone is a long-acting opioid and requires a complex dosing schedule. Methadone relieves pain for 4–8 hours, but remains in the body for up to 59 hours. A lack of knowledge about the unique properties of methadone was identified as contributing to some deaths.

Knowing whether other drugs are involved with opioid analgesics in poisoning deaths helps in developing prevention strategies. The data suggest that multiple drugs were involved in at least one-half of the opioid analgesic-related deaths. The involvement of benzodiazepines—sedatives used to treat anxiety, insomnia, and seizures—is particularly troubling as previous studies have shown that people who were prescribed both methadone and benzodiazepine were at greater risk of overdose than those prescribed only one of these drugs.

State variation in opioid analgesic-related death rates provides an opportunity to study factors associated with deaths involving opioid analgesics. States vary widely in their prescription and other drug policies. For instance, 32 states have operational drug monitoring programs with statewide databases that monitor the prescribing and dispensing of prescription drugs.

Opioid analgesics have abuse potential and are, therefore, a controlled substance under the U.S. Drug Enforcement Administration (DEA). Recent studies have shown a rise in distribution and prescription of opioids. It could not be determined from death certificates whether the opioid analgesics involved in poisoning deaths were prescribed for the decedent or obtained in another way. Several regional studies have shown that at least some decedents obtained opioid analgesics illegally.

The importance of opioid analgesics in the management of pain is unquestioned. However, increasing opioid analgesic-related poisoning deaths pose a serious public health risk.

Definitions

Narcotic refers to both opioid analgesics and illicit drugs including opium, heroin, and cocaine.

Opioid analgesics are drugs that are usually prescribed to relieve pain and include: methadone, which is used to treat opioid dependency as well as pain; other opioids, such as oxycodone and hydrocodone; and synthetic narcotics such as fentanyl and propoxyphene. Opium, heroin, and cocaine are not included in this class.

Poisoning deaths include those resulting from accidental or intentional overdoses of a drug, being given the wrong drug, taking the wrong drug in error, or taking a drug inadvertently. Poisoning deaths also include those involving biological or other toxic substances, gases, or vapors.

Chapter 4

The Controlled Substances Act

Drugs of Abuse

The Controlled Substances Act (CSA), Title II and Title III of the Comprehensive Drug Abuse Prevention and Control Act of 1970, is the legal foundation of the United States (U.S.) government's fight against the abuse of drugs and other substances. This law is a consolidation of numerous laws regulating the manufacture and distribution of narcotics, stimulants, depressants, hallucinogens, anabolic steroids, and chemicals used in the illicit production of controlled substances.

Controlling Drugs or Other Substances

Formal scheduling: The Controlled Substances Act (CSA) places all substances which were in some manner regulated under existing federal law into one of five schedules. This placement is based upon the substance's medical use, potential for abuse, and safety or dependence liability. The Act also provides a mechanism for substances to be controlled, or added to a schedule; decontrolled, or removed from control; and rescheduled or transferred from one schedule to another. The procedure for these actions is found in Section 201 of the Act (21 U.S.C. 811).

This chapter includes text from "Drugs of Abuse," U.S. Department of Justice, 2005; and from "Congress Passes Ryan Haight Online Pharmacy Consumer Protection Act," Drug Enforcement Administration (DEA), October 1, 2008.

Proceedings to add, delete, or change the schedule of a drug or other substance may be initiated by the Drug Enforcement Administration (DEA), the Department of Health and Human Services (HHS), or by petition from any interested person: the manufacturer of a drug, a medical society or association, a pharmacy association, a public interest group concerned with drug abuse, a state or local government agency, or an individual citizen. When a petition is received by the DEA, the agency begins its own investigation of the drug. The DEA also may begin an investigation of a drug at any time based upon information received from law enforcement laboratories, state and local law enforcement and regulatory agencies, or other sources of information.

Once the DEA has collected the necessary data, the DEA Administrator, by authority of the Attorney General, requests from HHS a scientific and medical evaluation and recommendation as to whether the drug or other substance should be controlled or removed from control. This request is sent to the Assistant Secretary of Health of HHS. HHS solicits information from the Commissioner of the Food and Drug Administration (FDA), evaluations and recommendations from the National Institute on Drug Abuse, and on occasion from the scientific and medical community at large. The Assistant Secretary, by authority of the Secretary, compiles the information and transmits back to the DEA a medical and scientific evaluation regarding the drug or other substance, a recommendation as to whether the drug should be controlled, and in what schedule it should be placed.

The medical and scientific evaluations are binding on the DEA with respect to scientific and medical matters and form a part of the scheduling decision. The recommendation on the initial scheduling of a substance is binding only to the extent that if HHS recommends that the substance not be controlled, the DEA may not add it to the schedules.

Once the DEA has received the scientific and medical evaluation from HHS, the Administrator will evaluate all available data and make a final decision whether to propose that a drug or other substance should be removed or controlled and into which schedule it should be placed.

The threshold issue is whether the drug or other substance has potential for abuse. If a drug does not have a potential for abuse, it cannot be controlled. Although the term "potential for abuse" is not defined in the CSA, there is much discussion of the term in the legislative history of the Act.

The following items are indicators that a drug or other substance has a potential for abuse:

1. There is evidence that individuals are taking the drug or other substance in amounts sufficient to create a hazard to their health or to the safety of other individuals or to the community.

2. There is significant diversion of the drug or other substance from legitimate drug channels.

3. Individuals are taking the drug or other substance on their own initiative rather than on the basis of medical advice from a practitioner licensed by law to administer such drugs.

4. The drug is a new drug so related in its action to a drug or other substance already listed as having a potential for abuse to make it likely that the drug will have the same potential for abuse as such drugs, thus making it reasonable to assume that there may be significant diversions from legitimate channels, significant use contrary to or without medical advice, or that it has a substantial capability of creating hazards to the health of the user or to the safety of the community. Of course, evidence of actual abuse of a substance is indicative that a drug has a potential for abuse.

In determining into which schedule a drug or other substance should be placed, or whether a substance should be decontrolled or rescheduled, certain factors are required to be considered. Specific findings are not required for each factor. These factors are listed in Section 201 (c), [21 U.S.C. 811 (c)] of the CSA as follows:

1. The drug's actual or relative potential for abuse.

2. Scientific evidence of the drug's pharmacological effects.

3. The state of all current scientific knowledge regarding the substance.

4. Its history and current pattern of abuse.

5. The scope, duration, and significance of abuse.

6. What, if any, risk there is to the public health.

7. The drug's psychic or physiological dependence liability.

8. Whether the substance is an immediate precursor of a substance already controlled.

After considering the listed factors, the Administrator must make specific findings concerning the drug or other substance. This will determine into which schedule the drug or other substance will be placed. These schedules are established by the CSA. They are as follows:

Schedule I

- The drug or other substance has a high potential for abuse.

- The drug or other substance has no currently accepted medical use in treatment in the United States.

- There is a lack of accepted safety for use of the drug or other substance under medical supervision.

- Examples of schedule I substances include heroin, lysergic acid diethylamide (LSD), marijuana, and methaqualone.

Schedule II

- The drug or other substance has a high potential for abuse.

- The drug or other substance has a currently accepted medical use in treatment in the United States or a currently accepted medical use with severe restrictions.

- Abuse of the drug or other substance may lead to severe psychological or physical dependence.

- Examples of schedule II substances include morphine, phencyclidine (PCP), cocaine, methadone, and methamphetamine.

Schedule III

- The drug or other substance has less potential for abuse than the drugs or other substances in schedules I and II.

- The drug or other substance has a currently accepted medical use in treatment in the United States.

- Abuse of the drug or other substance may lead to moderate or low physical dependence or high psychological dependence.

- Anabolic steroids, codeine and hydrocodone with aspirin or Tylenol®, and some barbiturates are examples of schedule III substances.

Schedule IV

- The drug or other substance has a low potential for abuse relative to the drugs or other substances in schedule III.

- The drug or other substance has a currently accepted medical use in treatment in the United States.

- Abuse of the drug or other substance may lead to limited physical dependence or psychological dependence relative to the drugs or other substances in schedule III.

- Examples of drugs included in schedule IV are Darvon®, Talwin®, Equanil®, Valium®, and Xanax®.

Schedule V

- The drug or other substance has a low potential for abuse relative to the drugs or other substances in schedule IV.

- The drug or other substance has a currently accepted medical use in treatment in the United States.

- Abuse of the drug or other substances may lead to limited physical dependence or psychological dependence relative to the drugs or other substances in schedule IV.

- Cough medicines with codeine are examples of schedule V drugs.

When the DEA Administrator has determined that a drug or other substance should be controlled, decontrolled, or rescheduled, a proposal to take action is published in the *Federal Register*. If a hearing is requested, the DEA will enter into discussions with the party or parties requesting a hearing in an attempt to narrow the issue for litigation. The DEA Administrator then publishes a final order in the *Federal Register* either scheduling the drug or other substance or declining to do so. Once the final order is published in the *Federal Register*, interested parties have 30 days to appeal to a U.S. Court of Appeals to challenge the order. Findings of fact by the Administrator are deemed conclusive if supported by "substantial evidence." The order imposing controls is not stayed during the appeal, however, unless so ordered by the Court.

Emergency or temporary scheduling: The CSA was amended by the Comprehensive Crime Control Act of 1984. This Act included a provision which allows the DEA Administrator to place a substance, on a temporary basis, into schedule I when necessary to avoid an imminent hazard to the public safety.

Controlled substance analogues: A new class of substances was created by the Anti-Drug Abuse Act of 1986. Controlled substance analogues are substances which are not controlled substances, but may be found in the illicit traffic. They are structurally or pharmacologically similar to schedule I or II controlled substances and have no legitimate medical use. A substance which meets the definition of a controlled substance analogue and is intended for human consumption is treated under the CSA as if it were a controlled substance in schedule I. [21U.S.C.802(32), 21U.S.C.813]

International treaty obligations: United States treaty obligations may require that a drug or other substance be controlled under the CSA, or rescheduled if existing controls are less stringent than those required by a treaty. The United States is a party to the Single Convention on Narcotic Drugs of 1961, designed to establish effective control over international and domestic traffic in narcotics, coca leaf, cocaine, and cannabis. A second treaty, the Convention on Psychotropic Substances of 1971, which entered into force in 1976, is designed to establish comparable control over stimulants, depressants, and hallucinogens. Congress ratified this treaty in 1980.

Regulation: The CSA creates a closed system of distribution for those authorized to handle controlled substances. The cornerstone of this system is the registration of all those authorized by DEA to handle controlled substances. All individuals and firms that are registered are required to maintain complete and accurate inventories and records of all transactions involving controlled substances, as well as security for the storage of controlled substances.

Distribution: The keeping of records is required for distribution of a controlled substance from one manufacturer to another, from manufacturer to distributor, and from distributor to dispenser. In the case of schedule I and II drugs, the supplier must have a special order form from the customer. This order form (DEA Form 222) is issued by DEA only to persons who are properly registered to handle schedules I and II. Distributors of controlled substances must report the quantity and form of all their transactions of controlled drugs listed in schedules I and II and narcotics listed in schedule III. Both manufacturers and distributors are required to provide reports of their annual inventories of these controlled substances. This data is entered into a system called the Automated Reports and Consolidated Orders System (ARCOS). It enables the DEA to monitor the distribution of controlled substances throughout the country, and to identify retail level registrants that receive unusual quantities of controlled substances.

Dispensing to patients: The dispensing of a controlled substance is the delivery of the controlled substance to the ultimate user, who may be a patient or research subject. Special control mechanisms operate here as well.

Quotas: DEA limits the quantity of schedule I and II controlled substances which may be produced in the United States in any given calendar year. The DEA establishes annual aggregate production quotas for schedule I and II controlled substances. DEA also allocates the amount of bulk drug which may be procured by those companies which prepare the drug into dosage units.

Security: DEA registrants are required by regulation to maintain certain security for the storage and distribution of controlled substances. All registrants are required to make every effort to ensure that controlled substances in their possession are not diverted into the illicit market. This requires operational as well as physical security.

Ryan Haight Online Pharmacy Consumer Protection Act

In October 2008, Congress passed the Ryan Haight Online Pharmacy Consumer Protection Act of 2007, which addresses the problems of online prescription drug trafficking, abuse, and availability. This legislation amends the Controlled Substances Act (CSA) in the following key respects:

1. **Face-to-face requirement for prescribing:** The Act prohibits dispensing controlled substances via the internet without a valid prescription. For a prescription to be valid, it must be issued for a legitimate medical purpose in the usual course of professional practice, meaning that, with limited exceptions, a doctor must conduct at least one in-person medical evaluation of the patient.

2. **Endorsement requirement:** The Act requires an endorsement from DEA before a pharmacy could dispense controlled substances via the internet. This endorsement would

supplement the existing registration a pharmacy holds for its brick-and-mortar operation, and allow law enforcement to clearly identify internet sites where controlled substances can be sold.

3. **Enhanced penalties for schedule III through V:** The Ryan Haight Act will enhance penalties for unlawfully dispensing controlled substances in schedules III through V. These enhanced penalties would apply equally to all unlawful distributors and dispensers of controlled substances (not just those who do so by means of the internet).

4. **Prohibition on advertising illegal sales:** The Ryan Haight Act will make it a crime to use the internet to advertise the illegal sale of a controlled substance by means of the internet.

5. **Requirement that internet pharmacies post certain information on their websites:** The Ryan Haight Act will require online pharmacies to post truthful information about their location, identity, and licensure of the pharmacy, pharmacists and prescribers, and states in which they are located.

6. **State Cause of Action:** The Ryan Haight Act will give the Attorney General of each state the ability to bring a civil action in a federal district court to enjoin the actions of an online pharmacy or person which/who is operating in violation of this statute. To bring such an action, the state must have served prior written notice on the Attorney General of the United States, giving the Attorney General the opportunity to intervene in the litigation. This provision would help ensure that state and federal enforcement authorities can work in partnership with each other and that individual states are able to take effective enforcement action.

Chapter 5

Purchasing Controlled Substances

Chapter Contents

Section 5.1—Prescriptions for Controlled Substances 30

Section 5.2—Online Dispensing and Purchasing of
Controlled Substances 33

Section 5.3—Facts about Medical Marijuana 36

Section 5.1

Prescriptions for Controlled Substances

Text in this section is from "General Questions and Answers," Office of Diversion Control, Drug Enforcement Administration (DEA), January 2009.

What is a prescription?

A prescription is an order for medication which is dispensed to or for an ultimate user. A prescription is not an order for medication which is dispensed for immediate administration to the ultimate user (for example, an order to dispense a drug to an inpatient for immediate administration in a hospital is not a prescription). To be valid, a prescription for a controlled substance must be issued for a legitimate medical purpose by a registered practitioner acting in the usual course of sound professional practice.

What information is required on a prescription for a controlled substance?

A prescription for a controlled substance must include the following information:

- Date of issue
- Patient's name and address
- Practitioner's name, address, and Drug Enforcement Administration (DEA) registration number
- Drug name
- Drug strength
- Dosage form
- Quantity prescribed
- Directions for use
- Number of refills (if any) authorized
- Manual signature of prescriber

A prescription must be written in ink or indelible pencil or typewritten and must be manually signed by the practitioner. An individual may be designated by the practitioner to prepare the prescriptions for his or her signature. The practitioner is responsible for making sure that the prescription conforms in all essential respects to the law and regulation.

Prescriptions for schedule II controlled substances must be written and be signed by the practitioner. In emergency situations, a prescription for a schedule II controlled substance may be telephoned to the pharmacy and the prescriber must follow up with a written prescription being sent to the pharmacy within seven days. Prescriptions for schedules III through V controlled substances may by written, oral, or transmitted by fax.

Can controlled substance prescriptions be refilled?

Prescriptions for schedule II controlled substances cannot be refilled. A new prescription must be issued. Prescriptions for schedules III and IV controlled substances may be refilled up to five times in six months. Prescriptions for schedule V controlled substances may be refilled as authorized by the practitioner.

Can controlled substance prescriptions for hospice patients be faxed to a pharmacy?

A prescription written for a schedule II narcotic substance for a patient enrolled in a hospice care program certified and/or paid for by Medicare under Title XVIII or a hospice program which is licensed by the state may be transmitted by the practitioner or the practitioner's agent to the dispensing pharmacy by facsimile.

A pharmacist may dispense directly a controlled substance listed in schedules III, IV, or V pursuant to either a written prescription signed by a practitioner or a facsimile of a written, signed prescription transmitted by the practitioner or the practitioner's agent to the pharmacy, or pursuant to an oral prescription made by an individual practitioner and promptly reduced to writing by the pharmacist.

Is it permissible to dispense a prescription for a quantity less than the face amount prescribed resulting in a greater number of dispensations than the number of refills indicated on the prescription?

Yes. Partial refills of schedules III and IV controlled substance prescriptions are permissible under federal regulations provided that each partial filling is dispensed and recorded in the same manner as a refilling (for example: date refilled, amount dispensed, initials of dispensing pharmacist, and so forth), the total quantity dispensed in all partial fillings does not exceed the total quantity prescribed, and no dispensing occurs after six months past the date of issue.

What changes may a pharmacist make to a prescription written for a controlled substance in schedules III–V?

The pharmacist may add or change the patient's address upon verification. The pharmacist may add or change the dosage form, drug strength, drug quantity, directions for use, or issue date only after consultation with and agreement of the prescribing practitioner. Such consultations and corresponding changes should be noted by the pharmacist on the prescription. Pharmacists and practitioners must comply with any state or local laws, regulations, or policies prohibiting any of these changes to controlled substance prescriptions.

The pharmacist is never permitted to make changes to the patient's name, controlled substance prescribed (except for generic substitution permitted by state law), or prescriber's signature.

Can a practitioner prescribe methadone for the treatment of pain?

Federal law and regulations do not restrict the prescribing, dispensing, or administering of any schedule II, III, IV, or V narcotic medication, including methadone, for the treatment of pain, if such treatment is deemed medically necessary by a registered practitioner acting in the usual course of professional practice.

Confusion often arises due to regulatory restrictions concerning the use of methadone for the maintenance or detoxification of opioid addicted individuals, in which case the practitioner is required to be registered with the DEA as a narcotic treatment program (NTP).

Can an individual return his or her controlled substance prescription medication to a pharmacy?

No. An individual patient may not return his or her unused controlled substance prescription medication to the pharmacy. Federal laws and regulations make no provisions for an individual to return the controlled substance prescription medication to a pharmacy for further dispensing or for disposal. There are no provisions in the Controlled Substances Act or Code of Federal Regulations (CFR) for a DEA registrant (retail pharmacy) to acquire controlled substances from a non-registrant (an individual patient).

The CFR does have a provision for an individual to return his or her unused controlled substance medication to the pharmacy in the event of the controlled substance being recalled or a dispensing error has occurred.

An individual may dispose of his or her own controlled substance medication without approval from DEA. Medications should be disposed of in such a manner that does not allow for the controlled substances to be easily retrieved. In situations where an individual has died, a caregiver or hospice staff member may assist the family with the proper disposal of any unused controlled substance medications.

Section 5.2

Online Dispensing and Purchasing of Controlled Substances

This section includes text from "Summary Record of the Ryan Haight Online Pharmacy Consumer Protection Act of 2008," Global Legal Information Network, Law Library of Congress, April 30, 2009; and "Don't Put Your Health in the Hands of Crooks: Illegal Online Pharmacies," Federal Bureau of Investigation (FBI), March 3, 2009.

Ryan Haight Online Pharmacy Consumer Protection Act of 2008

The Ryan Haight Online Pharmacy Consumer Protection Act of 2008 (Public Law 110–425, 122 Stat. 4820–4834) amends the Controlled Substances Act to prohibit the delivery, distribution, or dispensing of a controlled substance that is a prescription drug over the internet without a valid prescription. It exempts telemedicine practitioners.

It defines valid prescription as a prescription that is issued for a legitimate medical purpose in the usual course of professional practice by a practitioner who has conducted at least one in-person medical evaluation of a patient.

It defines online pharmacy as a person, entity, or internet site, whether in the United States or abroad, that knowingly or intentionally delivers, distributes, or dispenses a controlled substance by means of the internet. It excludes from such definition: (1) manufacturers or distributors who do not dispense controlled substances to an unregistered individual or entity; (2) non-pharmacy practitioners; (3) certain hospitals or medical facilities operated by the federal government or by an Indian tribe or tribal organization; (4) mere advertisements that do not attempt to facilitate an actual transaction involving a controlled substance; and (5) other persons or entities the exclusion of which the Attorney General and the Secretary of Health and Human Services find to be consistent with effective controls against diversion and with the public health and safety.

It imposes registration and reporting requirements on online pharmacies that dispense 100 or more prescriptions or 5,000 or more dosage units of all controlled substances combined in one month.

It requires an online pharmacy to: (1) display specified information on its internet home page, including a statement that it complies with the requirements of the Ryan Haight Online Pharmacy Consumer Protection Act, the pharmacy name, address, and telephone number, the qualifications of its pharmacist-in-charge, and a certification of its registration under this Act; (2) comply with state laws for the licensure of pharmacies in each state in which it operates or sells controlled substances; and (3) notify the Attorney General and applicable state boards of pharmacy 30 days prior to offering to sell, deliver, distribute, or dispense controlled substances over the internet.

It authorizes the Attorney General to issue a special registration under this Act for telemedicine practitioners. It requires practitioners who issue a prescription for a controlled substance under the authorization to conduct telemedicine during a medical emergency to report to the Secretary of Veterans Affairs the authorization of that emergency prescription.

It increases criminal penalties involving controlled substances in Schedules III, IV, and V of the Controlled Substances Act.

It authorizes states to apply for injunctions or obtain damages and other civil remedies against online pharmacies that are deemed a threat to state residents.

It requires the Drug Enforcement Administration (DEA) to report to Congress not later than 180 days after the enactment of this Act and annually for two years after such initial report on: (1) the foreign supply chains and sources of controlled substances offered for sale without a valid prescription on the internet; (2) DEA efforts and strategy to decrease such foreign supply chains; and (3) DEA efforts to work with domestic and multinational pharmaceutical companies and others in combating the sale of controlled substances over the internet without a valid prescription. (Bill: H.R. 6353)

Don't Put Your Health in the Hands of Crooks

It couldn't be easier—ordering prescription drugs online with a few clicks of the mouse and having them delivered right to your door, without ever having to see a doctor. But is it safe? Is it legal? You need to know the risks.

Yes, there are plenty of legitimate U.S. pharmaceutical companies and pharmacies (including online ones) that follow all the laws and regulations and put public safety first. But there are many that don't—they are just out to make a fast buck at your expense. These shady businesses fill orders without prescriptions. They pay doctors just to take a quick glance at your brief medical questionnaire. They don't know if you are drug-addicted, underage, or have another condition that their medications could make worse. And they don't care.

Worse yet, the products they peddle are questionable, at best. The drugs may be way past their expiration date. They may be counterfeit, mislabeled, adulterated, or contaminated. And they may well be made from suspect raw materials in underground laboratories in the U.S. and abroad, far from the safety-conscious eyes of the Food and Drug Administration.

Part of the problem is that these illegal pharmacies are all over the internet. More than 80,000 portal websites currently sell ad space for these medications and link to one of more than 1,400 anchor websites that allow customers to place orders through illegal pharmacies. You don't even have to search for these offers—they often come straight to your inbox as e-mail spam, enticing you with a cornucopia of drugs on the cheap.

Are there ways to tell whether an online pharmacy is legal?

Definitely, and here's what to look for. Legitimate pharmacies:

- require a prescription from a licensed doctor, usually by mail (if they accept a fax copy, they will always call your doctor to verify the prescription);
- make you submit a detailed medical history;

- clearly state their payment, privacy, and shipping fees on their sites; and

- use secure or encrypted website connections for transactions.

Many legitimate online pharmacies are also certified by the National Association of Boards of Pharmacy—check its website for a listing. Bear in mind, some of the larger internet pharmacies may not be certified because of their already well-recognized names. Remember: Do your homework and steer clear of illegal internet pharmacies, even if the prices are tempting. It's your health, after all.

Section 5.3

Facts about Medical Marijuana

This section includes text from "Medical Marijuana Reality Check," Office of National Drug Control Policy, February 2007; and "Medical Marijuana: The Facts," an undated document from the U.S. Drug Enforcement Administration.

Reality Check: What Is Wrong with Permitting the Use of Smoked Marijuana?

Simply put, the smoked form of marijuana is not considered modern medicine. On April 20, 2006, the U.S. Food and Drug Administration (FDA) issued an advisory concluding that no sound scientific studies have supported medical use of smoked marijuana for treatment in the United States, and no animal or human data support the safety or efficacy of smoked marijuana for general medical use. A number of states have passed voter referenda or legislative actions making smoked marijuana available for a variety of medical conditions upon a doctor's recommendation. According to the FDA, these measures are inconsistent with efforts to ensure medications undergo the rigorous scientific scrutiny of the FDA approval process and are proven safe and effective under the standards of the Federal Food, Drug, and Cosmetic (FD&C) Act.

While smoking marijuana may allow patients to temporarily feel better, the medical community makes an important distinction between inebriation and the controlled delivery of pure pharmaceutical medication. The raw (leaf) form of marijuana contains a complex mixture of compounds in uncertain concentrations, the majority of which have unknown pharmacological effects.

The Institute of Medicine (IOM) has concluded that smoking marijuana is not recommended for any long-term medical use, and a subsequent IOM report declared that, "marijuana is not modern medicine."

Smoking Marijuana May Unintentionally Cause Serious Harm to Patients

The delicate immune systems of seriously ill patients may become compromised by the smoking of marijuana. Additionally, the daily use of marijuana compromises lung function and increases the risk for respiratory diseases, similar to those associated with nicotine cigarettes. Marijuana has a high potential for abuse and can incur addiction. Frequent use of marijuana leads to tolerance to the psychoactive effects and smokers compensate by smoking more often or seeking higher potency marijuana. Also, in people with psychotic or other problems, the use of marijuana can precipitate severe emotional disorders. Chronic use of marijuana may increase the risk of psychotic symptoms in people with a past history of schizophrenia. Marijuana smoking by young people may lead to severe impairment of higher brain function and neuropsychiatric disorders, as well as a higher risk for addiction and polydrug abuse problems.

Existing Legal Drugs Provide Superior Treatment for Serious Medical Conditions

The FDA has approved safe and effective medication for the treatment of glaucoma, nausea, wasting syndrome, cancer, and multiple sclerosis. Marinol, the synthetic form of THC (tetrahydrocannabinol, the psychoactive ingredient contained in marijuana), is already legally available for prescription by physicians whose patients suffer from pain and chronic illness. "Medical marijuana was supposed to be for the truly ill cancer victims and AIDS [acquired immunodeficiency syndrome] patients who could use the drug to relieve pain or restore their appetites. Yet the number of dispensaries has skyrocketed from five in 2005 to 143 by the end of 2006. In North Hollywood alone, there are more pot clinics than Starbucks." *Pasadena Star-News*, January 21, 2007.

What the Experts Say

The American Academy of Ophthalmology: "Based on reviews by the National Eye Institute (NEI) and the Institute of Medicine and on available scientific evidence, the Task Force on Complementary Therapies believes that no scientific evidence has been found that demonstrates increased benefits and/or diminished risks of marijuana use to treat glaucoma compared with the wide variety of pharmaceutical agents now available." (Source: *Complementary Therapy Assessment: Marijuana in the Treatment of Glaucoma*, American Academy of Ophthalmology, May 2003.)

The American Medical Association (AMA): "…AMA recommends that marijuana be retained in Schedule I of the Controlled Substances Act…AMA believes that the NIH (National Institutes of Health) should use its resources and influence to support the development of a smoke-free inhaled delivery system for marijuana or delta-9-tetrahydrocannabinol (THC) to reduce the health hazards associated with the combustion and inhalation of marijuana…" (Source: Policy Statement H-95.952, American Medical Association, http://www.ama-assn.org.)

The National Multiple Sclerosis Society: "Studies completed thus far have not provided convincing evidence that marijuana or its derivatives provide substantiated benefits for symptoms of MS." (Source: *The MS Information Sourcebook*, Marijuana (Cannabis), National Multiple Sclerosis Society, September 18, 2006.)

The Institute of Medicine (IOM): "Because of the health risks associated with smoking, smoked marijuana should generally not be recommended for long-term medical use." (Source: *Marijuana and Medicine: Assessing the Science Base*, Institute of Medicine, 1999.)

Medical Marijuana—The Facts

Medical marijuana already exists. It's called Marinol. A pharmaceutical product, Marinol, is widely available through prescription. It comes in the form of a pill and is also being studied by researchers for suitability via other delivery methods, such as an inhaler or patch. The active ingredient of Marinol is synthetic tetrahydrocannabinol (THC), which has been found to relieve the nausea and vomiting associated with chemotherapy for cancer patients and to assist with loss of appetite with acquired immunodeficiency (AIDS) patients.

Unlike smoked marijuana—which contains more than 400 different chemicals, including most of the hazardous chemicals found in tobacco smoke—Marinol has been studied and approved by the medical community and the Food and Drug Administration (FDA), the nation's watchdog over unsafe and harmful food and drug products. Since the passage of the 1906 Pure Food and Drug Act, any drug that is marketed in the United States must undergo rigorous scientific testing. The approval process mandated by this act ensures that claims of safety and therapeutic value are supported by clinical evidence and keeps unsafe, ineffective, and dangerous drugs off the market.

There are no FDA-approved medications that are smoked. For one thing, smoking is generally a poor way to deliver medicine. It is difficult to administer safe, regulated dosages of medicines in smoked form. Secondly, the harmful chemicals and carcinogens that are byproducts of smoking create entirely new health problems. For example, the level of tar in a marijuana cigarette is four times greater than what is in a tobacco cigarette. Morphine, for example, has proven to be a medically valuable drug, but the FDA does not endorse the smoking of opium or heroin. Instead, scientists have extracted active ingredients from opium, which are sold as pharmaceutical products like morphine, codeine, hydrocodone, or oxycodone. In a similar vein, the FDA has not approved smoking marijuana for medicinal purposes, but has approved the active ingredient THC—in the form of scientifically regulated Marinol.

The Drug Enforcement Administration (DEA) helped facilitate the research on Marinol. The National Cancer Institute approached the DEA in the early 1980s regarding their study of THC in relieving nausea and vomiting. As a result, the DEA facilitated the registration and provided regulatory support and guidance for the study.

The DEA recognizes the importance of listening to science. That's why the DEA has registered seven research initiatives to continue researching the effects of smoked marijuana as medicine. For example, in one program established by the state of California, researchers are studying the potential use of marijuana and its ingredients on conditions such as multiple sclerosis and pain. At this time, however, neither the medical community nor the scientific community has found sufficient data to conclude that smoked marijuana is the best approach to dealing with these important medical issues.

The most comprehensive, scientifically rigorous review of studies of smoked marijuana was conducted by the Institute of Medicine, an organization chartered by the National Academy of Sciences. In a report released in 1999, the Institute did not recommend the use of

Chapter 6

Combat Methamphetamine Epidemic Act

Methamphetamine (meth) is an addictive stimulant drug that strongly activates certain areas in the brain. It is chemically related to amphetamine, but the central nervous system effects of methamphetamine are greater, resulting in a high potential for abuse and addiction.

Methamphetamine has become a tremendous challenge for the entire nation. Street names include: meth, speed, ice, chalk, crystal, crank, and fire. A clandestine meth lab has been found in every state across the country. Labs have been found in homes, cars, hotel rooms, storage facilities—these are generally referred to as small toxic labs. Ephedrine (EPH), pseudoephedrine (PSE), and phenylpropanolamine (PPA) are precursor chemicals used in the illicit manufacture of methamphetamine or amphetamine.

The Combat Methamphetamine Epidemic Act (CMEA) of 2005 was signed into law on March 9, 2006 to regulate, among other things, retail over-the-counter sales of EPH, PSE, and PPA products which are common ingredients found in cold and allergy products. The Drug Enforcement Administration (DEA) is committed to working with state and local law enforcement partners to ensure that streets and neighborhoods are safe and the methamphetamine problem is brought to an end. DEA's focus is to dismantle clandestine methamphetamine labs and trafficking organizations and to monitor the products that are illegally used to produce methamphetamine.

This chapter includes text from "Combat Methamphetamine Act of 2005," Drug Enforcement Administration (DEA), 2008; and excerpts from "The Combat Meth Act of 2005: Questions and Answers," an undated document from DEA.

Preventing Diversion

Per the CMEA, retailers must store products containing EPH, PSE, or PPA where customers do not have direct access to the product: either behind the counter or in a locked cabinet. Preventing diversion involves the coordination and cooperation of law enforcement officials, retailers, and individual consumers.

The seller must: Enforce daily sales and monthly purchase limits; store stock behind the counter or in a locked cabinet; maintain written or electronic logbook of sales; keep logbook for minimum of two years after date of sale; and confirm identification of purchaser.

The purchaser must: Enter his or her name, address, date and time of sale; provide photo identification issued by a state or federal government; and sign the logbook.

The logbook must: Document products by name, quantity sold, names and addresses of purchasers, date and time of sales, and contain the federal warning notice.

The Combat Methamphetamine Epidemic Act of 2005 established retail sales and purchase transaction limits in grams for scheduled listed chemical products which include pseudoephedrine drug products. Daily retail sales limit of PSE HCL is 3.6 grams per purchaser. Under the thirty day retail purchase limit, it is unlawful for any person to knowingly or intentionally purchase more than nine grams of PSE HCL per purchaser.

Why was the CMEA passed?

Ephedrine, pseudoephedrine, and phenylpropanolamine are precursor chemicals used in the illicit manufacture of methamphetamine or amphetamine. They are also common ingredients used to make cough, cold, and allergy products. Passage of the CMEA was accomplished to curtail the illicit production of methamphetamine and amphetamine.

Is methamphetamine production and abuse a nationwide problem?

Methamphetamine or "meth" has become a tremendous challenge for the entire nation. A clandestine methamphetamine laboratory has been found in every state over the past five years. A July 18, 2006,

National Association of Counties Survey found that meth is the leading drug-related local law enforcement problem in the country. The survey of 500 county law enforcement officials in 44 states found that meth continues to be the number one drug problem—more counties (48%) report that meth is the primary drug problem—more than cocaine (22%), marijuana (22%), and heroin (3%) combined. In addition, according to the survey, crimes related to meth continue to grow—55% of law enforcement officials report an increase in robberies or burglaries in the last year and 48% report an increase in domestic violence.

Chapter 7

Initiation of Substance Use

Information on substance use initiation, also known as incidence or first-time use, is important for policy makers and researchers. Measures of initiation are often leading indicators of emerging patterns of substance use. They provide valuable information that can be used in the assessment of the effectiveness of current prevention programs and in focusing prevention efforts.

With its large sample size and oversampling of youths aged 12 to 17 and young adults aged 18 to 25, the National Survey on Drug Use and Health (NSDUH) provides a variety of estimates related to substance use initiation based on questions on age, year, and month at first use. Using this information, along with the interview date and the respondent's date of birth, a date of first use is determined for each substance used by a respondent. Estimates of the number of initiates, rates of initiation, and average age at first use can be constructed for specific time periods.

Because of concerns about the validity of trend estimates of incidence based on long recall periods (Gfroerer, Hughes, Chromy, Heller, and Packer, 2004), this report only presents estimates of initiation occurring in the 12 months prior to the interview date. Individuals who initiated use within the past 12 months are defined as recent or

This chapter is excerpted from "Results from the 2007 National Survey on Drug Use and Health: National Findings, Chapter 5: Initiation of Substance Use," Substance Abuse and Mental Health Services Administration (SAMHSA), September 2008.

past year initiates. Estimates for each year are produced independently based on the data from the survey conducted that year. One caveat of this approach is that because the survey interviews persons aged 12 or older and asks about the past 12 months, the initiation estimates will represent some, but not all of initiation at age 11, and no initiation occurring at age ten or younger. This underestimation problem primarily affects estimates of initiation for cigarettes, alcohol, and inhalants because they tend to be initiated at a younger age than other substances.

There are some important issues that readers need to be aware of when interpreting these NSDUH incidence estimates. First, note that some tables and analyses are based on the ages of initiates at the time of interview, while others focus on the age at the time of first substance use. This can have a large impact on estimates, so readers should pay close attention to the approach used in each situation. Titles and notes on tables document which method applies.

An important consideration in looking at incidence estimates across different drug categories is that substance users typically initiate use of different substances at different times in their lives. Thus, the estimates for specific illicit drugs cannot be added to obtain the number of illicit drug initiates, because, for example, most of the cocaine initiates had previously used marijuana or other drugs and therefore would be represented in the illicit drug initiate estimates for a prior year. Similarly, the estimates of crack initiation are not a subset of the estimates of cocaine initiation, as some persons would have used powder cocaine prior to using crack. To help clarify this aspect of the incidence data, additional tables have been generated to identify which specific illicit drug was used at the time of first use of any illicit drug.

The drug use initiation estimates in this chapter, however, are based on data only from the core section of the questionnaire and do not take account of data from new items on the initiation of methamphetamine use that were added to the non-core section in 2007 following up on the additional methamphetamine users identified in the questions introduced in 2005 and 2006.

Initiation of Illicit Drug Use

In 2007, an estimated 2.7 million persons aged 12 or older used an illicit drug for the first time within the past 12 months; this averages to more than 7,000 initiates per day. This estimate was not significantly different from the number in 2006 (2.8 million). Three-fifths of initiates (60.1%) were younger than age 18 when they first used, and 54.1% of new users were female. The average age at initiation among persons aged 12 to 49 was 18.0 years.

In 2007, of the 2.7 million persons aged 12 or older who used illicit drugs for the first time within the past 12 months, a majority reported that their first drug was marijuana (56.%), see Figure 7.1. Nearly one-third initiated with psychotherapeutics (30.6%, including 19.0% with pain relievers, 6.5% with tranquilizers, 4.1% with stimulants, and 1.1% with sedatives). A sizable proportion reported inhalants (10.7%) as their first drug, and a small proportion used hallucinogens as their first illicit drug (2.0%). The percentage of past year illicit drug initiates whose first drug was tranquilizers increased from 2.4% in 2002 to 6.5% in 2007, while the percentage whose first drug was ecstasy decreased from 1.9% in 2002 to 0.6% in 2007.

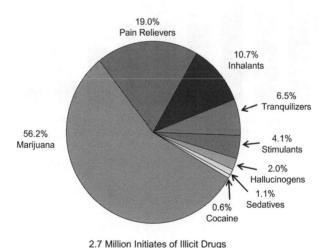

2.7 Million Initiates of Illicit Drugs

Figure 7.1. Specific Drug Used When Initiating Illicit Drug Use among Past Year Initiates of Illicit Drugs Aged 12 or Older: 2007. Note: The percentages add to greater than 100% because of a small number of respondents initiating multiple drugs on the same day.

Comparison, by Drug

The specific drug categories with the largest number of recent initiates among persons aged 12 or older were nonmedical use of pain relievers (2.1 million) and marijuana use (2.1 million), followed by nonmedical use of tranquilizers (1.2 million), cocaine (0.9 million), ecstasy (0.8 million), inhalants (0.8 million), and stimulants (0.6 million), see Figure 7.2.

Among persons aged 12 to 49, the average age at first use of inhalants in 2007 was 17.1 years; it was 17.6 years for marijuana, 20.2 years for cocaine, 20.2 years for ecstasy, 21.2 years for pain relievers, and 24.5 years for tranquilizers.

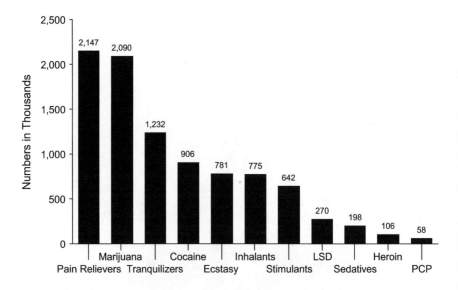

Figure 7.2. *Past Year Initiates for Specific Illicit Drugs among Persons Aged 12 or Older: 2007*

Marijuana

In 2007, there were 2.1 million persons who had used marijuana for the first time within the past 12 months; this averages to approximately 6,000 initiates per day. This estimate of past year initiates in 2007 was about the same as the number in 2006 (2.1 million), 2005 (2.1 million), 2004 (2.1 million), 2003 (2.0 million), and 2002 (2.2 million).

Most (62.2%) of the 2.1 million recent marijuana initiates were younger than age 18 when they first used. Among youths aged 12 to 17, an estimated 4.6% had used marijuana for the first time within the past year, similar to the rate in 2006 (4.7%).

As a percentage of those aged 12 to 17 who had not used marijuana prior to the past year, the youth marijuana initiation rate in 2007 (5.2%) was similar to the rate in 2006 (5.4%).

In 2007, the average age at first marijuana use among recent initiates aged 12 to 49 was 17.6 years, which was similar to the average in 2006 (17.4 years). Among recent initiates aged 12 or older who initiated use prior to the age of 21, the mean age at first use was 16.2 years in 2007, which was not significantly different from the estimate (16.1 years) in 2006.

Cocaine

In 2007, there were 906,000 persons aged 12 or older who had used cocaine for the first time within the past 12 months; this averages to approximately 2,500 initiates per day. This estimate was not significantly different from the number in 2006 (977,000).

Most (66.5%) of the 0.9 million recent cocaine initiates were 18 or older when they first used. The average age at first use among recent initiates aged 12 to 49 was 20.2 years, which was similar to the average age in 2006 (20.3 years).

Heroin

In 2007, there were 106,000 persons aged 12 or older who had used heroin for the first time within the past 12 months. The average age at first use of heroin among recent initiates aged 12 to 49 was 21.8 years in 2007. There were no significant changes in the number of initiates or in the average age at first use from 2006 to 2007.

Hallucinogens

In 2007, there were 1.1 million persons aged 12 or older who had used hallucinogens for the first time within the past 12 months. This estimate was not significantly different from the estimate in 2002, 2004, 2005, and 2006. However, the estimate was significantly higher than the estimate in 2003 (886,000).

There was no significant change between 2006 and 2007 in the number of past year initiates of lysergic acid diethylamide (LSD), 264,000 and 270,000, respectively.

There was no significant change in the past year initiates of ecstasy between 2006 (860,000) and 2007 (781,000). The number of past year ecstasy initiates in 2007, however, was significantly lower than the estimate in 2002 (1.2 million), but higher than the estimate in 2003 (642,000), 2004 (607,000), and 2005 (615,000). Most (61.2%) of the recent ecstasy initiates in 2007 were aged 18 or older at the time they first used ecstasy. The corresponding figure was 70.1% in 2006. Among past year initiates aged 12 to 49, the average age at initiation of ecstasy in 2007 was 20.2 years, similar to the average age in 2006 (20.6 years).

Inhalants

In 2007, there were 775,000 persons aged 12 or older who had used inhalants for the first time within the past 12 months; 66.3% were under age 18 when they first used. There was no significant difference in the number of inhalant initiates between 2006 and 2007. However, there was a significant increase in the average age at first use among recent initiates aged 12 to 49 from 2006 (15.7 years) to 2007 (17.1 years).

Psychotherapeutics

Psychotherapeutics include the nonmedical use of any prescription-type pain relievers, tranquilizers, stimulants, or sedatives. Over-the-counter substances are not included. In 2007, there were 2.5 million persons aged 12 or older who used psychotherapeutics nonmedically for the first time within the past year, which averages out to around 7,000 initiates per day. The numbers of new users of specific classes of psychotherapeutics in 2007 were 2.1 million for pain relievers, 1.2 million for tranquilizers, 642,000 for stimulants, and 198,000 for sedatives. There was a significant decrease in the number of past year initiates of stimulants from 2006 (845,000) to 2007 (642,000), but there were no significant changes in the estimates for the remaining psychotherapeutics between these years. The estimated number of past year initiates of nonmedical pain reliever use declined from 2.5 million in 2003 to 2.1 million in 2007.

The average age at first nonmedical use of any psychotherapeutics among recent initiates aged 12 to 49 was 21.8 years. More specifically, it was 21.2 years for pain relievers, 21.9 years for stimulants, 24.5 years for tranquilizers, and 24.2 years for sedatives.

In 2007, the number of new nonmedical users of OxyContin® aged 12 or older was 554,000, with an average age at first use of 24.0 years among those aged 12 to 49. These estimates are similar to those for 2006 (533,000 and 22.6 years, respectively).

The number of recent new users of methamphetamine among persons aged 12 or older was 157,000 in 2007. This estimate was significantly lower than the estimate in 2002 (299,000), 2003 (260,000), 2004 (318,000), and 2006 (259,000). The average age of new methamphetamine users aged 12 to 49 in 2007 was 19.1 years, not significantly different from the average ages in 2002 through 2006.

Chapter 8

Substance Abuse and Children

Chapter Contents

Section 8.1—Prenatal Exposure to
        Illicit Drugs and Alcohol 54

Section 8.2—Drug Endangered Children 59

Section 8.1

Prenatal Exposure to Illicit Drugs and Alcohol

Excerpted from "Family Matters: Substance Abuse and The American Family," March 2005, National Center on Addiction and Substance Abuse (CASA) at Columbia University, http://www.casacolumbia.org. © 2005. All rights reserved. Reprinted with permission. The complete document is available at http://www.casacolumbia.org/absolutenm/articlefiles/380-Family%20Matters.pdf.

Health Effects of Parental Substance Abuse

Family members living with a chronic substance abuser often suffer from psychological and emotional stress, as well as physical problems such as insomnia, headaches, allergies, asthma, gastrointestinal problems, cardiovascular disease, and even cancer.

Children of substance abusers face three main sources of risk to their health. Prenatal exposure to tobacco, alcohol, and drugs can impair their physical and mental development. Growing up in a substance-abusing environment can expose them to environmental tobacco smoke, rides in a car with a parent who is under the influence of alcohol or drugs, or to neglect or abuse. It also puts them at risk for conduct disorders, depression, anxiety, and academic difficulties. The prenatal and environmental effects of exposure to parental substance abuse are known pathways to children's own substance use and abuse.

Prenatal Exposure to Tobacco, Alcohol, and Illicit Drug Use

Prenatal exposure to tobacco, alcohol, and drugs is associated with a host of physical, mental, and cognitive disorders. The problems faced by children exposed prenatally to substances of abuse often continue into adolescence and adulthood, burdening them with ailments that may be as bad as or worse than those experienced by the actual substance abuser.

Smoking: Nearly one-third (31.1%) of women of reproductive age report smoking cigarettes in the past month, as do 17.3% of pregnant women. Among those who are pregnant, younger women ages 18 to 25 are more likely to report smoking cigarettes than women ages 26 to 44 (26.4% versus 10.2%).

Nicotine exposure during pregnancy increases the flow of carbon monoxide to the fetus and decreases placental flow, putting the infant at risk for growth retardation, low birth weight, premature delivery, spontaneous abortion, and other complications of pregnancy and delivery. As many as 14% of premature deliveries and 10% of all infant deaths can be linked to tobacco use during pregnancy. In 2002, 12.2% of smoking mothers (versus 7.5% of non-smoking mothers) had a low birth-weight baby. Low birth weight can lead to an infant's death, often from sudden infant death syndrome (SIDS).

Children exposed prenatally to smoking may suffer from a variety of cognitive and behavioral developmental problems that could increase their vulnerability to substance abuse. Long-term cognitive effects include lower intelligence quotient (IQ) and poor verbal, reading, and math skills. Long-term behavioral effects include an increased risk for conduct disorders, attention deficit hyperactivity disorder, and drug dependence. One decade-long study found that, compared to children of nonsmoking mothers, male children of mothers who smoked more than ten cigarettes nearly every day while pregnant were over three times likelier to have conduct disorder in their lifetime. Female children of mothers who smoked the same amount were over five times likelier to develop drug abuse or dependence.

The extent of the negative effects that a child experiences due to prenatal exposure to smoking is dependent on the frequency and quantity of that exposure; the greater the exposure, the more likely the child is to suffer.

Alcohol: More than half (53.4%) of women of reproductive age report drinking alcohol in the past month, as do 9.1% of pregnant women. Younger pregnant women, ages 18 to 25, are more likely to report drinking alcohol than older pregnant women ages 26 to 44 (10% versus 8.3%). Younger women of childbearing age also have higher rates than women of other ages of alcohol abuse and dependence (nearly 10% for women ages 18 to 29 versus 4% for women ages 30 to 44).

Prenatal exposure to alcohol increases the risk of a wide range of physical and mental health problems in children. The full range of possible outcomes resulting from maternal alcohol use during pregnancy is referred to as fetal alcohol spectrum disorder (FASD). The most severe is fetal alcohol syndrome (FAS). Children with FAS are small for their age, and are born with facial anomalies, and damage to the central nervous system. Other possible FAS characteristics are cardiac problems, skeletal malformations, visual and auditory deficits, and altered immunological function. These problems may be due to poor blood flow, hormonal imbalances, and the direct effects of alcohol on cellular processes during the prenatal period. The time of greatest likelihood of damage to the fetus' brain occurs during the final trimester of pregnancy when the brain is developing rapidly.

Other problems that have been associated with FAS and prenatal exposure to alcohol—all of which make the child more susceptible to difficulties in schooling and put him or her at risk for substance abuse—include hyperactivity and attention deficits, memory difficulties, poor problem solving skills, significant weakness in arithmetic skills, lower IQ scores, and problems with language, perception, and motor development.

FAS is the leading cause of preventable mental retardation in the Western world. Approximately 6% of the offspring of alcohol-abusing women have FAS, with up to 8,000 babies born with it each year in the U.S. The actual rate of FAS probably is even higher than these estimates, given the difficulty in making the diagnosis and because many physicians are reluctant to label children as having FAS and their mothers as being alcoholics due to the attached stigma.

Many children born with FAS continue to suffer into adulthood. One study found that the majority of adults with FAS or fetal alcohol effects (FAE, a more mild form of FAS) suffer from substantial mental illness, including drug and alcohol dependence, depression, bipolar disorder, anxiety disorder, and eating disorders, as well as avoidant, antisocial, and dependent personality disorders. In this study, 72% of the participants born with FAS had received some form of psychiatric treatment, with 24% requiring hospitalization in a psychiatric institution.

Even moderate levels of prenatal exposure to alcohol can have detrimental effects on children's learning and behavior. Prenatal exposure to alcohol is associated with antisocial and delinquent behavioral problems during adolescence and young adulthood, including poor impulse control, poor social adaptation, inappropriate sexual behavior, trouble with the law, problems with employment, and alcohol or drug problems.

Many factors can contribute to the severity of effects experienced by a child prenatally exposed to alcohol, such as how much alcohol he or she is exposed to, the pattern of the mother's drinking, the stage of pregnancy during which the drinking occurred, the use of other drugs, and the mother's nutrition and prenatal care. The duration of alcohol exposure during pregnancy influences the extent of impairment in children's attention, language, and memory skills up to early adolescence. The mother's age, the presence of maternal psychiatric disorders, and the family's socioeconomic status also all influence the extent of the problems resulting from prenatal exposure to alcohol.

Illicit drugs: Approximately 10.3% of women of reproductive age report using illicit drugs in the past month, as do 3.3% of pregnant women. Younger pregnant women ages 18 to 25 are more likely to report using illicit drugs than older pregnant women ages 26 to 44 (6.6% versus 0.5%).

More than half of the pregnant women who use illicit drugs also drink and smoke during pregnancy. Pregnant women are likelier to use marijuana (2.9%) or misuse prescription drugs (0.8%) than they are to use cocaine (0.3%) or hallucinogens (0.2%).

The majority of children who have been exposed prenatally to illicit drugs also have been exposed to other risk factors during childhood, including parental use of tobacco or alcohol, poverty, neglect, or abuse. Because of financial limitations or fear of legal repercussions, drug abusing women seldom receive adequate prenatal care. This lack of adequate prenatal care may account for some of the physiological and psychological problems found in children born to drug-abusing women.

Marijuana: Some of the effects of prenatal exposure to marijuana use are similar to those of tobacco, including increased carbon monoxide levels and reduced oxygen flow that place the fetus at risk for future verbal and memory problems. Heavy marijuana use has been associated with low birth weight, premature delivery, and complications in delivery.

Opiates: Prenatal exposure to opiates, such as heroin or methadone, has been associated with premature delivery, miscarriages, low birth weight, and increased risk for sudden infant death syndrome (SIDS). In most cases, prenatal exposure to opiates produces withdrawal symptoms in the newborn soon after birth, including respiratory problems, restlessness, disturbed sleep, feeding problems, vomiting, diarrhea, fever, and excessive crying. The duration of these symptoms can last anywhere from eight weeks to several months. Up to 90% of opioid-exposed infants require special handling and medical intervention. Many children who are exposed prenatally to opiates suffer from attention problems and developmental delays.

Cocaine: Cocaine use results in increased blood pressure and respiration. In pregnant women, these effects translate into decreased oxygen and nutrition flow to the fetus placing the fetus at greater risk for growth retardation, low birth weight, premature delivery, spontaneous abortion, premature detachment of the placenta, and stillbirth. Infants prenatally exposed to cocaine are at increased risk for intracranial hemorrhage, seizures, and respiratory distress, are likelier to demonstrate movement problems at birth, and may experience symptoms of irritability, hyperactivity, and problems with sleep and feeding.

Other stimulants: Many of the effects of prenatal exposure to amphetamines and methamphetamines are similar to those found in children prenatally exposed to cocaine or heroin, including withdrawal symptoms, irritability, sleep problems, and developmental delays.

Other Health Consequences Associated with Prenatal Exposure to Substances

Mothers who abuse substances may expose their babies to infectious diseases. A mother who has multiple sexual partners, a history of prostitution, or a history of injection drug use (all behaviors associated with drug abuse) puts her fetus at risk for gonorrhea, syphilis, herpes, chlamydia, hepatitis B, multiple drug-resistant tuberculosis (TB), human immunodeficiency virus (HIV), and/or acquired immunodeficiency syndrome (AIDS).

Section 8.2

Drug Endangered Children

This section includes text from "Drug Endangered Children," Office of National Drug Control Policy, 2009; and excerpts from "Family Matters: Substance Abuse and The American Family," March 2005, National Center on Addiction and Substance Abuse (CASA) at Columbia University, http://www.casacolumbia.org. © 2005. All rights reserved. Reprinted with permission. The complete document is available at http://www.casacolumbia.org/absolutenm/articlefiles/380-Family%20Matters.pdf.

Background

Innocent children are sometimes found in homes and other environments (hotels, automobiles, apartments) where methamphetamine and other illegal substances are produced. Around the country, Drug endangered children (DEC) programs have been developed to coordinate the efforts of law enforcement, medical services, and child welfare workers to ensure that children found in these environments receive appropriate attention and care.

Children who live at or visit drug-production sites or are present during drug production face a variety of health and safety risks, including: inhalation, absorption, or ingestion of toxic chemicals, drugs, or contaminated foods that may result in nausea, chest pain, eye and tissue irritation, chemical burns, and death; fires and explosions; abuse and neglect; and hazardous lifestyle (presence of booby traps, firearms, code violations, poor ventilation).

Prevalence

According to the El Paso Intelligence Center's (EPIC) National Clandestine Laboratory Seizure System, there were an estimated 1,025 children injured at or affected by methamphetamine labs during calendar year 2008 (report generated February 3, 2009—data are subject to change). A child affected by labs includes children who were residing at the labs but may not have been present at the time of the lab seizure as well as children who were visiting the site.

Table 8.1. Number of Children Affected by Methamphetamine Labs, 2004–2008

	2004	2005	2006	2007	2008
Child injured	13	11	—	7	6
Child killed	3	2	—	1	—
Children affected	3,088	1,647	—	778	1,019
Total injured/ killed/affected	3,104	1,660	1,222	786	1,025

Federal Response

In October 2008, the President signed the Drug Endangered Children Act of 2007 into law. This legislation will provide for funds to be used for DEC-related grants. A variety of agencies are called for response when drug laboratories are identified. When children are found at the laboratories, additional agencies and officials should be called in to assist, including emergency medical personnel, social services, and physicians. Actions of the responding agencies should include taking children into protective custody and arranging for child protective services, immediately testing the children for methamphetamine exposure, conducting medical and mental health assessments, and ensuring short- and long-term care.

Living with a Substance-Abusing Parent Can Put Children's Physical and Mental Health at Risk

Many aspects of the environment in which the children of substance-abusing parents are reared can be detrimental to children's physical and mental health and increase their own risk for substance use and abuse. In 2002, almost five million adults who abused or were dependent on alcohol had at least one child younger than 18 living with them. Many of these alcohol abusing adults also smoked cigarettes (57.9%) or used illicit drugs (35.5%).

Exposure to Environmental Tobacco Smoke

Environmental tobacco smoke (ETS) is present in just over 25% of households with children under the age of 18. Children of smokers have a disproportionate number of medical conditions compared to children of non-smokers. Non-smokers who are exposed to ETS absorb nicotine and other carcinogenic materials just as smokers themselves do, although the smoke is less concentrated. One study found that 87.9% of children and adult non-users of tobacco had detectable levels of serum cotinine (a metabolite of nicotine) in their blood, indicating the widespread exposure to ETS. Exposure to ETS has both short- and long-term effects on the child. Because the respiratory tract of a young child is not fully developed, children exposed to tobacco smoke are at greater risk than non-exposed children for respiratory illness, cough, asthma and sudden infant death syndrome (SIDS). In addition, these children are more likely to suffer from ear infections and to have their tonsils and/or adenoids surgically removed. The longer-term effects include higher risks of lung and other forms of cancer, atherosclerosis (hardening of the arteries due to the build-up of fatty deposits called plaque, which can lead to stroke), and coronary heart disease.

Every year, ETS exposure among children living in the United States is associated with an estimated 700,000 to 1.6 million visits to the doctor for ear infections; 14,000 to 21,000 tonsillectomies and/or adenoidectomies; 8,000 to 26,000 new cases of asthma, 400,000 to one million cases of exacerbations of asthma symptoms and 529,000 physician visits for asthma; 1.3 to two million visits for coughs; and 150,000 to 300,000 cases of bronchitis or pneumonia (primarily among younger children). ETS exposure also is associated with 280 to 360 childhood deaths from respiratory illness, more than 300 fire-related injuries, and 1,900 to 2,700 deaths due to SIDS.

Mothers who smoke and breast feed their babies put their children at even greater risk for ETS exposure. Cotinine levels are five to ten times higher in breast-fed infants of smoking mothers than among bottle-fed infants of smoking mothers, indicating higher levels of ETS exposure. Cotinine levels also are elevated among both breast-fed and bottle-fed children of non-smoking mothers who live in a household with a smoker. Thus, infants can be exposed to nicotine and cotinine from ETS via both inhalation and ingestion.

Accidents and Injuries Due to Parents' Alcohol or Drug Use

Alcohol is found in the blood of up to 60% of motor vehicle crash victims, up to 50% of suicides, up to 46% of homicide victims, up to 50% of drowning victims, and up to 64% of fire and burn fatalities. In 2002, there were 17,419 alcohol-related traffic fatalities (41% of total traffic fatalities) and 258,000 alcohol-related injuries due to automobile crashes alone. Thirty-two percent of the people who were killed in alcohol-related crashes were non-intoxicated occupants and non-occupants of the car. There is little doubt that many of the non-intoxicated occupants were family members of a substance abuser who drove while under the influence of alcohol or other drugs. Recent research reveals that between 1997 and 2002, 2,355 children died in alcohol-related crashes; 68% of those children were riding with a driver who had been drinking. Drugs other than alcohol (for example, marijuana and cocaine) have been identified as factors in 18% of motor vehicle driver deaths.

Children of substance abusers may experience accidental injuries and may suffer from malnutrition or live in unhygienic conditions, increasing their risk of illness.

Children of Alcohol and Drug Abusers Are at Greater Risk for Mental Health Problems

Children of substance-abusing parents tend to have two types of psychiatric disorders: behavioral problems that are directed outward toward others such as attention deficit hyperactivity disorder, conduct disorder, and oppositional defiant disorder; or, problems that are directed inward such as depression or anxiety. Outwardly directed disorders are more commonly found in boys and inwardly directed disorders are more commonly found in girls. Both types of disorders have been linked to increased risk for substance use in children and teens.

Children of alcoholics (COAs): COAs are at increased risk for a range of mental health problems. The extent to which these problems develop depends on the severity of the family dysfunction and the extent to which other family members can compensate. Many alcoholics suffer from co-occurring psychiatric disorders, such as anxiety disorders or mood disorders. COAs (particularly sons of alcoholics) tend to exhibit more stress and anxiety than that found in non-COAs, increasing the likelihood that they will drink alcohol or use other substances in order to reduce their feelings of anxiety.

COAs also have lower self-esteem than non-COAs, and tend to have more impulsive personality traits, demonstrating greater sensation seeking and aggressiveness than non-COAs. Preschool-aged COAs are likelier than non-COAs to be shy, perhaps due to a biological predisposition to anxiety or a home life that promotes fear and uncertainty.

The link between parental alcoholism and their children's mental health disorders could be due to the fact that alcoholism interferes with healthy parenting or that COAs are genetically predisposed to psychiatric disorders. The frequency of psychiatric disorders among children with two alcoholic parents is distinctly higher than among those with one alcoholic parent.

Children of illicit drug users: Children of illicit drug abusers are likelier than children of non-drug abusers to demonstrate immature, impulsive, or irresponsible behavior, to have lower intelligence quotient (IQ) scores, more absences from school, and to have behavioral problems, depression, and anxiety—all signs of risk for substance abuse. Children of drug-abusing parents, particularly drug-abusing mothers, are more likely to be disobedient, aggressive, withdrawn, and detached. These children also tend to have fewer friends, lower confidence in their ability to make friends, and a greater likelihood of being avoided by their peers.

Children of Substance Abusers Are at Increased Risk for Substance Abuse

A large body of research indicates that all types of parental substance use, including smoking, drinking, and illicit drug use, are associated with an increased risk that their children also will be substance abusers.

Environment and genetics: Through studies of adopted children and twins who have grown up in different environments, researchers have established that genetic factors play a role in the transmission of tobacco use, alcohol abuse, and illicit drug use from parent to child. Adopted children with alcohol-dependent biological parents are at least twice as likely as other adopted children to develop alcoholism, providing evidence of a genetic link.

Family, friends, and the community have much to do with whether a child decides to use or experiment with substances. However, once a child has begun to smoke, drink, or use drugs, genetic factors influence the transition from use to abuse. Similarly, the ability to tolerate a substance, for example, without becoming impaired may be strongly influenced by genetic makeup, and may in turn contribute to a propensity to abuse that substance. Early-onset alcoholism with severe symptoms and the need for extensive treatment has a substantial genetic basis.

Children of alcoholics: There are an estimated five million children living with their alcohol-abusing or dependent parent in the

United States. Other research suggests that almost ten million children under age 18 live with an adult with a past-year diagnosis of alcohol abuse or dependence and more than 28 million live with an adult who has at one point in his or her lifetime been diagnosed with alcohol abuse or dependence. In this study, 70 to 83% of the children were the biological, foster, adopted, or stepchildren of the alcohol-abusing or dependent adults. Ten to 20% were adult siblings or other biological relatives, and the rest were non-relatives or had an unspecified relationship with the alcohol-abusing or dependent adult.

COAs are approximately four times likelier than non-COAs to use alcohol or develop alcohol-related problems. COAs tend to initiate alcohol use earlier and engage in problem drinking at a younger age than non-COAs. It is not clear from existing research the extent to which COAs' greater susceptibility to alcohol problems is a function of parental alcoholism or a result of other mental health problems.

COAs have more positive beliefs and expectations than non-COAs about the effects of alcohol and experience increased feelings of pleasure and relaxation, decreased muscle tension, and decreased feelings of intoxication at the same blood alcohol levels as non-COAs. This reduced impairment from drinking often is associated with future problems with alcohol.

Chapter 9

Adolescents at Risk for Substance Use Disorders

Adolescence is the developmental period of highest risk for the onset of problematic alcohol and other drug (AOD) use. Some experimentation with alcohol may be considered normal during adolescence; however, people who engage in binge drinking or who have developed alcohol use disorders typically also engage in other drug use, most frequently cigarettes and marijuana. AOD use behaviors are multifaceted and complex and are influenced by a multiplicity of genetic and environmental liabilities. Risk factors for adolescent AOD use and substance use disorders (SUD) can be conceptually divided into heritable, environmental, and phenotypic factors (Clark and Winters 2002). Heritable risk factors are reflected in familial patterns of SUD and other psychiatric disorders. Environmental risk factors include family-related characteristics, such as family functioning, parenting practices, and child maltreatment, as well as other contextual factors, such as peer influences, substance availability, and consumption opportunities. These heritable and environmental factors then interact to determine a person's observable characteristics and behaviors (for example, phenotypes), such as AOD use.

Text in this chapter is excerpted from "Adolescents at Risk for Substance Use Disorders," *Alcohol Research and Health Journal*, Vol. 31, No. 2, National Institute on Alcohol Abuse and Alcoholism (NIAAA), 2008. The complete text, including references, is available online at http://pubs.niaaa.nih.gov/publications/arh312/168-176.pdf.

Recent studies (for example, Tarter et al. 1999, 2003) have identified a construct referred to as childhood psychological dysregulation as a behavioral phenotype that reflects a person's general liability of developing AOD problems in adolescence. For people with this liability, adverse environmental characteristics often lead to the development of SUD. Furthermore, researchers have identified other, covert characteristics known as endophenotypes that link a specific genotype with a behavioral phenotype or disease. For example, specific neurobiological endo-phenotypes, such as a type of brain wave known as the P300 event-related potential (ERP), may constitute the underpinnings of psychological dysregulation.

Heritable Risks

Historically, a person's genetic risk for developing a certain disorder has been estimated by establishing a family history of the disorder, and this approach remains important for research on SUD. Presence of a SUD in a parent has consistently been shown to be a strong risk factor for adolescent AOD use and SUD. However, the transmission of SUD from parent to offspring occurs through both genetic and environmental influences (Sartor et al. 2006).

In general, children of alcoholic parents (COA) have been studied more extensively than children of parents with other addictive disorders. The existing studies identified both common and distinct features between COA and children of parents with other SUD. For example, compared with children whose parents have no SUD (reference children), COA exhibit increased rates of alcohol use disorders (Schuckit and Smith 1996). Similarly, children of parents with SUD involving cocaine, heroin, or other illicit drugs tend to start using tobacco earlier than reference children and to have increased rates of illicit drug use and SUD symptoms (Clark et al. 1999).

Psychological Dysregulation

Psychological dysregulation is defined as deficiency in three domains—cognitive, behavioral, and emotional—when adapting to environmental challenges. These three domains of dysregulation are statistically related to one overall dimension, conceptualized as psychological dysregulation (Tarter et al. 2003). An increasing number of studies indicate that childhood psychological dysregulation predicts adolescent SUD (such as Tarter et al. 1999). Furthermore, childhood psychological dysregulation significantly discriminates boys with and without parental SUD (Tarter et al. 2003).

In its more severe forms, psychological dysregulation during child-hood manifests as disruptive behavior disorders, such as conduct dis-order (CD), oppositional defiant disorder (ODD), and attention deficit/ hyperactivity disorder (ADHD). However, psychological dysregulation in different manifestations can be observed at all developmental stages, including CD and ADHD during childhood, SUD during ado-lescence, and borderline personality disorder or antisocial personal-ity disorder during adulthood.

Conduct disorder during childhood is one of the most important predictors of adolescent SUD (Bukstein 2000; Clark et al. 2002; Sartor et al. 2006). In a study of 177 adolescent boys with and 203 boys with-out paternal SUD, Clark and colleagues (1999) demonstrated that antisocial disorders, including CD and ODD, partially were respon-sible for the relationship between paternal SUD and substance-related problems during adolescence. However, it is not only psychological dysregulation found in a child that may predict SUD when that child reaches adolescence. Psychological dysregulation in that child's par-ents during their childhood also may contribute to the heritable risks for SUD (Clark et al. 2004a).

The cognitive dimension of psychological dysregulation, also known as executive cognitive dysfunction, is particularly relevant for under-standing SUD (Giancola and Tarter 1999). For example, in a study of 66 high-risk adolescents, Tapert and colleagues (2002) demonstrated that a high level of executive cognitive dysfunction predicted AOD use and SUD eight years later, even when controlling for other factors, such as level of baseline AOD use, family history of SUD, and CD in the child. Executive cognitive function might be one of the primary components underlying the relationship between psychological dysregulation and AOD involvement.

Brain Structures Related to Psychological Dysregulation as Endo-Phenotypes

Chambers and colleagues (2003) have described adolescence as the "critical period of addiction vulnerability" (p. 1042), because during this period the brain pathways (neural circuits) that enable people to experience motivation and rewarding experiences still are developing. Variations in how these neural pathways develop may contribute to the risk for AOD drug use during adolescence. Specifically, researchers have suggested that psychological dys-regulation may be related to the function of the prefrontal cortex (Dawes et al. 2000).

Endo-phenotypes are characteristics that cannot be observed with the naked eye but can be measured using other techniques and which are part of the pathway from a person's genotype to an observable behavioral phenotype or outcome (Gottesman and Gould 2003). A well-accepted endo-phenotype in psychiatry is a certain brain wave called the P300 event-related potentials (ERP). ERP are a series of changes in normal electrical brain activity that occur after a person is exposed to a sudden stimulus, such as a sound or light, and are a measure of brain activity during the processing of new information. They can be recorded using an electroencephalograph (EEG). One of the most consistent components of the ERP occurs approximately 300 milliseconds after a novel and rare stimulus and is therefore called P300 (Bauer and Hesselbrock 1999). It is one of the most commonly used ERP components in the study of the effects of AOD on cognitive functions.

Studies found that in adolescent boys a reduced P300 amplitude is associated with disorders reflecting psychological dysregulation in the father and predicts the development of SUD by young adulthood (Iacono et al. 2002). The relationship between low P300 amplitudes during childhood and increased risk of SUD in young adulthood appears to be mediated by behavioral problems during childhood and adolescence—that is, adolescents with lower P300 amplitudes also had more behavioral problems during childhood and adolescence and were also more likely to develop SUD during young adulthood (Habeych et al. 2005).

A large study of identical and fraternal twins—the Minnesota Twin Family Study—has provided substantial support for the notion that the P300 response can serve as an endo-phenotype for adolescent SUD. For example, the study investigators found that the P300 response was strongly heritable and showed strong relationships to many other phenotypic predictors of adolescent SUD, such as early or frequent cannabis use (Yoon et al. 2006).

Environmental Influences on Risk of Adolescent SUDs

Several environmental influences have been identified that affect the risk of accelerated AOD involvement and the development of adolescent SUD. Major environmental influences include child maltreatment and other traumatic events; parental influences, such as parenting practices; and peer influences. Some of these also lead to manifestations of psychological dysregulation, such as CD, attention deficit/hyperactivity disorder (ADHD), and major depressive disorder.

Moreover, it is important to note that the risk factors that contribute to the initiation of AOD use likely are distinct from those factors that contribute to the progression from initial use to regular use and ultimately to diagnosed SUD (Clark and Winters 2002; Donovan 2004). This also applies to the relative importance of genetic versus environmental risk factors. In any case, early initiation of AOD use has been well established as a risk factor for adolescent SUD (for example, Clark et al. 2005a).

Maltreatment and Other Traumatic Events

The finding that child maltreatment has an impact on the development of adolescent SUD has been supported by several studies. For example, in a study by Clark and colleagues (1997), adolescents with SUD retrospectively reported higher incidences of childhood maltreatment, including physical and/or sexual abuse, than adolescents without SUD. Although child maltreatment is clearly associated with adolescent SUD, the mechanisms underlying this relationship are less clear. They likely involve both psychological and physiological responses. From a psychological perspective, traumatic events such as child maltreatment may lead directly to AOD use because the affected person attempts to self-medicate the anxiety and depression resulting from the traumatic event. Additionally, the effect of child maltreatment is related to and may be confounded by parental SUD—that is, parents with SUD may be more likely to mistreat their children and also are likely to pass on a genetic predisposition to AOD use.

Parenting Practices

Low levels of parental monitoring are a significant predictor of adolescent SUD. A study based on the Monitoring the Future data from 1994 to 1996 (Johnston et al. 2004) found that parental involvement significantly predicted AOD use in the past 30 days across all age, gender, and ethnic groups (Pilgrim et al. 2006). The association of parental monitoring and both alcohol and marijuana use also has been demonstrated in a sample of low-income teens in a health clinic setting (DiClemente et al. 2001). Moreover, this relationship is found regardless of whether parental monitoring is assessed based on adolescents' perceptions or on adult reports of monitoring (Griffin et al. 2000). Finally, in a prospective study, Clark and colleagues (2004a, 2005b) found that among community adolescents who had never had an SUD, those who reported low levels of parental supervision were more likely to subsequently develop an alcohol use disorder.

The relationship between parenting practices and adolescent SUDs may result, in part, from the effects of parental SUD, which contributes to such environmental influences as inadequate parental involvement and modeling of substance use. For example, Barnes and colleagues (2000) demonstrated that the effects of parental alcohol abuse on adolescent alcohol use were largely through inadequate monitoring and inadequate emotional support behaviors. In general, three types of factors have been found to contribute to the increased risk of AOD use observed among COA: genetic factors such as the ones described earlier in this article, alcohol-specific parenting factors, and non-alcohol-specific parenting factors (Ellis et al. 1997; Jacob and Johnson 1997). Alcohol-specific parenting factors include direct modeling of drinking and drug use behavior as well as shaping of alcohol expectancies. Non-alcohol-specific factors placing children at greater risk of AOD use include coexisting other psychological disorders or cognitive dysfunction in the parents, low socioeconomic status, and increased family aggression and violence.

Peer Influences

Peers are an important environmental factor in the development of adolescent SUD, although peers seem to have a more modest role relative to parents. Longitudinal studies have demonstrated that peer AOD use predicts adolescent alcohol use (Bray et al. 2003) and marijuana use (Brook et al. 1999). Moreover, affiliation with peers who generally engage in deviant behaviors predicted adolescent SUDs in a longitudinal study (Cornelius et al. 2007).

Prevention and Intervention

The available research shows that childhood manifestations of psychological dysregulation, including affective dysregulation and irritability, behavioral impulsivity and CD, and executive cognitive dysfunction, predict problematic AOD use during adolescence. These results have important implications for the design of prevention and intervention programs to be delivered during childhood and adolescence. Given the limited funds available for prevention programs, targeting children who exhibit early indicators of psychological dysregulation seems a reasonable starting point. Research has demonstrated that children with conduct problems or CD, early cigarette or other substance use, and parents who have SUD are extremely likely to engage in problematic AOD use by early adolescence. These three criteria are relatively straightforward to assess on an individual basis in schools or in primary care settings.

Briones and colleagues (2006) summarized the biopsychosocial model of adolescent SUD and made specific recommendations for prevention efforts. From a biological perspective, the investigators recommended that detection and treatment of early symptoms of CD and ADHD should be accomplished as early as possible by a primary care provider and/or child psychiatrist. Additionally, education of children and adolescents, their families, schools, and broader communities about the increased risk to children of parents with SUD is critical for effective prevention. Notably, Kelley and Fals-Stewart (2008) found secondary effects of treatment of parental SUD in terms of diminished externalizing behavior in their young children but not in adolescent children, supporting the notion that intervention is particularly effective in families with young children.

From a psychological perspective, Briones and colleagues (2006) recommended early and frequent screening for problematic alcohol use during late childhood and early adolescence using established screening instruments and established cutoff scores (for example, Chung et al. 2000). Finally, from a social perspective, Briones and colleagues (2006) noted that adolescents who engage in positive social activities such as organized sports, volunteer activities, and religious activities are less likely to engage in AOD use and develop SUD than adolescents who do not engage in such activities. However, these studies are cross-sectional in nature—that is, they assess a large group of adolescents at one time and do not follow specific adolescents over time to see which factors affect their development. Moreover, the causes underlying this observed relationship still are unclear.

Parental influences—particularly low levels of parental monitoring—are strongly associated with accelerated substance involvement among adolescents. These associations exist regardless of the SUD status of the parents, and parenting behaviors seem to be a significant environmental mechanism mediating the association between parental alcohol use disorders and adolescent alcohol involvement and problems. Accordingly, parental involvement has been shown to be critical to the success of adolescent alcohol prevention and treatment programs. Specifically, high levels of parental supervision and communication are associated with better outcomes after treatment (Thatcher and Clark 2004).

In summary, effective treatment programs for adolescent SUD are likely to be multimodal, to involve the family to the extent possible, and to focus on aspects of AOD involvement as well as related problems.

Chapter 10

Adolescent Drug Abuse

Chapter Contents

Section 10.1—Teen Use of Illicit Drugs Is Declining 74

Section 10.2—Prescription and Over-the-Counter
                 Drug Abuse 75

Section 10.3—Impact of Nonmedical Stimulant Use 80

Section 10.4—Teen Marijuana Use Worsens Depression 83

Section 10.1.

Teen Use of Illicit Drugs Is Declining

Text in this section is from "Teen Substance Abuse Continues to Decline," *NIDA Notes*, Volume 21, Number 5, National Institute on Drug Abuse (NIDA), March 2008.

Use of illicit drugs by students in the 8th, 10th, and 12th grades declined 24% over the past six years, according to the *2007 Monitoring the Future* (MTF) survey. The rate of past-month illicit drug use dropped from 19.4% in 2001 to 14.8% in 2007, which indicates that an estimated 860,000 fewer teenagers are current users.

Table 10.1. Change in Illicit Drug Use by 8th, 10th, and 12th Graders Since 2001

Percent Reporting Past Month Use

	2001	2007	Change as a percent of 2001
Any illicit drug	19.4%	14.8%	-24*
Marijuana	16.6%	12.4%	-25*
MDMA (ecstasy)	2.4%	1.1%	-54*
LSD (lysergic acid diethylamide)	1.5%	0.6%	-60*
Amphetamines	4.7%	3.2%	-32*
Inhalants	2.8%	2.6%	-7
Methamphetamine	1.4%	0.5%	-64*
Steroids	0.9%	0.6%	-33*
Cocaine	1.5%	1.4%	-7
Heroin	0.4%	0.4%	0
Alcohol	35.5%	30.1%	-15*
Cigarettes	20.2%	13.6%	-33*

*Denotes statistically significant change from 2001.
Note: Past month use, 8th, 10th, and 12th grades combined; percent change calculated from figures having more precision than shown.

Source: University of Michigan, *2007 Monitoring the Future* survey.

Declines among 8th graders were particularly noteworthy. Illicit drug use and cigarette smoking declined significantly not only in the past six years, but also since 2006. Typically, year-to-year changes are within a margin of error and therefore not large enough to be considered significant.

Marijuana, methamphetamine, and amphetamines are among the drugs most responsible for the overall decline in abuse of illicit drugs over the past six years. Although marijuana continued to be the most widely abused illicit drug, past-month abuse rates fell 25%, from 16.6% to 14.8%, since 2001. Past-month meth abuse dropped 64% (from 1.4% to 0.5%) and abuse of amphetamines fell 32% (from 4.7% to 3.2%).

Section 10.2

Prescription and Over-the-Counter Drug Abuse

Text in this section is from "Teens and Prescription Drugs: An Analysis of Recent Trends on the Emerging Drug Threat," Office of National Drug Control Policy, February 2007.

Teens and Prescription Drugs

A number of national studies and published reports indicate that the intentional abuse of prescription drugs, such as pain relievers, tranquilizers, stimulants, and sedatives, to get high is a growing concern in the United States—particularly among teens. In fact, among young people ages 12–17, prescription drugs have become the second most abused illegal drug, behind marijuana. Though overall teen drug use is down nationwide and the percentage of teens abusing prescription drugs is still relatively low compared to marijuana use, there are troubling signs that teens view abusing prescription drugs as safer than illegal drugs and parents are unaware of the problem. This section examines this emerging threat by seeking to identify trends in the intentional abuse of prescription drugs among teens.

Prevalence and incidence: Next to marijuana, the most common illegal drugs teens are using to get high are prescription medications.

Teens are turning away from street drugs and using prescription drugs to get high. Indeed, new users of prescription drugs have caught up with new users of marijuana. For the first time, there are just as many new abusers (12 and older) of prescription drugs as there are for marijuana. (Substance Abuse and Mental Health Services Administration [SAMHSA], 2006)

- Three percent, or 840,000 teens ages 12–17, reported current abuse of prescription drugs in 2005, making this illegal drug category the second most abused next to marijuana (7%). (National Survey on Drug Use and Health [NSDUH], 2006)

- Prescription drugs are the most commonly abused drug among 12–13-year-olds. (NSDUH, 2006)

Myth versus reality: Teens are abusing prescription drugs because they believe the myth that these drugs provide a medically safe high.

- Nearly one in five teens (19% or 4.5 million) report abusing prescription medications that were not prescribed to them. (Partnership Attitude Tracking Study [PATS], 2006)

- Teens admit to abusing prescription medicine for reasons other than getting high, including to relieve pain or anxiety, to sleep better, to experiment, to help with concentration or to increase alertness. (Boyd, McCabe, Cranford and Young, 2006)

- When teens abuse prescription drugs, they often characterize their use of the drugs as responsible, controlled, or safe, with the perception that the drugs are safer than street drugs. (Friedman, 2006)

- More than one-third of teens say they feel some pressure to abuse prescription drugs, and nine percent say using prescription drugs to get high is an important part of fitting in with their friends. (*Seventeen*, 2006)

- Four out of ten teens agree that prescription medicines are much safer to use than illegal drugs, even if they are not prescribed by a doctor. (PATS, 2006)

- One-third of teens (31% or 7.3 million) believe there's nothing wrong with using prescription medicines without a prescription once in a while. (PATS, 2006)

- Nearly three out of ten teens (29% or 6.8 million) believe prescription pain relievers—even if not prescribed by a doctor—are not addictive. (PATS, 2006)

Availability and accessibility: The majority of teens get prescription drugs easily and for free, often from friends and relatives.

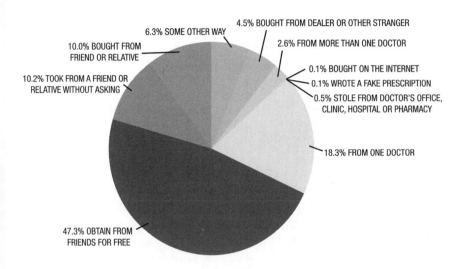

Figure 10.1. *Source Where Pain Relievers Were Obtained for Most Recent Nonmedical Past-Year Users Aged 12–17 (Percentage) Source: 2005 National Survey on Drug Use and Health, SAMHSA 2006.*

- Nearly half (47%) of teens who use prescription drugs say they get them for free from a relative or friend. Ten percent say they buy pain relievers from a friend or relative, and another ten percent say they took the drugs without asking. (NSDUH, 2006)

- More than three in five (62% or 14.6 million) teens say prescription pain relievers are easy to get from parents' medicine cabinets; half of teens (50% or 11.9 million) say they are easy to get through other people's prescriptions; and more than half (52% or 12.3 million) say prescription pain relievers are available everywhere. (PATS, 2006)

- The majority of teens (56% or 13.4 million) agree that prescription drugs are easier to get than illegal drugs. (PATS, 2006)

- More teens have been offered prescription drugs than other illicit drugs, excluding marijuana. Fourteen percent of 12–17-year-olds have been offered prescription drugs at some point in their lives, compared to 10% of teens who have been offered cocaine, ecstasy (9%), methamphetamine (6%), and lysergic acid diethylamide (LSD) (5%). (National Center on Addiction and Substance Abuse [CASA], 2006)

- Fourteen-year-olds are four times more likely than 13-year-olds to be offered prescription drugs. (CASA, 2006)

- Thirty-nine percent of 14–20-year-olds say it is easy to get prescription drugs online or by phone. Of that total, more girls than boys said it was easy (48% versus 31%). (Teenage Research Unlimited [TRU], 2006)

Gender differences: Girls are more likely than boys to intentionally abuse prescription drugs to get high. Among 12–17-year-olds, girls are more likely than boys to have abused prescription drugs (9.9% of girls versus 8.2% of boys), pain relievers (8.1% versus 7.0%), tranquilizers (2.6% versus 1.9%), and stimulants (2.6% versus 1.9%) in the past year. (SAMHSA, 2006)

Types of prescription drugs abused by teens: Pain relievers such as OxyContin® and Vicodin® are the most commonly abused prescription drugs by teens. Pain relievers are currently the most abused type of prescription drugs by 12–17-year-olds, followed by stimulants, tranquilizers, and sedatives. (NSDUH, 2006) On average, almost four percent (3.5%) of 8th–12th graders reported using OxyContin®, and six percent reported using Vicodin® in the past year. (Monitoring the Future [MTF], 2006) Almost two out of five teens reported having friends who abused prescription pain relievers and nearly three out of ten reported having friends who abused prescription stimulants in the past year. (PATS, 2006)

Dependence and treatment: Adolescents are more likely than young adults to become dependent on prescription medication.

- In 2004, more than 29% of teens in treatment were dependent on tranquilizers, sedatives, amphetamines, and other stimulants. (TEDS, 2004)

- More 12–17-year-olds than young adults (18–25) (15.9% versus 12.7%) became dependent on or abused prescription drugs in the past year. (SAMHSA, 2006)

- Abusing prescription drugs for the first time before age 16 leads to a greater risk of dependence later in life. (SAMHSA, 2006)

- In the past year, nearly half (48%) of all emergency department (ED) visits resulting from dextromethorphan abuse were patients 12–20 years old. (DAWN, 2006)

- Prescription drug abuse dramatically increased during the past decade. In the last ten years, the number of teens going into treatment for addiction to prescription pain relievers has increased by more than 300%. (TEDS, 2006)

- Between 2004 and 2005, the proportion of those seeking treatment for prescription pain medication increased nine percent, to more than 64,000 admissions. (TEDS, 2006)

Section 10.3

Impact of Nonmedical Stimulant Use

This section includes text from "Nonmedical Stimulant Use, Other
Drug Use, Delinquent Behaviors, and Depression among Adolescents,"
Substance Abuse and Mental Health Services Administration
(SAMHSA), February 2008.

The National Survey on Drug Use and Health (NSDUH) asks
youths aged 12 to 17 questions related to their use of illicit drugs in
the past year, including nonmedical use of stimulants. Nonmedical use
is defined as the use of prescription-type psychotherapeutic drugs not
prescribed for the respondent by a physician or used only for the experience or feeling they caused. Nonmedical use of prescription-type
stimulants does not include use of over-the-counter drugs, but it does
include use of methamphetamine as well as other stimulants. Illicit
drugs refer to marijuana/hashish, cocaine (including crack), inhalants,
hallucinogens, heroin, or prescription-type drugs used nonmedically.

NSDUH also asks youths aged 12 to 17 how often they engaged in
the following delinquent activities during the past year: (a) getting into
a serious fight at school or work, (b) taking part in a fight where a group
of friends fought against another group, (c) carrying a handgun, (d) selling illegal drugs, (e) stealing or trying to steal anything worth more than
$50, and (f) attacking someone with the intent to seriously hurt them.

NSDUH also includes questions for youths aged 12 to 17 to assess
lifetime and past year major depressive episode (MDE). For these estimates, MDE is defined using the diagnostic criteria set forth in the 4th
edition of the *Diagnostic and Statistical Manual of Mental Disorders*
(DSM-IV),[2] which specifies a period of two weeks or longer during which
there is either depressed mood or loss of interest or pleasure and at
least four other symptoms that reflect a change in functioning, such
as problems with sleep, eating, energy, concentration, and self-image.[3]

* This section examines past year nonmedical use of stimulants
  among youths aged 12 to 17 and its association with other illicit
  drug use, delinquent activity, and MDE. All findings presented
  in this report are annual averages based on combined 2005 and
  2006 NSDUH data.

Nonmedical Use of Stimulants and Other Illicit Drug Use

In 2005 and 2006, youths aged 12 to 17 who used stimulants nonmedically in the past year were more likely to have used other illicit drugs in the past year compared with youths who did not use stimulants nonmedically in the past year. For example, 70.2% of youths who used stimulants nonmedically in the past year also used marijuana compared with 12.1% of youths who did not use stimulants nonmedically in the past year.

Table 10.2. Percentages of Youths Aged 12 to 17 Using Illicit Drugs in the Past Year, by Past Year Nonmedical Stimulant Use: 2005 and 2006

Illicit drug	Among youths who used stimulants nonmedically	Among youths who did not use stimulants nonmedically
Marijuana	70.2%	12.1%
Pain relievers	56.5%	6.0%
Hallucinogens	34.2%	1.9%
Tranquilizers	29.8%	1.4%
Inhalants	27.5%	4.0%
Cocaine	24.1%	1.2%
Sedatives	7.5%	0.3%
Heroin	3.2%	0.1%

Source: SAMHSA, 2005 and 2006 NSDUH.

Nonmedical Use of Stimulants and Delinquent Behavior

In 2005 and 2006, an estimated 8.7 million (34.5%) youths aged 12 to 17 reported that they engaged in at least one of the six queried types of delinquent behavior in the past year. Over 71% (approximately 360,000) of youths who used stimulants nonmedically in the past year reported any type of delinquent behavior compared with approximately 34% of youths who did not use stimulants nonmedically in the past year.

Youths who engaged in nonmedical stimulant use in the past year were more likely to have participated in each of the six delinquent behaviors in the past year compared with other youths. For example, almost 30% of youths who used stimulants nonmedically in the past year sold drugs compared with 2.8% of youths who did not use stimulants nonmedically in the past year.

Table 10.3. Percentages of Youths Aged 12 to 17 Engaging in Delinquent Behaviors[1] in the Past Year, by Past Year Nonmedical Stimulant Use: 2005 and 2006

Delinquent behavior	Among youths who used stimulants nonmedically	Among youths who did not use stimulants nonmedically
Got into a serious fight	47.2%	22.5%
Took part in a group fight against another group	36.4%	16.5%
Sold drugs	29.8%	2.8%
Stole anything valued more than $50.00	26.1%	4.1%
Attacked someone	24.4%	7.3%
Carried a handgun	8.6%	3.1%

Source: SAMHSA, 2005 and 2006 NSDUH.

Nonmedical Use of Stimulants and Major Depressive Episode

In 2005 and 2006, an estimated 2.1 million (8.3%) youths aged 12 to 17 experienced at least one MDE in the past year. Youths who used stimulants nonmedically in the past year were more likely to have experienced MDE in the past year than youths who did not use stimulants nonmedically in the past year (22.8% versus 8.1%).

Table 10.4. Percentages of Youths Aged 12 to 17 with Past Year Major Depressive Episode (MDE), by Past Year Nonmedical Stimulant Use: 2005 and 2006

Nonmedical stimulant use	Percentage
Among youths who used stimulants nonmedically	22.8%
Among youths who did not use stimulants nonmedically	8.1%

Source: SAMHSA, 2005 and 2006 NSDUH.

End Notes

1. Youths aged 12 to 17 were asked how many times in the past 12 months they had participated in each delinquent behavior. The response options were (a) 0 times, (b) 1–2 times, (c) 3–5 times, (d) 6–9 times, and (e) 10 or more times. For this report, youths were counted as engaging in the behavior if they reported participating one or more times. Youths with unknown or missing data of delinquent behavior were excluded from this analysis.

2. American Psychiatric Association. (1994). *Diagnostic and statistical manual of mental disorders (4th ed.)*. Washington, DC: Author.

3. In assessing MDE, no exclusions were made for MDE caused by medical illness, bereavement, or substance use disorders.

Section 10.4

Teen Marijuana Use Worsens Depression

Text in this section is excerpted from "Teen Marijuana Use Worsens Depression," Office of National Drug Control Policy, May 2008.

Millions of American teens report experiencing weeks of hopelessness and loss of interest in normal daily activities, and many of these depressed teens are making the problem worse by using marijuana and other drugs. Some teens use marijuana to relieve the symptoms of depression (self-medicate), wrongly believing it may alleviate these depressed feelings.

Alarmingly, the majority of teens who report feeling depressed aren't getting professional help. They have not seen or spoken to a medical doctor or other professional about their feelings. For parents, this means they need to pay closer attention to their teen's behavior and mood swings, and recognize that marijuana and other drugs could be playing a dangerous role in their child's life.

In this section, references to teens, youth, and children include youth ages 12 to 17 unless otherwise noted.

Drugs and Depression

According to recent national surveys, two million youths (8%) felt depressed at some point in the course of a year. Another survey of high school students shows that percentage even higher (29%). There are indications that many teens are using drugs to self-medicate (deal with problems of depression and anxiety by using drugs to alleviate the symptoms). Many teens say they use drugs to make them feel good or feel better.

However, research shows that using marijuana and other illicit drugs puts a teen at even greater risk for more serious mental illnesses. A teen who has been depressed at some point in the past year is more than twice as likely to have used marijuana (25%) as teens who have not reported being depressed (12%). Similarly, 35% of depressed teens used an illicit drug (including marijuana) during the year, compared to 18% of teens who did not report being depressed. Depressed teens are more likely to engage in other risky behaviors, as well. They are more likely than non-depressed teens to report daily cigarette use (5% versus 3%) and heavy alcohol use (5% versus 2%).

Link between Marijuana Use, Depression, and Other Mental Health Problems

Teens who use marijuana can end up making tough times worse. Mental health risks associated with recent and long-term marijuana use include schizophrenia, other forms of psychosis, and even suicide. Recent research makes a strong case that cannabis smoking itself may be a causal agent in psychiatric symptoms, particularly schizophrenia.

Research shows that teens who smoke marijuana at least once a month in the past year are three times more likely to have suicidal thoughts than non-users during the same period. Yet another study found that marijuana use was associated with depression, suicidal thoughts, and suicide attempts. One 16-year study showed that individuals who were not depressed and then used marijuana were four times more likely to be depressed at follow up. Another study conducted over a 14-year period found that marijuana use was a predictor of later major depressive disorder.

An extensive analysis of longitudinal studies on marijuana use and risk of mental illness later in life showed that marijuana use increases the risk of developing mental disorders by 40%. The risk of psychosis increases with frequency of marijuana use, from 50% to 200% among frequent users. The authors conclude that "there is now sufficient evidence to warn young people that using cannabis could increase their risk of developing a psychotic illness later in life."

Other studies also show a strong relationship between marijuana and schizophrenia. A study from New Zealand showed "a clear increase in rates of psychotic symptoms after the start of regular use" of marijuana. Another 21-year longitudinal study showed that marijuana use was associated with psychotic symptoms and suggested a causal relationship. A study published in *Schizophrenia Research* found that cannabis use seems to be a specific risk factor for future psychotic symptoms.

Another study of young adults from birth to age 21 found a relationship between early initiation and frequent use of cannabis and symptoms of anxiety and depression, regardless of a history of mental illness.

Teens who smoke marijuana when feeling depressed are also more likely to become addicted to marijuana or other illicit drugs. Eight percent of depressed teens abused or became dependent on marijuana during the year they experienced depression, compared with only 3% of non-depressed teens. Overall, more teens are in treatment for marijuana dependence than for any other illicit drug.

Depressed Teens More Likely to Use Drugs than Depressed Adults

The percentage of teens reporting being depressed is similar to the percentage of adults reporting depression. Depressed teens, however, are more likely than depressed adults to use drugs. In the course of a year, seven percent of adults reported feeling depressed, compared to eight percent of teens. But a quarter (25%) of depressed teens used marijuana in the course of a year, while only 19% of depressed adults did. Additionally, 35% of depressed teens used other illicit drugs (including marijuana), compared to 28% of depressed adults.

Girls at Greater Risk

Teen girls are especially at risk. In fact, three times as many girls (12%) as boys (4%) experienced depression during the year. Another study confirms that girls are more likely than boys to report feelings of sadness or hopelessness (37% versus 29%). Substance abuse can compound the problem. Girls who smoke marijuana daily are significantly more likely to develop symptoms of depression and anxiety: their odds are more than five times higher than those of girls who do not smoke marijuana.

Parental Involvement

Parents should not dismiss changes in their teen's behavior as a phase. Their teen could be depressed, using drugs—or both. Parents can help their teen understand the risks of marijuana use, and should be on the lookout for signs of depression.

It has been shown that parents who make an effort to understand the pressures and influences on young people are more likely to keep their teen healthy and drug-free. Teens who report having conversations with their parents about alcohol and drug use are more likely to stay drug-free, compared to teens who do not talk about substance abuse with their parents.

Chapter 11

Women, Girls, and Drugs

A three-year study on women and young girls (ages 8–22) from the National Center on Addiction and Substance Abuse (CASA) at Columbia University revealed that girls and young women use substances for reasons different than boys and young men. The study also found that the signals and situations of higher risk are different and that girls and young women are more vulnerable to abuse and addiction, they get hooked faster and suffer the consequences sooner than boys and young men.

According to the 2008 National Survey on Drug Use and Health (NSDUH), approximately 42.9% of women ages 12 or older reported using an illicit drug at some point in their lives. Approximately 12.2% of females ages 12 and older reported past year use of an illicit drug and 6.3% reported past month use of an illicit drug.

The rate of substance dependence or abuse for males aged 12 or older in 2008 was nearly twice as high as the rate for females (11.5% versus 6.4%). Among youths aged 12 to 17, however, the rate of substance dependence or abuse was higher among females than males (8.2% versus 7.0%).

According to the Centers for Disease Control and Prevention (CDC), approximately 34.5% of female high school students surveyed nationwide in 2007 used marijuana during their lifetime. This is down from 35.9% in 2005 and 37.6% in 2003. Inhalant abuse among

Excerpted from "Women and Drugs: Facts and Figures," Office of National Drug Control Policy, 2009.

surveyed high school females has increased from 11.4% in 2003, to 13.5% in 2005, and 14.3% in 2007.

Table 11.1. Percent of High School Females Reporting Drug Use, 2003–2007

Drug type	2003	2005	2007
Lifetime marijuana	37.6	35.9	34.5
Current marijuana	19.3	18.2	17.0
Lifetime cocaine	7.7	6.8	6.5
Current cocaine	3.5	2.8	2.5
Lifetime inhalant	11.4	13.5	14.3
Lifetime heroin	2.0	1.4	1.6
Lifetime methamphetamine	6.8	6.0	4.1
Lifetime ecstasy	10.4	5.3	4.8
Lifetime steroid	5.3	3.2	2.7

Health Effects

A National Vital Statistics Report found that 38,396 persons died of drug-induced causes in 2006. Of the drug-induced deaths, 13,889 were females. Drug-induced deaths include deaths from dependent and nondependent use of drugs (legal and illegal use) and poisoning from medically prescribed and other drugs. It excludes unintentional injuries, homicides, and other causes indirectly related to drug use. Also excluded are newborn deaths due to mother's drug use.

The Drug Abuse Warning Network (DAWN) collects data on drug-related visits to emergency departments (ED) nationwide. In 2006, there were 1,742,887 drug related ED episodes. The rates of ED visits involving cocaine, marijuana, and heroin were higher for males than females, but the rates for stimulants did not differ by gender during 2006.

The impact of drug use and addiction can be far reaching. Cardiovascular disease, stroke, cancer, human immunodeficiency virus/acquired immunodeficiency syndrome (HIV/AIDS), hepatitis, and lung disease can all be affected by drug abuse. Some of these effects occur when drugs are used at high doses or after prolonged use, while some may occur after just one use. Drug abuse not only weakens the immune system but is also linked to risky behaviors like needle sharing and unsafe sex. The combination greatly increases the likelihood of acquiring human immunodeficiency virus/acquired immunodeficiency syndrome (HIV/AIDS), hepatitis, and many other infectious diseases.

Effects on Pregnancy

Alcohol and drug use by pregnant women is a public health problem with potentially severe consequences. Combined data from the 2002 to 2007 National Surveys on Drug Use and Health shows that past month alcohol use was highest among women who were not pregnant and did not have children living in the household (63.0%) and lowest for women in the second and third trimesters (7.8% and 6.2%, respectively). Similar patters were seen among women for marijuana, cigarette and binge alcohol use.

Research has shown that babies born to women who used marijuana during their pregnancies display altered responses to visual stimuli, increased tremulousness, and a high-pitched cry, which may indicate problems with neurological development. Heroin abuse during pregnancy and its many associated environmental factors (for example, lack of prenatal care) have been associated with adverse consequences including low birth weight, an important risk factor for later developmental delay. Knowledge of the effects of methamphetamine during pregnancy is limited. However, the few human studies that exist on the subject have shown increased rates of premature delivery, placental abruption, fetal growth retardation, and heart and brain abnormalities. These studies, though, are difficult to interpret due to methodological issues, such as small sample size and maternal use of other drugs.

Treatment

Of the approximately 1.8 million admissions to drug or alcohol treatment in the U.S. during 2007, 32.3% were female. For 18% of the female admissions in 2007, alcohol only was the primary substance of abuse. Fifteen percent involved alcohol along with a secondary drug.

According to the Substance Abuse and Mental Health Services Administration's (SAMHSA) 2007 National Survey of Substance Abuse Treatment Services (N-SSATS), which presents data from more than 13,000 facilities, approximately 32% of the facilities offered special programs or groups for adult women and 14% offered programs or groups for pregnant or postpartum women.

Table 11.2. Female Admissions by Primary Substance, 2007

Drug type	% of Total
Alcohol	18.0
Alcohol with secondary drug	15.0
Heroin	13.2
Other opiates	7.2
Cocaine-smoked	12.1
Cocaine-other route	4.0
Marijuana	13.0
Methamphetamine/amphetamine	11.1
Other stimulants	0.1
Tranquilizers	0.9
Sedatives	0.4
Hallucinogens	0.1
Phencyclidine (PCP)	0.2
Inhalants	0.1
Other/none specified	4.8

Arrests and Sentencing

According to the Federal Bureau of Investigation's Uniform Crime Reporting Program, during 2007, there were a total of 1,033,203 state and local arrests for drug abuse violations in the United States where gender information was available. Of these drug abuse violation arrests, 199,262 involved females.

At year end 2005, there were approximately 88,200 sentenced female prisoners under state jurisdiction. Approximately 28.7% of incarcerated females were sentenced for drug offenses compared to 18.9% of incarcerated males.

During FY 2008, there were 25,332 federal defendants whose gender was reported to the U.S. Sentencing Commission who were charged with a drug offense. Approximately 12.3% of these defendants were female. For 17.4% of the female defendants, methamphetamine was the type of drug involved in the case.

A Bureau of Justice Statistics (BJS) report found that about half of women offenders confined in state prisons had been using alcohol, drugs, or both at the time of the offense for which they had been incarcerated. About six in ten women in state prison described themselves as using drugs in the month before the offense and five in ten described themselves as a daily user of drugs. Nearly one in three women serving time in state prisons said they had committed the offense which brought them to prison in order to obtain money to support their need for drugs.

A report from the Office of Juvenile Justice and Delinquency Prevention (OJJDP) summarized research on female gangs finding that drug offenses are among the most common offenses committed by female gang members.

Chapter 12

Minorities and Drugs

According to the 2006 American Community Survey, the estimated the population of the United States was 299,398,485. The population breakdown was 73.9% White, 12.4% Black/African American, 0.8% American Indian/Alaska Native, 4.4% Asian, 0.1% Native Hawaiian/other Pacific Islander, 6.3% some other race, 2.0% two or more races. An estimated 14.8% of the population was of Hispanic/Latino origin (of any race).

Extent of Drug Use by Ethnicity

The 2008 National Survey on Drug Use and Health showed that the highest rate of current (past month) illicit drug use was among persons reporting two or more races (14.7%), followed by Blacks/African Americans (10.1%), American Indian/Alaska Natives (9.5%), Whites (8.2%), Native Hawaiian or other Pacific Islander (7.3%); and Hispanics (6.2%). The lowest rate of current illicit drug use was among Asians (3.6%).

The Youth Risk Behavior Surveillance System (YRBSS) study by the Centers for Disease Control and Prevention (CDC) surveys high school students on several risk factors including drug and alcohol use. The 2007 report showed that 21.5% of Black, 19.9% of White, 18.5% of Hispanic, and 17.2% of "other" race high school students were current marijuana users.

Excerpted from "Minorities and Drugs: Facts and Figures," Office of National Drug Control Policy, 2009.

Table 12.1. Reported Drug Use by High School Students, by Race/ Ethnicity, 2007

Drug use	White	Black	Hispanic	Other
Lifetime marijuana	38.0%	39.6%	38.9%	32.9%
Current marijuana	19.9	21.5	18.5	17.2
Lifetime cocaine	7.4	1.8	10.9	6.5
Current cocaine	3.0	1.	5.3	4.0
Lifetime inhalant	14.4	8.5	14.1	12.6
Lifetime heroin	1.7	1.8	3.7	2.9
Lifetime methamphetamine	4.5	1.9	5.7	5.2
Lifetime ecstasy	5.6	3.7	7.4	5.8
Lifetime illegal steroid	4.1	2.2	4.6	3.1
Marijuana before age 13	7.2	9.5	9.8	9.9

According to 2006 findings from the Monitoring the Future study, African-American 8th, 10th, and 12th grade students have substantially lower usage rates for most illicit drugs when compared to White students. Hispanics generally have rates of use for many drugs that tend to fall between usage rates for Whites and Blacks. However, Hispanic seniors have the highest rate of lifetime usage for powder cocaine, crack cocaine, heroin with and without a needle, methamphetamine, and crystal methamphetamine (ice).

According to data from the Bureau of Justice Statistics, more than half of Black state and federal prisoners surveyed in 2004 indicated that they used drugs in the month before their offense. According to additional data from the Bureau of Justice Statistics, approximately half of Black prisoners in state prisons and more than 40% in federal prisons surveyed in 2004 met drug dependence or abuse criteria.

Health effects: A National Vital Statistics Report found that 30,711 persons died of drug-induced causes in 2004. Of the drug-induced deaths, 3,633 were Black, 26,474 were White, and 604 were another race. Drug-induced deaths include deaths from dependent and nondependent use of drugs (legal and illegal use) and poisoning from medically prescribed and other drugs. It excludes unintentional injuries, homicides, and other causes indirectly related to drug use. Also excluded are newborn deaths due to mother's drug use.

Treatment: According to the Treatment Episode Data Set (TEDS), more than 20% of those admitted to treatment facilities in the U.S. during 2006 were Black (non-Hispanic).

Arrests and Sentencing

According to the Federal Bureau of Investigation's Uniform Crime Reporting Program, there were a total of 1,382,783 state and local arrests for drug abuse violations in the United States during 2007 where the race of the offender was reported. Of these drug abuse violation arrests, 63.7% of those arrested were White, 35.1% were Black, 0.6% were Asian or Pacific Islander, and 0.6% were American Indian or Alaskan Native.

In fiscal year (FY) 2004, the U.S. Marshals Service arrested and booked 140,755 total suspects for federal offenses, 23.6% of which were for drug offenses. Of these arrestees booked by the U.S. Marshals Service for drug offenses, 66.1% were White, 31.0% were Black/African American, 0.1% were Indian/Alaska Natives, and 1.9% were Asian/Native Hawaiian or other Pacific Islander. Also in FY 2004, the Drug Enforcement Administration (DEA) arrested 27,454 individuals. Of those arrested by the DEA, 67.7% were White, 29.2% were Black/African American, 0.6% were Indian/Alaska Natives and 2.5% were Asian/Native Hawaiian, or other Pacific Islander. Additionally, 42.4% of those arrested by the DEA in FY 2004 were Hispanic or Latino of any race.

Table 12.2. DEA Arrests, by Race/Ethnicity and Type of Drug, FY 2004

Drug category	White	Black	Indian	Asian	Hispanic
Powered cocaine	4,648	2,273	26	49	3,943
Crack cocaine	695	3,161	22	25	300
Marijuana	4,573	1,017	56	122	2,882
Methamphetamine	5,367	141	60	191	2,197
Opiates	1,398	833	5	18	1,311
Other or non-drug	1,726	500	5	272	497

During FY 2007, there were 25,457 federal defendants charged with a drug offense whose race was reported to the U.S. Sentencing Commission. Approximately one-quarter (24.3%) of these defendants were White, 29.5% were Black, and 42.7% were Hispanic. Individuals of another race made up 3.5% of these drug cases. Hispanic defendants were sentenced for the majority of powder cocaine, heroin, and marijuana cases. White defendants were sentenced for the majority of methamphetamine cases and Blacks were sentenced for the majority of crack cocaine offenses.

At year end 2004, there were an approximate total of 1,274,600 sentenced state prison inmates, 249,400 of whom were incarcerated for drug offenses. The majority of drug offenders held in state prisons were Black (112,500), followed by Whites (65,900), and Hispanics (51,800).

During 1995 there were a total of 2,065,896 state and local probationers; of that total, 20% (414,832) were on probation for a drug offense. White probationers (73%) had the highest rate of prior drug use, followed by Black probationers (68%) and Hispanics (56%). Drug use at the time of the offense was similar for White (14%) and Black (15%) probationers, and lowest for Hispanics (11%).

Chapter 13

Substance Use in the Workplace

General Workplace Impact

Substance use and abuse is a concern for employers. Most drug users, binge and heavy drinkers, and people with substance use disorders are employed. In 2007, of the 17.4 million current illicit drug users age 18 and over, 13.1 million (75.3%) were employed. Also, of the 20.4 million adults classified with substance dependence or abuse, 12.3 million (60.4%) were employed full-time.

The prevalence of substance use among workers is lower than the prevalence among the unemployed, but a sizable number of employed individuals use drugs and alcohol. For example, in 2007, 8.4% of those employed full-time were current illicit drug users, and 8.8% reported heavy alcohol use.

Substance Use Disorder: Worker Age May Be a Factor

According to 2002–2004 data, among full-time employed persons diagnosed with a substance use disorder, those ages 18–25 had the highest rates of substance use disorder relative to those in other age categories. Illicit drug use for the ages 18–25 group (not accounting for employment) has remained relatively stable from 2004 (19.4 million)

This chapter includes text from "General Workplace Impact," U.S. Department of Labor, March 2009; and "Worker Substance Use, by Industry Category," Substance Abuse and Mental Health Services Administration (SAMHSA), August 23, 2007.

to 2007 (19.7 million) while specific rates of use dropped significantly from 2006 to 2007 for several drugs: methamphetamine use fell 33% from 0.6% to 0.4%, ecstasy use fell 30% from 1% to 0.7%, stimulant use fell 21% from 1.4% to 1.1%, and cocaine use fell by 23% from 2.2% to 1.7%. Declining rates of use for methamphetamine and cocaine have been noted in the workplace, with drug test positives for methamphetamine declining 50% since 2005 and cocaine dropping 19% in 2007 to the lowest levels in the history of this testing system. At the same time that these positive indicators are noted among the age 18–25 group, the rate of nonmedical use of prescription pain relievers rose 12% to 4.6% in 2007. In the ages 50–59 group (not accounting for employment), illicit drug use has grown substantially from 2004 (3.8%) to 2007 (5.0%).

America's Workplaces at Risk

Substance use and abuse is not necessarily limited to after work hours, leading to the risk of impairment on the job. An estimated 3.1% of employed adults actually used illicit drugs before reporting to work or during work hours at least once in the past year, with about 2.9% working while under the influence of an illicit drug.

Regardless of where illicit drug use or heavy alcohol use takes place, workers reporting substance use and abuse have higher rates of turnover and absenteeism. Workers reporting heavy alcohol use or illicit drug use, as well as workers reporting dependence on or abuse of alcohol or illicit drugs, are more likely to have worked for more than three employers in the past year. Likewise, those workers are more likely to have skipped work more than two days in the past month. Workers reporting illicit drug use or dependence on or abuse of alcohol or illicit drugs were also more likely to have missed more than two days of work due to illness or injury.

Furthermore, the impact of employee substance use and abuse is a problem that extends beyond the substance-using employee. There is evidence that co-worker job performance and attitudes are negatively affected. Workers have reported being put in danger, having been injured, or having had to work harder, to redo work, or to cover for a co-worker as a result of a fellow employee's drinking.

Small Businesses Most Vulnerable

Smaller firms may be particularly disadvantaged by worker substance use and abuse. For example, while about half of all United States (U.S.) workers work for small and medium sized businesses (those with fewer than 500 employees), about nine in ten employed current illicit drug users and almost nine in ten employed heavy drinkers work for small and medium sized firms. Likewise, about nine in ten full-time workers with alcohol or illicit drug dependence or abuse work for small and medium size firms. However, smaller firms are generally less likely to test for substance use.

Smaller businesses are less likely to have programs in place to combat the problem, yet they are more likely to be the employer-of-choice for illicit drug users. Individuals who can't adhere to a drug-free workplace policy seek employment at firms that don't have one, and the cost of just one error caused by an impaired employee can devastate a small company.

The good news is that there are steps businesses can take to minimize the risks of worker alcohol use, and there are resources to help them do so. The U.S. Department of Labor can help employers develop drug-free workplace programs that educate employees about the dangers of alcohol and encourage those with alcohol problems to seek help.

Worker Substance Use, by Industry Category

Substance use in the workplace negatively affects U.S. industry through lost productivity, workplace accidents and injuries, employee absenteeism, low morale, and increased illness. The loss to U.S. companies due to employees' alcohol and drug use and related problems is estimated at billions of dollars a year. Research shows that the rate of substance use varies by occupation and industry. Studies also have indicated that employers vary in their treatment of substance use issues and that workplace-based employee assistance programs (EAPs) can be a valuable resource for obtaining help for substance-using workers. The National Survey on Drug Use and Health (NSDUH) asks persons aged 12 or older to report on their use of alcohol and illicit drugs during the past month. NSDUH defines illicit drugs as marijuana/hashish, cocaine (including crack), inhalants, hallucinogens, heroin, or prescription-type drugs used nonmedically. Heavy alcohol use is defined as drinking five or more drinks on the same occasion (at the same time or within a couple of hours of each other) on five or more days in the past 30 days. NSDUH also asks respondents about their current employment situation and the type of business or industry in which they worked. NSDUH defines full-time employed respondents as those who usually work 35 or more hours per week and who worked in the past week or had a job despite not working in the past week. This information from the NSDUH

Report uses data from the combined 2002 to 2004 surveys to present estimates of current (past month) heavy alcohol use and illicit drug use among full-time workers aged 18 to 64 by industry category. The data are abstracted from a more extensive report available online at http://www.oas.samhsa.gov/analytic.htm.

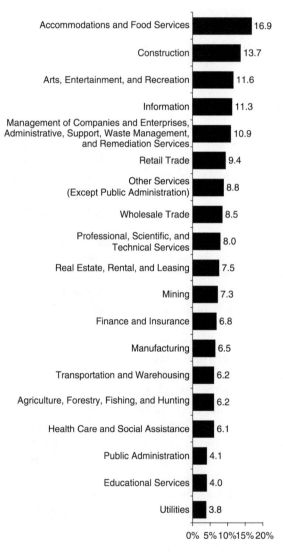

Figure 13.1. *Past Month Illicit Drug Use among Full-Time Workers Aged 18 to 64, by Industry Categories: 2002–2004 Combined (Source: SAMHSA, 2002, 2003, 2004 NSDUHs).*

Chapter 14

Drug Use and Crime

Drug-Related Crime

In 2004, 17% of state prisoners and 18% of federal inmates said they committed their current offense to obtain money for drugs. In 2002, about a quarter of convicted property and drug offenders in local jails had committed their crimes to get money for drugs, compared to 5% of violent and public order offenders. Among state prisoners in 2004 the pattern was similar, with property (30%) and drug offenders (26%) more likely to commit their crimes for drug money than violent (10%) and public-order offenders (7%). In federal prisons property offenders (11%) were less than half as likely as drug offenders (25%) to report drug money as a motive in their offenses.

The Uniform Crime Reporting Program (UCR) of the Federal Bureau of Investigation (FBI) reported that in 2007, 3.9% of the 14,831 homicides in which circumstances were known were narcotics related. Murders that occurred specifically during a narcotics felony, such as drug trafficking or manufacturing, are considered drug related.

This chapter includes text from "Drug Use and Crime," U.S. Department of Justice (DOJ), reviewed August 17, 2009; "Co-Occurrence of Substance Use Behaviors in Youth," DOJ, November 2008; and "Drugs and Gangs Fast Facts: Questions and Answers," DOJ, 2005.

Drug Use at Time of Offense Reported by Prisoners

In the 2004 Survey of Inmates in State and Federal Correctional Facilities, 32% of state prisoners and 26% of federal prisoners said they had committed their current offense while under the influence of drugs. Among state prisoners, drug offenders (44%) and property offenders (39%) reported the highest incidence of drug use at the time of the offense. Among federal prisoners, drug offenders (32%) and violent offenders (24%) were the most likely to report drug use at the time of their crimes. (Source: Bureau of Justice Statistics (BJS), "Drug Use and Dependence, State and Federal Prisoners, 2004," NCJ 213530, October 2006.)

About 74% of state prisoners who had a mental health problem and 56% of those without were dependent on or abused alcohol or drugs. By specific type of substance, inmates who had a mental health problem had higher rates of dependence or abuse of drugs than alcohol. Among state prisoners who had a mental health problem, 62% were dependent on or abused drugs and 51% alcohol.

Over a third (37%) of state prisoners who had a mental health problem said they had used drugs at the time of the offense, compared to over a quarter (26%) of state prisoners without a mental problem. (Source: BJS, "Mental Health Problems of Prison and Jail Inmates," NCJ 213600, September 2006.)

Prisoners who are parents: A third of the parents in state prison reported committing their current offense while under the influence of drugs. Parents were most likely to report the influence of cocaine-based drugs (16%) and marijuana (15%) while committing their crime. About equal percentages of parents in state prison reported the use of opiates (6%) and stimulates (5%) at the time of their offense, while 2% used depressants or hallucinogens.

Thirty-two percent of mothers in state prison reported committing their crime to get drugs or money for drugs, compared to 19% of fathers. (Source: BJS, "Incarcerated Parents and Their Children," NCJ 182335, August 2000.)

Jail inmates: Of inmates held in jail, only convicted offenders were asked if they had used drugs at the time of the offense. In 2002, 29% of convicted inmates reported they had used illegal drugs at the time of the offense, down from 35% in 1996. Marijuana and cocaine or crack were the most common drugs convicted inmates said they had used at the time of the offense with 14% reporting use of marijuana in 2002, down from 18% in 1996; and 11% reporting use of cocaine or crack, down from 14% in 1996. In 2002, jail inmates convicted of robbery (56%), weapons violations (56%), burglary (55%), or motor vehicle theft (55%) were most likely to have reported to be using drugs at the time of the offense. (Source: BJS, "Substance Dependence, Abuse, and Treatment of Jail Inmates, 2002," NCJ 209588, July 2005.)

Inmates with a mental health problem: Seventy-six percent of jail inmates who had a mental health problem were dependent on or abused alcohol or drugs, compared to 53% of inmates without a mental health problem. This was the highest rate of substance dependence or abuse among all inmates, including state and federal prisoners.

By specific type of substance, jail inmates who had a mental health problem had higher rates of dependence or abuse of drugs than alcohol. An estimated 63% of local jail inmates who had a mental health problem were dependent on or abused drugs, while about 53% were dependent on or abused alcohol. Over a third (34%) of local jail inmates who had a mental health problem said they had used drugs at the time of the offense, compared to a fifth (20%) of jail inmates without a mental problem

State prisoners who had a mental health problem (62%) had a higher rate of drug use in the month offense compared to those without a mental health problem (49%). Marijuana was the most common drug inmates said they had used in the month before the offense. Among state prisoners who had a mental health problem in the month before the offense: 46% had used marijuana or hashish, 24% had used cocaine or crack, and 13% had used methamphetamines. (Source: BJS, "Mental Health Problems of Prison and Jail Inmates," NCJ 213600, September 2006.)

Domestic disputes: Domestic disputes were also one of the most commonly reported experiences associated with drug use with 25% of jail inmates reporting they had arguments with their family, friends, spouse, or boyfriend or girlfriend while under the influence of drugs.

Co-Occurrence of Substance Use Behaviors in Youth

This section reviews the prevalence and overlap of substance-related behaviors among youth, with comparisons by age group, gender, and race/ethnicity. It uses data from the first two waves of the 1997 National Longitudinal Survey of Youth (NLSY97)—self-reports gathered in 1997 and 1998 from a nationally representative sample of youth ages 12–17. The data are from questions asking about drinking alcohol during the previous 30 days, using marijuana during the previous 30 days, and ever selling or helping to sell marijuana (pot, grass), hashish (hash), or other hard drugs such as heroin, cocaine, or lysergic acid diethylamide (LSD).

The central finding of the analysis is that, given one substance-related behavior, other substance-related behaviors became much more likely. For example, 9% of all youth ages 12–17 reported marijuana use and 8% said they had sold drugs. Among youth who reported drinking alcohol (23% of all youth ages 12–17), the level of marijuana use was 32% and the level of drug selling was 23%. In contrast, among youth ages 12–17 who did not report recent alcohol use, the level of marijuana use was 2% and the level of drug selling was 3%. Other findings include the following:

- Of youth who reported marijuana use, 81% said they drank alcohol and 45% said they had sold drugs.

- Of youth who reported drug selling, 68% said they drank alcohol and 54% reported marijuana use. In contrast, among youth who said they had not sold drugs, 19% reported drinking alcohol and 6% reported using marijuana.

- Among those who sold drugs, both White and Hispanic youth were more likely than African Americans to also report alcohol use; White youth who sold drugs were also more likely than African Americans who sold drugs to report using marijuana.

Prevalence of substance-related behaviors was tied to age: In general, the levels of reported substance-related behaviors climbed steadily with increasing age. From age 12 to age 17, alcohol use in the previous 30 days increased more than eight-fold, from 5% to 43% of youth, as did marijuana use in the previous 30 days (from 2% to 17%). The lifetime prevalence of reported drug selling rose from 1% at age 12 to 16% at age 17.

Drugs and Gangs: Fast Facts

What is the relationship between drugs and gangs?

Street gangs, outlaw motorcycle gangs, and prison gangs are the primary distributors of illegal drugs on the streets of the United States (U.S.). Gangs also smuggle drugs into the United States and produce and transport drugs within the country.

Street gang members convert powdered cocaine into crack cocaine and produce most of the phencyclidine (PCP) available in the United States. Gangs, primarily outlaw motorcycle gangs, also produce marijuana and methamphetamine. In addition, gangs increasingly are involved in smuggling large quantities of cocaine and marijuana and lesser quantities of heroin, methamphetamine, and MDMA (also known as ecstasy) into the United States from foreign sources of supply. Gangs primarily transport and distribute powdered cocaine, crack cocaine, heroin, marijuana, methamphetamine, MDMA, and PCP in the United States.

Located throughout the country, street gangs vary in size, composition, and structure. Large, nationally affiliated street gangs pose the greatest threat because they smuggle, produce, transport, and distribute large quantities of illicit drugs throughout the country and are extremely violent. Local street gangs in rural, suburban, and urban areas pose a low but growing threat. Local street gangs transport and distribute drugs within very specific areas. These gangs often imitate the larger, more powerful national gangs in order to gain respect from rivals.

Some gangs collect millions of dollars per month selling illegal drugs, trafficking weapons, operating prostitution rings, and selling stolen property. Gangs launder proceeds by investing in real estate, recording studios, motorcycle shops, and construction companies. They also operate various cash-based businesses, such as barbershops, music stores, restaurants, catering services, tattoo parlors, and strip clubs, in order to commingle drug proceeds with funds generated through legitimate commerce.

What is the extent of gang operation and crime in the United States?

There are at least 21,500 gangs and more than 731,000 active gang members in the United States. Gangs conduct criminal activity in all 50 states and U.S. territories. Although most gang activity is concentrated in major urban areas, gangs also are proliferating in rural and suburban areas of the country as gang members flee increasing law enforcement pressure in urban areas or seek more lucrative drug markets. This proliferation in non-urban areas increasingly is accompanied by violence and is threatening society in general.

According to a 2001 Department of Justice survey, 20% of students aged 12 through 18 reported that street gangs had been present at their school during the previous six months. More than a quarter (28%) of students in urban schools reported a street gang presence, and 18% of students in suburban schools and 13% in rural schools reported the presence of street gangs. Public schools reported a much higher percentage of gang presence than private schools.

What are the dangers associated with gang activity?

Large street gangs readily employ violence to control and expand drug distribution activities, targeting rival gangs and dealers who neglect or refuse to pay extortion fees. Members also use violence to ensure that members adhere to the gang' s code of conduct or to prevent a member from leaving. In November 2004, a 19-year-old gang member in Fort Worth, Texas was sentenced to 30 years in prison for fatally shooting a childhood friend who wanted to leave their local street gang.

Authorities throughout the country report that gangs are responsible for most of the serious violent crime in the major cities of the United States. Gangs engage in an array of criminal activities including assault, burglary, drive-by shooting, extortion, homicide, identification fraud, money laundering, prostitution operations, robbery, sale of stolen property, and weapons trafficking.

What are some signs that young people may be involved in gang activity?

Changes in behavior such as skipping school, hanging out with different friends, or in certain places, spray-painting graffiti, and using hand signals with friends can indicate gang affiliation. In addition, individuals who belong to gangs often dress alike by wearing clothing of the same color, wearing bandannas, or even rolling up their pant legs in a certain way. Some gang members wear certain designer labels to show their gang affiliation. Gang members often have tattoos. Also, because gang violence frequently is glorified in rap music, young people involved in gangs often try to imitate the dress and actions of rap artists. Finally, because substance abuse is often a characteristic of gang members, young people involved in gang activity may exhibit signs of drug or alcohol use.

Chapter 15

Drugged Driving

"Have one [drink] for the road" was, until recently, a commonly used phrase in American culture. It has only been within the past 20 years that as a nation, we have begun to recognize the dangers associated with drunk driving. Through a multi-pronged and concerted effort involving many stakeholders, including educators, media, legislators, law enforcement, and community organizations such as Mothers Against Drunk Driving (MADD), the nation has seen a decline in the numbers of people killed or injured as a result of drunk driving. It is now time that we recognize and address the similar dangers that can occur with drugged driving.

In 15 states (Arizona, Georgia, Indiana, Illinois, Iowa, Michigan, Minnesota, Nevada, North Carolina, Ohio, Pennsylvania, Rhode Island, Utah, Virginia, and Wisconsin), it is illegal to operate a motor vehicle if there is any detectable level of a prohibited drug, or its metabolites, in the driver's blood. Other state laws define drugged driving as driving when a drug renders the driver incapable of driving safely or causes the driver to be impaired.

The principal concern regarding drugged driving is that driving under the influence of any drug that acts on the brain could impair one's motor skills, reaction time, and judgment. Drugged driving is a public health concern because it puts not only the driver at risk, but also passengers and others who share the road.

This chapter includes "NIDA InfoFacts: Drugged Driving," National Institute on Drug Abuse (NIDA), April 2008; and "Some Medications and Driving Don't Mix," U.S. Food and Drug Administration (FDA), December 11, 2008.

How many people take drugs and drive?

The National Highway Traffic Safety Administration (NHTSA) reports that more than 17,000 people were killed in alcohol-related crashes in 2006. Studies also have found that drugs are used by 10–22% of drivers involved in crashes, often in combination with alcohol.

According to the 2006 National Survey on Drug Use and Health, an estimated 10.2 million people age 12 and older reported driving under the influence of illicit drugs during the year prior to being surveyed. This corresponds to 4.2% of the population age 12 and older, similar to the rate in 2005 (4.3%), but lower than the rate in 2002 (4.7%). In 2006, the rate was highest among young adults age 18 to 25 (13.0%). In addition:

- In 2006, an estimated 13.3% of persons age 12 and older drove under the influence of an illicit drug or alcohol at least once in the past year. This percentage has dropped since 2005, when it was 14.1%. The 2006 estimate corresponds to 32.8 million persons.

- Driving under the influence of an illicit drug or alcohol was associated with age. In 2006, an estimated 7.3% of youth age 16 drove under the influence. This percentage steadily increased with age to reach a peak of 31.8% among young adults age 22. Beyond the age of 22, these rates showed a general decline with increasing age.

- Also in 2006, among persons age 12 and older, males were nearly twice as likely as females (17.6% versus 9.3%) to drive under the influence of an illicit drug or alcohol in the past year.

In recent years, drugs other than alcohol that act on the brain have increasingly been recognized as hazards to road traffic safety. Some of this research has been done in other countries or in specific regions within the United States, and the prevalence rates for different drugs vary accordingly. Overall, the research indicates that marijuana is the most prevalent illegal drug detected in impaired drivers, fatally injured drivers, and motor vehicle crash victims. Other drugs also implicated include benzodiazepines, cocaine, opiates, and amphetamines.

A number of studies have examined illicit drug use in drivers involved in motor vehicle crashes, reckless driving, or fatal accidents. For example: Studies conducted in several localities have found that approximately 4–14% of drivers who sustained injury or died in traffic accidents tested positive for delta-9-tetrahydrocannabinol (THC), the active ingredient in marijuana.

Teens and Drugged Driving

According to the NHTSA, vehicle accidents are the leading cause of death among young people age 16 to 20. It is generally accepted that because teens are the least experienced drivers as a group, they have a higher risk of being involved in an accident compared with more experienced drivers. When this lack of experience is combined with the use of marijuana or other substances that impact cognitive and motor abilities, the results can be tragic. Results from NIDA's Monitoring the Future survey indicate that, in 2006, more than 13 percent of high school seniors admitted to driving under the influence of marijuana in the two weeks prior to the survey. The 2004 State of Maryland Adolescent Survey indicates that 13.5% of Maryland's licensed adolescent drivers reported driving under the influence of marijuana on three or more occasions.

Why is drugged driving hazardous?

Drugs act on the brain and can alter perception, cognition, attention, balance, coordination, reaction time, and other faculties required for safe driving. The effects of specific drugs of abuse differ depending on their mechanisms of action, the amount consumed, the history of the user, and other factors.

Marijuana: THC affects areas of the brain that control the body's movements, balance, coordination, memory, and judgment, as well as sensations. Because these effects are multifaceted, more research is required to understand marijuana's impact on the ability of drivers to react to complex and unpredictable situations. However, we do know that:

- a meta-analysis of approximately 60 experimental studies, including laboratory, driving simulator, and on-road experiments, found that behavioral and cognitive skills related to driving performance were impaired in a dose-dependent fashion with increasing THC blood levels;

- evidence from both real and simulated driving studies indicates that marijuana can negatively affect a driver's attentiveness, perception of time and speed, and the ability to draw on information obtained from past experiences;

- research shows that impairment increases significantly when marijuana use is combined with alcohol; and

- studies have found that many drivers who test positive for alcohol also test positive for THC, making it clear that drinking and drugged driving are often linked behaviors.

Prescription drugs: Many medications (for example, benzodiazepines and opiate analgesics) act on systems in the brain that could impair driving ability. In fact, many prescription drugs come with warnings against the operation of machinery—including motor vehicles—for a specified period of time after use. Also, when prescription drugs are taken without medical supervision, impaired driving and other harmful reactions can result.

Remember: Drugged driving is a dangerous activity that puts us all at risk.

Some Medications and Driving Don't Mix

If you are taking a medication, is it okay to drive?

Most likely, yes. But the Food and Drug Administration (FDA) advises that it's best to be absolutely sure before you get behind the wheel. While most medications don't affect driving ability, some prescription and over-the-counter (OTC) medicines can cause reactions that may make it unsafe to drive. These reactions may include: sleepiness/drowsiness, blurred vision, dizziness, slowed movement, fainting, inability to focus or pay attention, nausea, and excitability.

Driving while on medications can also be a legal issue. State laws differ, but being found driving under the influence of certain medications (prescription and OTC products) could get you in the same kind of trouble as people caught driving under the influence of alcohol.

Products That Require Caution

Knowing how your medications—or any combination of them—affect your ability to drive is clearly a safety measure involving you, your passengers, and others on the road. Products that could make it dangerous to drive include:

- prescription drugs for anxiety,
- some antidepressants,
- products containing codeine,
- some cold remedies and allergy products,

- tranquilizers,
- sleeping pills,
- pain relievers, and
- diet pills, stay awake drugs, and other medications with stimulants (for example, caffeine, ephedrine, pseudoephedrine).

Products that contain stimulants may cause excitability or drowsiness. Also, never combine medication and alcohol while driving.

If You Have to Drive

Let's say that you must take medications that could affect your driving. But you also have to get to work, pick up the kids from school or sports practice, or run errands. Here are some tips for what to do:

Don't stop using your medicine unless your doctor tells you to. Take medications at prescribed levels and dosages.

Talk to your health care professionals about side effects. Doctors and pharmacists can tell you about known side effects of medications, including those that interfere with driving. Request printed information about the side effects of any new medicine.

Inform health care professionals about all of the products you are taking, including prescription, OTC, and herbal products. Also, let them know about any reactions you may experience. Health care professionals may be able to adjust the dose, adjust the timing of doses or when you use the medicine, add an exercise or nutrition program to lessen the need for medicine, or change the medicine to one that causes less drowsiness.

Monitor yourself. Learn to know how your body reacts to the medicine and supplements. Keep track of how you feel, and when the effects occur.

Carry a medication list. In case of an emergency, carry a list of all medications you are taking, including product names and dosages.

Alternatives to Driving Yourself

Planning ahead will help get you to the places you want to go. Consider the following alternatives to driving yourself: rides with family and friends, taxi cabs, shuttle buses or vans; public buses, trains, and subways, and walking. Also, senior centers and religious and other local service groups often offer transportation services for older adults in the community.

Part Two
Drugs of Abuse

Chapter 16

2C-I

Drug name: 4-Iodo-2,5-Dimethoxyphenethylamine

Street names: 2C-I, i

Introduction: 4-Iodo-2,5-dimethoxyphenethylamine (2C-I, 4-iodo-2,5-DMPEA) is a synthetic drug abused for its hallucinogenic effects. It has been encountered in a number of states by federal, state, and local law enforcement agencies.

Licit uses: 2C-I has no approved medical uses in the United States.

Chemistry and pharmacology: 4-Iodo-2,5-dimethoxyphenethylamine is closely related to the phenylisopropylamine hallucinogens, 1-(4-bromo-2, 5-dimethoxyphenyl)-2-aminopropane (DOB) and 2,5-dimethoxy-4-methylamphetamine (DOM). Like DOM and DOB, 2C-I displays high affinity for central serotonin receptors. 2C-I selectively binds to the 5-HT receptor system.

Drug discrimination studies in animals indicate that 2C-I produces discriminative stimulus effects that are similar to those of several schedule I hallucinogens such as lysergic acid diethylamide (LSD), N,N-dimethyltryptamine (DMT), and methylene-dioxymethamphetamine (MDMA). In rats trained to discriminate LSD, DMT, or MDMA from saline, 2C-I fully substituted for these schedule I hallucinogens.

"4-Iodo-2,5-Dimethoxyphenethylamine," Drug Enforcement Administration (DEA), June 2009.

In humans, 2C-I produces dose dependent psychoactive effects. User reports have mentioned oral doses between three and twenty-five milligrams (mg), producing LSD-like hallucinations and visual distortions, and MDMA-like empathy. Onset of subjective effects following 2C-I ingestion is around forty minutes with peak effects occurring at approximately two hours. Effects of 2C-I can last up to eight hours. Various users reported delayed desired effects compared to related drugs, which may result in some users taking additional doses or other drugs which may increase the risk of toxicity or accidental over dosage.

Radioimmunoassay detection system that is commonly used for testing amphetamine and hallucinogens is not expected to detect 2C-I. In the Marquis Reagent Field Test, 2C-I produces a dark green to black color.

Illicit uses: 2C-I is abused for its hallucinogenic effects. 2C-I is taken orally in tablet or capsule forms or snorted in its powder form. It has also been found impregnated on small squares of blotter paper for oral administration, which is a technique often seen for the distribution and abuse of LSD. The drug has been misrepresented by distributors and sold as other hallucinogens such as MDMA and LSD.

User population: 2C-I is used by the same population as those using ecstasy and other club drugs, high school and college students, and other young adults in dance and nightlife settings.

Illicit distribution: 2C-I is distributed as capsules, tablets, in powder form, or in liquid form. The Drug Enforcement Administration (DEA) identified occurrences of the drug being purchased through internet retailers. In one instance, it was purchased in powder form through the internet and encapsulated for retail, at a street value of $6 per capsule. In Europe, 2C-I has often been seized in tablet form with an "I" logo which may be to signify that it is not ecstasy (MDMA).

In the past five years, 2C-I has been encountered by law enforcement in many states including Arkansas, California, Florida, Illinois, North Dakota, New Jersey, New York, Ohio, Pennsylvania, South Carolina, Texas, and Virginia. According to the National Forensic Laboratory Information system, law enforcement officials submitted 25 2C-I exhibits/items to DEA laboratories from 2004 to 2008 and submitted 27 exhibits/items to state and local forensic laboratories during the same time period.

Control status: Currently, 2C-I is not a scheduled drug under the Controlled Substances Act (CSA). However, 2C-I can be considered an analogue of 2C-B, which is a schedule I hallucinogen under the CSA (60 FR 28718). As such, 2C-I can be treated on a case-by-case basis as if it were a schedule I controlled substance, if it is distributed with the intention for human consumption [21 U.S.C. 802 (32), 21 U.S.C. 813].

Chapter 17

Anabolic Steroids

Drug name: Anabolic steroids

Street names: Arnolds, gym candy, pumpers, roids, stackers, weight trainers, gear, and juice

Introduction: Anabolic steroids are a class of drugs with a basic steroid ring structure that produce anabolic effects and androgenic effects. Athletes, bodybuilders, and others abuse anabolic steroids with the intent to improve athletic performance, muscle strength, and appearance.

Licit uses: In the United States (U.S.), only a small number of anabolic steroids are approved for either human or veterinary use. Testosterone and several of its esters, as well as methyltestosterone, nandrolone decanoate, and oxandrolone are the main anabolic steroids currently prescribed in the U.S. Some of the approved medical uses include the treatment of testosterone deficiency, delayed puberty, anemia, breast cancer, and tissue wasting resulting from acquired immunodeficiency syndrome (AIDS). Trenbolone, boldenone, and mibolerone are used only in veterinary medicine.

Chemistry and pharmacology: Most anabolic steroids are synthetically manufactured variations of testosterone. No anabolic steroid is devoid of androgenic effects. Activation of androgen receptors in

This chapter includes "Anabolic Steroids," Drug Enforcement Administration (DEA), June 2009; and excerpts from "Anabolic Steroids: Hidden Dangers," DEA, March 2008.

various cells and tissues primarily mediate the anabolic and androgenic effects. The anabolic effects include the growth of skeletal and cardiac muscle, bone, and red blood cells, whereas the androgenic effects include the development of male secondary sexual characteristics.

The adverse effects associated with anabolic steroids are dependent on the age of the user, the sex of the user, the anabolic steroid used, the amount used, and the duration of use. In adolescents, use can permanently stunt growth. In women, use can induce permanent physical changes including deepening of the voice, increased facial and body hair growth, and the lengthening of the clitoris. In men, use can cause shrinkage of the testicles, enlargement of the male breast tissue, and sterility. Anabolic steroid use can damage the liver and can cause an increase in cholesterol levels. Anabolic steroid use can also induce psychological effects such as aggression, increased feelings of hostility, psychological dependence, and addiction. Upon abrupt termination of long-term anabolic steroid use, abusers may experience withdrawal symptoms including severe depression.

Illicit uses: Anabolic steroids are abused with the intent to enhance athletic performance, increase muscle strength, and improve appearance. The doses used are often 10–100 times higher than the doses used to treat medical conditions. Users typically take two or more anabolic steroids at the same time in a cyclic manner believing that this will improve their effectiveness and minimize the adverse effects. Anabolic steroid abuse is often accompanied by the use of other drugs.

User population: Anabolic steroids are abused by professional, amateur, recreational athletes, and bodybuilders. Adolescents and young adults in the general population also abuse steroids to improve their appearance.

In the 2008 Monitoring the Future Study (MTF), which surveys eighth, tenth, and twelfth grade students, 1.4%, of eighth graders, 1.4% of tenth graders, and 2.2% of twelfth graders reported using steroids at least once in their lifetimes. Regarding the ease by which steroids can be obtained, 16.8% of eighth graders, 24.5% of tenth graders, and 35.2% of twelfth graders reported that steroids were fairly easy, or very easy, to obtain. Although the percentage of students reporting ease of obtaining steroids in 2008 declined significantly from the percentage reported in 2007 for tenth and twelfth graders, illicit steroid use among those students did not decrease during the same period of time.

Illicit distribution: Anabolic steroids are available as injectable preparations, tablets and capsules, and gels and creams. Most anabolic steroids sold illegally in the U.S. come from abroad. The internet is the most widely used means of buying and selling anabolic steroids. However, there is also evidence of professional diversion through unscrupulous pharmacists, doctors, and veterinarians.

New steroids, which have not undergone safety or efficacy testing in the U.S., have appeared over the years. Some of these designer steroids were supplied to athletes to avoid detection. Commercially available dietary supplements are sold purporting to contain novel anabolic steroids. These products, which are advertised to build muscle and increase strength, are readily available on the internet.

The National Forensic Laboratory Information System (NFLIS) data indicate that the 12 most frequently encountered schedule III anabolic steroid items/exhibits submitted to Drug Enforcement Administration (DEA) laboratories declined from 2,107 in 2007 to 734 in 2008. Similarly, anabolic steroids submitted to state and local laboratories declined from 2,474 in 2007 to 2,196 in 2008. According to NFLIS, testosterone, nandrolone, methandrostenolone, and stanozolol are the four most frequently encountered steroids by the federal, state, and local forensic laboratories in 2007 and 2008.

Control status: After the Anabolic Steroid Control Acts of 1990 and 2004 passed, Congress placed a total of 59 anabolic steroids in schedule III of the Controlled Substances Act. The salts, esters, and ethers of these 59 anabolic steroids are also controlled. Congress provided a definition to administratively classify additional steroids as schedule III anabolic steroids.

Anabolic Steroids: Hidden Dangers

Steroid users are vulnerable to physical and psychological side effects, many of which are irreversible in women. The short-term adverse physical effects of anabolic steroid abuse are fairly well known. However, the long-term adverse physical effects of anabolic steroid abuse have not been studied and are not known.

Side effects of steroid use include the following:

- **For guys:** Baldness, development of breasts, painful erections, shrinkage of testicles, and loss of function of testicles

- **For girls:** Growth of facial and body hair, deepened voice, breast reduction, enlarged clitoris, and menstrual irregularities

- **For everyone:** Acne, jaundice (yellowing of the skin), swelling (fluid retention), stunted growth (closes the growth plates in the long bones and permanently stunts their growth), increase in bad cholesterol levels, decrease in good cholesterol levels, mood swings, increase in feelings of hostility, and increase in aggressive behavior

Laws and Penalties for Anabolic Steroid Abuse

Anabolic steroids as a class of drugs were placed in schedule III of the Controlled Substances Act (CSA) as of February 27, 1991. The possession or sale of anabolic steroids without a valid prescription is illegal. Simple possession of illicitly obtained anabolic steroids carries a maximum penalty up to one year in prison and a minimum fine of $1,000 if this is an individual's first drug offense. The maximum penalty for trafficking is five years in prison and a fine of $250,000 if this is the individual's first felony drug offense. If this is the second felony drug offense, the maximum period of imprisonment and the maximum fine both double. The period of imprisonment and the amount of fine are enhanced if the offense involves the distribution of an anabolic steroid and a masking agent or if the distribution is to an athlete. In addition, enhanced penalties exist for any athletic coach who uses his or her position to influence an athlete to use an anabolic steroid. While the listed penalties are for federal offenses, individual states have also implemented fines and penalties for illegal use of anabolic steroids.

The International Olympic Committee (IOC), National Collegiate Athletic Association (NCAA), and many professional sports leagues (Major League Baseball, National Basketball Association, National Football League , and National Hockey League) have banned the use of steroids by athletes, both because of their potential dangerous side effects and they give the user an unfair advantage. The IOC and professional sports leagues use urine testing to detect steroid use both in and out of competition.

What can you do to help a friend who is abusing steroids?

The most important aspect to curtailing abuse is education concerning dangerous and harmful side effects and symptoms of abuse. Athletes and others must understand they can excel in sports and have a great body without steroids. They should focus on a proper diet, rest, and good overall mental and physical health. These are all factors in how the body is shaped and conditioned. Millions of people have excelled in sports and look great without steroids.

Chapter 18

Blue Mystic

Drug name: 2,5-dimethoxy-4-(n)-propylthiophenethylamine (2C-T-7)

Street names: 2C-T-7, Blue Mystic, T7, Beautiful, Tripstay, Tweety-Bird Mescaline

In the fall of 2000, a young healthy male died following snorting an excessive amount of 2,5-dimethoxy-4-(n)-propylthiophenethylamine (2C-T-7). Since this initial 2C-T-7-related death, two additional deaths reported in April 2001 have been linked to 2C-T-7. These two deaths resulted from the co-abuse of 2C-T-7 with MDMA.

Licit uses: 2C-T-7 is not approved for marketing by the Food and Drug Administration (FDA) and is not sold legally in the United States.

Chemistry and pharmacology: 2,5-dimethoxy-4-(n)-propylthiophenethylamine (2C-T-7), is a phenethylamine hallucinogen that is structurally related to the schedule I phenethylamine hallucinogens, 4-bromo-2, 5-dimethoxyphenethylamine (2C-B, Nexus) and mescaline. Based on structural similarly to these compounds, the pharmacological profile of 2C-T-7 is expected to be qualitatively similar to these hallucinogens.

"2,5-Dimethoxy-4-(n)-Propylthiophenethylamine," Drug Enforcement Administration (DEA), June 2009.

Drug discrimination studies in animals indicate that 2C-T-7 produces discriminative stimulus effects similar to those of several schedule I hallucinogens. In rats trained to discriminate 2,5-dimethoxy-4-methylamphetamine (DOM), 2C-T-7 fully substituted for DOM and was slightly less potent than 2C-B in eliciting DOM-like effects. 2C-T-7 was also shown to share some commonality with lysergic acid diethylamide (LSD); it partially substituted for LSD up to doses that severely disrupted performance in rats trained to discriminate LSD. 2C-T-7 can also function as a discriminative stimulus in rats. Rats readily learned to discriminate 2C-T-7 from saline. When either 2C-B or LSD was substituted for 2C-T-7, each elicited 2C-T-7-like discriminative stimulus effects. The subjective effects of 2C-T-7, like those of 2C-B and DOM, appear to be mediated through central serotonin receptors. 2C-T-7 selectively binds to the 5-HT receptor system. According to one published case report, 2C-T-7 abuse has been associated with convulsions in humans.

Illicit uses: 2C-T-7 is abused orally and intranasally for its hallucinogenic effects. Information from a website about a variety of illicit drugs has suggested that 2C-T-7 produces effects similar to those of 2C-B. This information is based on individuals self-administering 2C-T-7 illicitly and self-reporting the effects. Its effects include visual hallucination, mood lifting, sense of well being, emotionality, volatility, increased appreciation of music, and psychedelic ideation. The oral and intranasal doses recommended by the website are 10–50 mg and 5–10 mg, respectively. 2C-T-7's onset and duration of actions are dependent upon the route of administration. Following oral administration, onset and duration of effects are 1–2.5 hours and 5–7 hours, respectively. After intranasal administration, the onset of action and duration of effects are 5–15 minutes and 2–4 hours, respectively.

User Population: Young adults are the main abusers of 2C-T-7.

Illicit distribution: According to National Forensic Laboratory Information System (NFLIS), law enforcement officials seized and submitted 38 items (nine cases) of 2C-T-7 to state and local forensic laboratories from 2004 to 2008. Seizures of 2C-T-7 have occurred in California, Florida, Minnesota, and Wisconsin in the last five years. A vast majority of the drugs (29 items from two cases) were seized in the state of Florida. There were no 2C-T-7 drug items submitted and analyzed by Drug Enforcement Administration (DEA) laboratories from 2004 to 2008.

2C-T-7 was being purchased over the internet from a company located in Indiana. This site was traced to an individual who had been selling large quantities of this substance since January 2000. Sales through this internet site were thought to be the major sources of 2C-T-7 in the United States. One clandestine laboratory was identified in Las Vegas, Nevada as the supplier of 2C-T-7 to the individual in Indiana. 2C-T-7 has been sold under the street names Blue Mystic, T7, Beautiful, Tweety-Bird Mescaline, or Tripstay.

Control status: 2C-T-7 has been placed in schedule I of the Controlled Substances Act of 1970.

Chapter 19

Buprenorphine

Drug name: Buprenorphine

Trade names: Buprenex®, Suboxone®, Subutex®

Introduction: Buprenorphine was first marketed in the United States in 1985 as a schedule V narcotic analgesic. Until recently, the only available buprenorphine product in the United States has been a low-dose (0.3 milligrams/milliliter [mg/ml]) injectable formulation under the brand name, Buprenex®. Diversion, trafficking, and abuse of other buprenorphine products have occurred in Europe and other areas of the world.

In October 2002, the Food and Drug Administration (FDA) approved two buprenorphine products (Suboxone® and Subutex®) for the treatment of narcotic addiction. Both products are high dose (2 mg and 8 mg) sublingual (under the tongue) tablets: Subutex® is a single entity buprenorphine product and Suboxone® is a combination product with buprenorphine and naloxone in a 4:1 ratio, respectively. After reviewing all the available data and receiving a schedule III recommendation from the Department of Health and Human Services (DHHS), the DEA placed buprenorphine and all products containing buprenorphine into schedule III in 2002. Since 2003, diversion, trafficking, and abuse of buprenorphine have become more common in the United States.

"Buprenorphine," Drug Enforcement Administration (DEA), June 2009.

Licit uses: Buprenorphine is intended for the treatment of pain (Buprenex®) and opioid addiction (Suboxone® and Subutex®). In 2001, 2005, and 2006, the Narcotic Addict Treatment Act was amended to allow qualified physicians, under certification of the DHHS, to prescribe schedule III–V narcotic drugs (FDA approved for the indication of narcotic treatment) for narcotic addiction, up to 30 patients per physician at any time, outside the context of clinic-based narcotic treatment programs (Pub. L. 106-310). This limit was increased to 100 patients per physician, for physicians who meet the specified criteria, under the Office of National Drug Control Policy Reauthorization Act (P.L. 69–469, ONDCPRA), which became effective on December 29, 2006.

Suboxone® and Subutex® are the only treatment drugs that meet the requirement of this exemption. Currently, there are nearly 15,700 physicians who have been approved by the Substance Abuse and Mental Health Services Administration (SAMHSA) and the Drug Enforcement Administration (DEA) for office-based narcotic buprenorphine treatment. Of those physicians, approximately 13,150 were approved to treat up to 30 patients per provider and about 2,500 were approved to treat up to 100 patients. More than 3,000 physicians have submitted their intention to treat up to 100 patients per provider. IMS Health National Prescription Audit Plus data indicate that 3.54 million buprenorphine prescriptions were dispensed in the United States in 2008, compared to 2.12 million prescriptions in 2007.

Chemistry and pharmacology: Buprenorphine has a unique pharmacological profile. It produces the effects typical of both pure mu agonists (morphine) and partial agonists (pentazocine) depending on dose, pattern of use, and population taking the drug. It is about 20–30 times more potent than morphine as an analgesic; and like morphine it produces dose-related euphoria, drug liking, pupillary constriction, respiratory depression, and sedation. However, acute, high doses of buprenorphine have been shown to have a blunting effect on both physiological and psychological effects due to its partial opioid activity.

Buprenorphine is a long-acting (24–72 hours) opioid that produces less respiratory depression at high doses than other narcotic treatment drugs. However, severe respiratory depression can occur when buprenorphine is combined with other central nervous system depressants, especially benzodiazepines. Deaths have resulted from this combination.

The addition of naloxone in the Suboxone® product is intended to block the euphoric high resulting from the injection of this drug by non-buprenorphine maintained narcotic abusers.

User population: In countries where buprenorphine has gained popularity as a drug of abuse, it is sought by a wide variety of narcotic abusers: young naive individuals, non-addicted opioid abusers, heroin addicts, and buprenorphine treatment clients.

Illicit uses: Like other opioids commonly abused, buprenorphine is capable of producing significant euphoria. Data from other countries indicate that buprenorphine has been abused by various routes of administration (sublingual, intranasal, and injection) and has gained popularity as a heroin substitute and as a primary drug of abuse. Large percentages of the drug abusing populations in some areas of France, Ireland, Scotland, India, Nepal, Bangladesh, Pakistan, and New Zealand have reported abusing buprenorphine by injection and in combination with a benzodiazepine.

According to the National Forensic Laboratory Information System (NFLIS), drug items/exhibits submitted and identified as buprenorphine in state and local laboratories increased from 229 in 2004 to 4,245 in 2008. DEA laboratories identified five buprenorphine items/exhibits in 2004 and 49 in 2008. Buprenorphine now ranks among the top 25 most frequently identified substances analyzed in federal, state, and local laboratories according to NFLIS. According to the 2006 Drug Abuse Warning Network (New DAWN ED) survey, an estimated 4,440 emergency room visits were associated with buprenorphine misuse.

Control status: Buprenorphine and all products containing buprenorphine are controlled in schedule III of the Controlled Substances Act.

Chapter 20

BZP

Drug name: N-benzylpiperazine (BZP)

Street names: BZP, A2, Legal E or Legal X

Introduction: N-benzylpiperazine (BZP) was first synthesized in 1944 as a potential antiparasitic agent. It was subsequently shown to possess antidepressant activity and amphetamine-like effects, but was not developed for marketing. The amphetamine-like effects of BZP attracted the attention of drug abusers. Since 1996, BZP has been abused by drug abusers; as evidenced by the encounters of this substance by law enforcement officials in various states and the District of Columbia. The Drug Enforcement Administration (DEA) placed BZP in schedule I of the Controlled Substances Act (CSA) because of its high abuse potential and lack of accepted medical use or safety.

Licit uses: BZP is used as an intermediate in chemical synthesis. It has no known medical use in the United States.

Chemistry and pharmacology: BZP is an N-monosubstituted piperazine derivative available as either base or the hydrochloride salt. The base form is a slightly yellowish-green liquid. The hydrochloride salt is a white solid. BZP base is corrosive and causes burns. The salt form of BZP is an irritant to eyes, respiratory system, and skin.

"N-Benzylpiperazine," Drug Enforcement Administration (DEA), August 2007.

Both animal studies and human clinical studies have demonstrated that the pharmacological effects of BZP are qualitatively similar to those of amphetamine. BZP has been reported to be similar to amphetamine in its effects on chemical transmission in brain. BZP fully mimics discriminative stimulus effects of amphetamine in animals. BZP is self-administered by monkeys indicating reinforcing effects. Subjective effects of BZP were amphetamine-like in drug-naive volunteers and in volunteers with a history of stimulant dependence. BZP acts as a stimulant in humans and produces euphoria and cardiovascular effects, namely increases in heart rate and systolic blood pressure. BZP is about 10–20 times less potent than amphetamine in producing these effects. Experimental studies demonstrate that the abuse, dependence potential, pharmacology, and toxicology of BZP are similar to those of amphetamine. Public health risks of BZP are similar to those of amphetamine.

Illicit uses: BZP is often taken in combination with 1-[3-(trifluoromethyl)phenyl]piperazine (TFMPP), a non-controlled substance, in order to enhance its spectrum of effects and has been promoted to youth population as substitute for MDMA at raves (all-night dance parties). It may also be abused alone for its stimulant effects. BZP is generally administered orally as either powder or tablets and capsules. Other routes of administration included smoking and snorting. In 2001, a report from University in Zurich, Switzerland described the death of a young female which was attributed to the combined use of BZP and MDMA.

User population: Youth and young adults are the main abusers of BZP.

Illicit distribution: According to System to Retrieve Information from Drug Evidence (STRIDE) and National Forensic Laboratory Information System (NFLIS), BZP has been encountered in a number of states including Alabama, Arizona, Arkansas, California, Colorado, Connecticut, District of Columbia, Florida, Georgia, Illinois, Indiana, Louisiana, Maryland, Massachusetts, Maine, Michigan, Minnesota, Missouri, Mississippi, North Carolina, Nevada, New Jersey, New Mexico, New York, Ohio, Oregon, Pennsylvania, South Carolina, Texas, Virginia, Washington, and Wisconsin.

Since 2001, according to the STRIDE database, DEA forensic laboratories analyzed 128 drug exhibits from 59 law enforcement cases pertaining to the trafficking, distribution, and abuse of BZP. The analyzed drug exhibits comprised of 66,645 tablets, 8,409 capsules and 356,997.1 grams of powder.

According to the NFLIS, state and local forensic laboratories analyzed 94 BZP drug items from 76 law enforcement cases during 2000 through 2006.

Illicit distributions occur through smuggling of bulk powder through drug trafficking organizations with connections to overseas sources of supply. The bulk powder is then processed into capsules and tablet. BZP is encountered as pink, white, off-white, purple, orange, tan, and mottle orange-brown tablets. These tablets bear imprints commonly seen on MDMA tablets such as housefly, crown, heart, butterfly, smiley face, or bull's head logos and are often sold as ecstasy. BZP has been found in powder or liquid form which is packaged in small convenience sizes and sold on the internet.

Control status: BZP was temporarily placed into schedule I of the CSA on September 20, 2002 (67 FR 59161). On March 18, 2004, the DEA published a Final Rule in the *Federal Register* permanently placing BZP in schedule I.

Chapter 21

Clenbuterol

Drug name: Clenbuterol

Street name: Clen

Introduction: Clenbuterol is a potent, long-lasting bronchodilator that is prescribed for human use outside of the United States (U.S.) It is abused generally by bodybuilders and athletes for its ability to increase lean muscle mass and reduce body fat (repartitioning effects). However, clenbuterol is also associated with significant adverse cardiovascular and neurological effects.

Licit uses: In the U.S., clenbuterol is not approved for human use; the only approved use is for horses. In 1998, the Food and Drug Administration (FDA) approved the clenbuterol-based Ventipulmin Syrup, manufactured by Boehringer Ingelheim Vetmedica, Inc., as a prescription-only drug for the treatment of airway obstruction in horses (0.8–3.2 micrograms per kilogram [μg/kg] twice daily). This product is not intended for human use or for use in food-producing animals.

Outside the U.S., clenbuterol is available by prescription for the treatment of bronchial asthma in humans. It is available in tablets (0.01 or 0.02 milligrams [mg] per tablet) and liquid preparations. The recommended dosage is 0.02–0.03 mg twice daily.

"Clenbuterol," Drug Enforcement Administration (DEA), August 2007.

Chemistry and pharmacology: Clenbuterol is a beta2-adrenergic agonist. Stimulation of the beta2-adrenergic receptors on bronchial smooth muscle produces bronchodilation. However, clenbuterol also stimulates beta2-adrenergic receptors in other tissues, as well as beta1-adrenergic receptors, producing adverse cardiovascular and neurological effects, such as heart palpitations, muscle tremors, and nervousness. Activation of beta-adrenergic receptors also accounts for clenbuterol's ability to increase lean muscle mass and reduce body fat, although the downstream mechanisms by which it does so have yet to be clearly defined.

After ingestion, clenbuterol is readily absorbed (70–80%) and remains in the body for awhile (25–39 hours). As a result of its long half life, the adverse effects of clenbuterol are often prolonged.

Illicit uses: Clenbuterol is abused for its ability to alter body composition by reducing body fat and increasing skeletal muscle mass. It is typically abused by athletes and bodybuilders at a dose of 60–120 µg per day. It is often used in combination with other performance enhancing drugs, such as anabolic steroids and growth hormone.

It is also illicitly administered to livestock for its repartitioning effects. This has resulted in several outbreaks of acute illness in Spain, France, Italy, China, and Portugal 0.5–3 hours after individuals ingested liver and meat containing clenbuterol residues. The symptoms, which included increased heart rate, nervousness, headache, muscular tremor, dizziness, nausea, vomiting, fever, and chills, typically resolved within 2–6 days. Consequently, the U.S. and Europe actively monitor urine and tissue samples from livestock for the presence of clenbuterol.

There have also been reports of clenbuterol-tainted heroin and cocaine. Although no deaths were attributed to the clenbuterol exposures, the individuals were hospitalized for up to several days due to clenbuterol intoxication.

User population: Clenbuterol is typically abused by athletes. It is thought to be more popular among female athletes as the repartitioning effects are not associated with the typical androgenic side effects (facial hair, deepening of the voice, and thickening of the skin) of anabolic steroids. Professional athletes in several different sports have recently tested positive for clenbuterol. Clenbuterol is also marketed and abused for weight-loss purposes.

Illicit distribution: Clenbuterol is readily available on the internet as tablets, syrup, and an injectable formulation. The drug is purportedly obtained by illegal importation from other countries where it is approved for human use.

According to the System to Retrieve Information on Drug Evidence (STRIDE) data, since 2000, Drug Enforcement Administration (DEA) forensic laboratories analyzed 109 clenbuterol drug items from 77 different law enforcement cases. The analyzed drug exhibits comprised of 39,643 tablets, 17,704.11 grams of powder, and 1,828.7 milliliters liquid. Since 2000, according to National Forensic Laboratory Information System (NFLIS), state and local forensic laboratories analyzed 68 clenbuterol drug items from 53 different law enforcement cases. These relatively small numbers are likely a reflection of the non-controlled status of clenbuterol in the U.S. Clenbuterol is often seized in cases that also involve anabolic steroids and other performance enhancing drugs (for example, human growth hormone.)

Control status: Clenbuterol is currently not controlled under the Controlled Substances Act (CSA). However, clenbuterol is listed by the World Anti-Doping Agency and the International Olympic Committee as a performance enhancing drug and therefore athletes are barred from its use. At present, no states have placed clenbuterol under control.

Chapter 22

Cocaine and Crack Cocaine

Drug name: Cocaine

Street names: Coke, snow, crack, rock

Introduction: Cocaine abuse has a long, deeply rooted history in United States (U.S.) drug culture, both urban and rural. It is an intense, euphorigenic drug with strong addictive potential. With the advent of the higher purity free-base form of cocaine (crack), and its easy availability on the street, cocaine continues to burden both law enforcement and health care systems in the U.S.

Licit uses: Cocaine hydrochloride (4% and 10%) solution is used primarily as a topical local anesthetic for the upper respiratory tract. The vasoconstrictor and local anesthetic properties of cocaine cause anesthesia and mucosal shrinkage. It constricts blood vessels and reduces blood flow, and is used to reduce bleeding of the mucous membranes in the mouth, throat, and nasal cavities. However, better products have been developed for these purposes and cocaine is rarely used medically in the U.S.

Chemistry and pharmacology: Cocaine is the principal alkaloid in the leaves of *Erythroxylon coca*, a shrub indigenous to the Andean

---

This chapter includes text from "Cocaine," Drug Enforcement Administration (DEA), September 2007; and excerpts from "Crack and Cocaine," National Institute on Drug Abuse (NIDA), revised June 2009.

region of South America. Cocaine is an ester of benzoic acid and methylecgonine. Ecgonine, an amino alcohol, is structurally similar to atropine and some local anesthetics. Cocaine is a local anesthetic and a strong central nervous system stimulant which produces intense euphoria. Inhalation of the vapors of cocaine base (crack), known as basing or free basing, became a popular practice in the 1980s because of its rapid onset of action (7–10 seconds), ease of repeat administration, and an unwarranted belief by users that smoking cocaine was less harmful and less likely to produce addiction than injecting cocaine. Smoking cocaine base produces a sudden and intense rush with an equally intense high or euphoria lasting from 2–20 minutes. Tolerance develops to the euphoric effects of cocaine. Physiological effects of cocaine include constricted peripheral blood vessels, dilated pupils, and increased blood pressure and heart rate. Cocaine also produces restlessness, irritability, and anxiety in some users. High doses of cocaine or prolonged use can cause paranoia.

Illicit uses: Cocaine can be packaged as a white crystalline powder (snow), or in paste, free-base, or rock form (crack). Crack can be sprinkled on marijuana or tobacco and smoked. It is also taken in combination with an opiate, like heroin; a practice commonly referred to as speedballing. Intravenous and intramuscular injections, snorting, and smoking are the common routes of administration. All mucous membranes readily absorb cocaine. Cocaine smugglers who transport the drug by ingestion have died from the rapid absorption of cocaine through the bowel mucosa after swallowed cocaine-packed balloons inadvertently rupture in transit.

The widespread abuse of street cocaine of high purity has led to many adverse health consequences such as cardiac arrhythmias, ischemic heart conditions, sudden cardiac arrest, convulsions, strokes, and death. The availability of crack cocaine led to an increase in inhalation as the preferred route of administration for many abusers. In order to avoid the discomfort associated with post-euphoric crash, crack or free base smokers continue to smoke often in marathon binges, until they become exhausted or run out of cocaine supply. The long-term use of inhaled cocaine has led to a unique respiratory syndrome in some abusers, and the chronic snorting of cocaine has led to the erosion of the upper nasal cavity.

Illicit distribution: Colombia produces about 90% of the cocaine powder reaching the U.S. The 2006 wholesale price for cocaine powder ranged from $9,000 to $52,000 per kilogram. The prices for crack cocaine ranged from $5 to $100 per rock. According to the 2005 Colombia Threat Assessment, 90% of the cocaine shipped to the U.S. comes from the Central America/Mexico corridor. According to the Federal-Wide Drug Seizure System, U.S. federal law enforcement seized 150,176 kilograms of cocaine in 2006. According to the System to Retrieve Information from Drug Evidence, DEA forensic laboratories analyzed a total of 21,783 cocaine exhibits in 2006. According to the National Forensic Laboratory Information System, state and local forensic laboratories analyzed 371,602 cocaine exhibits from 312,099 cases across the U.S. in 2006.

Control status: Cocaine is a schedule II substance under the federal Controlled Substances Act.

Facts about Crack and Cocaine

How is cocaine abused?

Three routes of administration are commonly used for cocaine: snorting, injecting, and smoking. Snorting is the process of inhaling cocaine powder through the nose, where it is absorbed into the bloodstream through the nasal tissues. Injecting is the use of a needle to insert the drug directly into the bloodstream. Smoking involves inhaling cocaine vapor or smoke into the lungs, where absorption into the bloodstream is as rapid as by injection. All three methods of cocaine abuse can lead to addiction and other severe health problems including increasing the risk of contracting human immunodeficiency virus (HIV) and other infectious diseases.

The intensity and duration of cocaine's effects—which include increased energy, reduced fatigue, and mental alertness—depend on the route of drug administration. The faster cocaine is absorbed into the bloodstream and delivered to the brain, the more intense the high. Injecting or smoking cocaine produces a quicker, stronger high than snorting. On the other hand, faster absorption usually means shorter duration of action: the high from snorting cocaine may last 15–30 minutes, but the high from smoking may last only 5–10 minutes. In order to sustain the high, a cocaine abuser has to administer the drug again. For this reason, cocaine is sometimes abused in binges—taken repeatedly within a relatively short period of time at increasingly higher doses.

How does cocaine affect the brain?

Cocaine is a strong central nervous system stimulant that increases levels of dopamine, a brain chemical (or neurotransmitter) associated with pleasure and movement, in the brain's reward circuit. Certain brain cells, or neurons, use dopamine to communicate. Normally, dopamine is released by a neuron in response to a pleasurable signal (for example, the smell of good food), and then recycled back into the cell that released it, thus shutting off the signal between neurons. Cocaine acts by preventing the dopamine from being recycled, causing excessive amounts of the neurotransmitter to build up, amplifying the message to and response of the receiving neuron, and ultimately disrupting normal communication. It is this excess of dopamine that is responsible for cocaine's euphoric effects. With repeated use, cocaine can cause long-term changes in the brain's reward system and in other brain systems as well, which may eventually lead to addiction. With repeated use, tolerance to the cocaine high also often develops. Many cocaine abusers report that they seek but fail to achieve as much pleasure as they did from their first exposure. Some users will increase their dose in an attempt to intensify and prolong the euphoria, but this can also increase the risk of adverse psychological or physiological effects.

What adverse effects does cocaine have on health?

Abusing cocaine has a variety of adverse effects on the body. For example, cocaine constricts blood vessels, dilates pupils, and increases body temperature, heart rate, and blood pressure. It can also cause headaches and gastrointestinal complications such as abdominal pain and nausea. Because cocaine tends to decrease appetite, chronic users can become malnourished as well.

Different methods of taking cocaine can produce different adverse effects. Regular intranasal use (snorting) of cocaine, for example, can lead to loss of the sense of smell; nosebleeds; problems with swallowing; hoarseness; and a chronically runny nose. Ingesting cocaine can cause severe bowel gangrene as a result of reduced blood flow. Injecting cocaine can bring about severe allergic reactions and increased risk for contracting HIV and other blood-borne diseases. Binge-patterned cocaine use may lead to irritability, restlessness, and anxiety. Cocaine abusers can also experience severe paranoia, a temporary state of full-blown paranoid psychosis, in which they lose touch with reality and experience auditory hallucinations.

Regardless of the route or frequency of use, cocaine abusers can experience acute cardiovascular or cerebrovascular emergencies, such as a heart attack or stroke, which may cause sudden death. Cocaine-related deaths are often a result of cardiac arrest or seizure followed by respiratory arrest.

Added Danger: Cocaethylene

Polydrug use—use of more than one drug—is common among substance abusers. When people consume two or more psychoactive drugs together, such as cocaine and alcohol, they compound the danger each drug poses and unknowingly perform a complex chemical experiment within their bodies. Researchers have found that the human liver combines cocaine and alcohol to produce a third substance, cocaethylene, which intensifies cocaine's euphoric effects. Cocaethylene is associated with a greater risk of sudden death than cocaine alone.

What treatment options exist?

Behavioral interventions—particularly, cognitive-behavioral therapy—have been shown to be effective for decreasing cocaine use and preventing relapse. Treatment must be tailored to the individual patient's needs in order to optimize outcomes—this often involves a combination of treatment, social supports, and other services.

Currently, there are no U.S. Food and Drug Administration (FDA)-approved medications for treating cocaine addiction. Current research suggests that while medications are effective in treating addiction, combining them with a comprehensive behavioral therapy program is the most effective method to reduce drug use in the long term.

How widespread is cocaine abuse?

According to the 2008 Monitoring the Future survey—a national survey of students in grades 8, 10, and 12—cocaine use among students did not change significantly, though it remained at unacceptable high levels: 3.0% of 8th-graders, 4.5% of 10th-graders, and 7.2% of 12th-graders have tried cocaine; 0.8% of 8th-graders, 1.2% of 10th-graders, and 1.9% of 12th-graders were current (past-month) cocaine users.

Chapter 23

Dextromethorphan (DXM)

Drug name: Dextromethorphan

Street names: DXM, CCC, triple C, skittles, robo, poor man's PCP

Introduction: Dextromethorphan (DXM) is an over-the-counter (OTC) cough suppressant commonly found in cold medications. DXM is often abused in high doses by adolescents to generate euphoria and visual and auditory hallucinations. Illicit use of DXM is referred to on the street as robo-tripping or skittling. These terms are derived from the most commonly abused products, Robitussin® and Coricidin®.

Licit uses: DXM is an antitussive found in more than 120 over-the-counter (OTC) cold medications either alone or in combination with other drugs such as analgesics (for example, acetaminophen), antihistamines (such as chlorpheniramine), decongestants (like pseudoephedrine) and/or expectorants (such as guaifenesin). The typical antitussive adult dose is 15–30 milligrams (mg) taken three to four times daily. The suppressant effects of DXM persist for 5–6 hours after oral administration. When taken as directed, side effects are rarely observed.

Illicit use: DXM is abused by individuals of all ages but its abuse by teenagers and young adults is of particular concern. This abuse is

---

"Dextromethorphan," Drug Enforcement Administration (DEA), September 2007.

fueled by DXM's OTC availability and extensive how-to abuse information on various websites. The sale of the powdered form of DXM over the internet poses additional risks due to the uncertainty of composition and dose.

DXM abusers report a heightened sense of perceptual awareness, altered time perception, and visual hallucinations. The typical clinical presentation of DXM intoxication involves hyperexcitability, lethargy, ataxia, slurred speech, sweating, hypertension, and/or nystagmus. Abuse of combination DXM products also results in health complications from the other active ingredient(s), which include increased blood pressure from pseudoephedrine, potential delayed liver damage from acetaminophen, and central nervous system toxicity, cardiovascular toxicity, and anticholinergic toxicity from antihistamines. The use of high doses of DXM in combination with alcohol or other drugs is particularly dangerous and deaths have been reported.

Chemistry and pharmacology: Dextromethorphan (DXM) (d-3-methoxy-N-methyl-morphinan) is the dextro isomer of levomethorphan, a semisynthetic morphine derivative. Although structurally similar to other narcotics, DXM does not act as a mu receptor opioid (such as morphine, heroin). DXM and its metabolite, dextrorphan, act as potent blockers of the N-methyl-d-aspartate (NMDA) receptor. At high doses, the pharmacology of DXM is similar to the controlled substances phencyclidine (PCP) and ketamine that also antagonize the NMDA receptor. High doses of DXM produce PCP-like behavioral effects. DXM may cause a false-positive test result with some urine immunoassays for PCP.

Table 23.1. Four Dose-Dependent Plateaus Described by DXM Abusers

Plateau	Dose (mg)	Behavioral Effects
1st	100–200	Mild stimulation
2nd	200–400	Euphoria and hallucinations
3rd	300–600	Distorted visual perceptions, Loss of motor coordination
4th	500–1500	Dissociative sedation

Approximately 5–10% of Caucasians are poor DXM metabolizers which increases their risk for overdoses and deaths. DXM should not be taken with antidepressants due to the risk of inducing a life-threatening serotonergic syndrome.

User population: The 2006 Monitoring the Future (MTF) showed that 4%, 5%, and 7% of 8th, 10th, and 12th grade students, respectively, reported nonmedical use of DXM during the previous year. This was the first year MTF added DXM to the survey for students.

A 6-year retrospective study from 1999 to 2004 of the California Poison Control System (CPCS) showed a ten-fold increase in the rate of CPCS DXM abuse cases in all ages and a fifteen-fold increase in the rate of CPCS DXM abuse cases in adolescents. In 2004, CPCS reports 1,382 DXM abuse cases. About 75% of CPCS DXM abuse cases are adolescents (ages 9–17) with a median age of 16.

Illicit distribution: DXM abuse has traditionally been with the OTC liquid cough preparations. More recently, abuse of tablet and gel capsule preparations has increased. DXM powder sold over the internet is also a source of DXM for abuse. DXM is also distributed in illicitly manufactured tablets containing only DXM or mixed with other illicit drugs such as ecstasy and/or methamphetamine.

Control status: DXM is neither a controlled substance nor a regulated chemical under the Controlled Substances Act (CSA). The CSA specifically excluded DXM from any of the schedules in 1970 because of a lack of significant opiate-like abuse potential [21 USC 811(g) (2)]. However the CSA provided that DXM could be added in the future to the CSA through the traditional scheduling process if warranted. DEA is currently reviewing DXM for possible control.

Chapter 24

DMT

Drug name: N,N-dimethyltryptamine (DMT)

Introduction: N,N-dimethyltryptamine (DMT) is the prototypical indolethylamine hallucinogen. The history of human experience with DMT probably goes back several hundred years since DMT usage is associated with a number of shamanic practices and rituals. As a naturally occurring substance in many species of plants, DMT is present in a number of South American snuffs and brewed concoctions, like Ayahuasca. In addition, DMT can be produced synthetically. The original synthesis was conducted by a British chemist, Richard Manske, in 1931.

DMT gained popularity as a drug of abuse in the 1960s and was placed under federal control in schedule I when the Controlled Substances Act was passed in 1971. Today, it is still encountered sporadically on the illicit market along with a number of other tryptamine hallucinogens.

Licit use: DMT has no approved medical use in the United States but can be used by researchers under a schedule I researcher registration that requires approval from both Drug Enforcement Administration (DEA) and the Food and Drug Administration (FDA).

"N,N-Dimethyltryptamine (DMT)," Drug Enforcement Administration (DEA), August 2007.

Chemical structure: All indolethylamine hallucinogens have the tryptamine molecule in their structural core. DMT is formed by substituting two methyl (CH3) groups for the two hydrogen (H) atoms on the terminal nitrogen of the ethylamine side chain of tryptamine.

Pharmacology: Administered alone, DMT is usually snorted, smoked, or injected because the oral bioavailability of DMT is very poor unless it is combined with a substance that inhibits its metabolism. For example, in ayahuasca, the presence of harmala alkaloids (harmine, harmaline, tetrahydro-harmaline) inhibits the enzyme, monoamine oxidase which normally metabolizes DMT. As a consequence, DMT remains intact long enough to be absorbed in sufficient amounts to affect brain function and produce psychoactive effects.

In clinical studies, DMT was fully hallucinogenic at doses between 0.2 and 0.4 milligrams per kilogram (mg/kg). The onset of DMT effects is very rapid but usually resolves within 30–45 minutes. Psychological effects include intense visual hallucinations, depersonalization, auditory distortions, and an altered sense of time and body image. Physiological effects include hypertension, increased heart rate, agitation, seizures, dilated pupils, nystagmus (involuntary rapid rhythmic movement of the eye), dizziness, and ataxia (muscular incoordination). At high doses, coma and respiratory arrest have occurred.

Illicit use: DMT is used for the psychoactive effects it produces. The intense effects and short duration of action are attractive to individuals who want the psychedelic experience but do not choose to experience the mind altering perceptions over an extended period of time as occurs with other hallucinogens, like lysergic acid diethylamide (LSD).

DMT is generally smoked or consumed orally in brews like Ayahuasca. Like most other hallucinogens, DMT is not associated with physical dependence or addiction.

Illicit distribution: DMT is found in a number of plant materials and can be extracted or synthetically produced in clandestine labs. Like other hallucinogens, internet sales and distribution have served as the source of drug supply in this country. According to the System to Retrieve Information from Drug Evidence (STRIDE), a federal database for the seized drugs samples analyzed by DEA forensic laboratories, there were 71 drug records and 31 cases involving DMT during 1996–2006. The amounts of drug seized included ten tablets, 157.562 kilograms of powder, and 462.9 liters of liquid containing DMT. According to the National Forensic Laboratory Information

System (NFLIS), there were a total of 65 state and local cases involving 82 DMT containing drug items during 1999–2006. According to STRIDE and NFLIS, DMT has been encountered in a number of states including Alaska, Arkansas, California, Colorado, Florida, Georgia, Hawaii, Idaho, Illinois, Indiana, Louisiana, Maryland, Missouri, Minnesota, Montana, New Mexico, New York, Oregon, Pennsylvania, Tennessee, Utah, Virginia, Washington, Wisconsin and District of Columbia

Control status: DMT is controlled in schedule I of the Controlled Substances Act.

Chapter 25

Downers

Drug name: Benzodiazepines

Street names: Benzos, downers, nerve pills, tranks

Introduction: Benzodiazepines are a class of drugs that produce central nervous system (CNS) depression and that are most commonly used to treat insomnia and anxiety. There is the potential for dependence on and abuse of benzodiazepines particularly by individuals with a history of multi-substance abuse. Alprazolam (Xanax®), lorazepam (Ativan®), clonazepam (Klonopin®), diazepam (Valium®), and temazepam (Restoril®) are the five most prescribed, as well as the most frequently encountered benzodiazepines on the illicit market.

Chemistry and pharmacology: All benzodiazepines are composed of a benzene ring and a seven-member diazepine ring. Most benzodiazepines also possess a phenyl ring attached at the 5-position of the diazepine ring. Small modifications of this basic structure account for the varied pharmacologic effects of these drugs.

Benzodiazepines produce central nervous system (CNS) depression by enhancing the effects of the major inhibitory neurotransmitter, gamma-aminobutyric acid, thereby decreasing brain activity. Benzodiazepines are classified by their duration of action that ranges from less than six hours to more than 24 hours. Some benzodiazepines have active metabolites that prolong their effects.

"Benzodiazepines," Drug Enforcement Administration (DEA), September 2007.

Adverse effects include increased reaction time, motor incoordination, anterograde amnesia, slurred speech, restlessness, delirium, aggression, depression, hallucinations, and paranoia. Unlike barbiturates, large doses of benzodiazepines are rarely fatal unless combined with other CNS depressant drugs, such as alcohol or opioids. Flumazenil can be administered by injection to reverse the adverse effects of benzodiazepines.

Tolerance often develops after long-term use requiring larger doses to achieve the desired effect. Physical and psychological dependence may develop, whether taken under a doctor's orders or used illicitly. Withdrawal symptoms, the severity of which is dependent on the dose, duration of use, and particular drug used, include anxiety, insomnia, dysphoria, tremors, and seizures. Withdrawal can be precipitated by the administration of flumazenil to individuals dependent upon benzodiazepines.

Illicit uses: Benzodiazepines, particularly those having a rapid onset, are abused to produce a euphoric effect often described as a high. Abuse of benzodiazepines is often associated with multiple-substance abuse. Diazepam and alprazolam are used in combination with methadone to potentiate methadone's euphoric effect. Cocaine addicts use benzodiazepines to relieve the side effects (for example, irritability and agitation) associated with cocaine binges. Benzodiazepines are also used to augment alcohol's effects and modulate withdrawal states. The doses of benzodiazepines taken by abusers are usually in excess of the recommended therapeutic dose. Benzodiazepines have been used to facilitate sexual assault.

Illicit distribution: Individuals abusing benzodiazepines obtain them by getting prescriptions from several doctors, forging prescriptions, or buying diverted pharmaceutical products on the illicit market. Domestic and foreign products are found in the illicit market. Alprazolam is one of the top three prescription drugs illegally encountered. In 2006, as reported by the National Forensic Laboratory Information System, state and local drug laboratories analyzed 24,057 alprazolam, 6,360 clonazepam, 5,886 diazepam, 1,444 lorazepam, and 333 temazepam exhibits. In 2006, the Drug Enforcement Administration (DEA) drug laboratories, as reported in the System to Retrieve Information from Drug Evidence system, analyzed 384 alprazolam, 107 clonazepam, 179 diazepam, 60 lorazepam, and 22 temazepam exhibits.

Control status: Benzodiazepines are classified as schedule IV depressants under the Controlled Substances Act. Flunitrazepam is unique among the benzodiazepines in being placed in schedule IV but having schedule I penalties.

Chapter 26

Ecstasy (MDMA)

Drug name: 3,4-methylenedioxymethamphetamine (MDMA)

Street name: Ecstasy

MDMA is an illegal drug that acts as both a stimulant and psychedelic, producing an energizing effect, as well as distortions in time and perception and enhanced enjoyment from tactile experiences. Typically, MDMA is taken orally, usually in a tablet or capsule, and its effects last approximately 3–6 hours. The average reported dose is one to two tablets, with each tablet typically containing between 60 and 120 milligrams of MDMA. It is not uncommon for users to take a second dose of the drug as the effects of the first dose begin to fade.

MDMA can affect the brain by altering the activity of chemical messengers, or neurotransmitters, which enable nerve cells in the brain to communicate with one another. Research in animals has shown that MDMA in moderate to high doses can be toxic to nerve cells that contain serotonin and can cause long-lasting damage to them. Furthermore, MDMA raises body temperature. On rare but largely unpredictable occasions, this has led to severe medical consequences, including death. Also, MDMA causes the release of another neurotransmitter, norepinephrine, which is likely the cause of the increase in heart rate and blood pressure that often accompanies MDMA use.

Text in this chapter is from "Research Report Series: MDMA (Ecstasy) Abuse," National Institute on Drug Abuse (NIDA), NIH Publication Number 06–4728, March 2006.

Although MDMA is known universally among users as ecstasy, researchers have determined that many ecstasy tablets contain not only MDMA but also a number of other drugs or drug combinations that can be harmful as well. Adulterants found in MDMA tablets purchased on the street include methamphetamine, caffeine, the over-the-counter cough suppressant dextromethorphan, the diet drug ephedrine, and cocaine. Also, as with many other drugs of abuse, MDMA is rarely used alone. It is not uncommon for users to mix MDMA with other substances, such as alcohol and marijuana.

What is the scope of MDMA abuse in the U.S.?

It is difficult to determine the exact scope of this problem because MDMA is often used in combination with other substances, and does not appear in some traditional data sources, such as treatment admission rates.

More than 11 million persons aged 12 or older reported using ecstasy at least once in their lifetimes, according to the 2004 National Survey on Drug Use and Health. The number of current (use in past month) users in 2004 was estimated to be 450,000.

Who is abusing MDMA?

MDMA first gained popularity among adolescents and young adults in the nightclub scene or weekend-long dance parties known as raves. However, the profile of the typical MDMA user has been changing. Reports also indicate that use is spreading beyond predominantly White youth to a broader range of ethnic groups.

What are the effects of MDMA?

MDMA has become a popular drug, in part because of the positive effects that a person may experience within an hour or so after taking a single dose. Those effects include feelings of mental stimulation, emotional warmth, empathy toward others, a general sense of well being, and decreased anxiety. In addition, users report enhanced sensory perception as a hallmark of the MDMA experience. Because of the drug's stimulant properties, when used in club or dance settings, MDMA can also enable users to dance for extended periods. However, there are some users who report undesirable effects immediately, including anxiety, agitation, and recklessness.

As noted, MDMA is not a benign drug. MDMA can produce a variety of adverse health effects, including nausea, chills, sweating, involuntary teeth clenching, muscle cramping, and blurred vision. MDMA overdose can also occur—the symptoms can include high blood pressure, faintness, panic attacks, and in severe cases, a loss of consciousness and seizures.

Because of its stimulant properties and the environments in which it is often taken, MDMA is associated with vigorous physical activity for extended periods. This can lead to one of the most significant, although rare, acute adverse effects—a marked rise in body temperature (hyperthermia). Treatment of hyperthermia requires prompt medical attention, as it can rapidly lead to muscle breakdown, which can in turn result in kidney failure. In addition, dehydration, hypertension, and heart failure may occur in susceptible individuals. MDMA can also reduce the pumping efficiency of the heart, of particular concern during periods of increased physical activity, further complicating these problems.

MDMA is rapidly absorbed into the human bloodstream, but once in the body, MDMA metabolites interfere with the body's ability to metabolize, or break down, the drug. As a result, additional doses of MDMA can produce unexpectedly high blood levels, which could worsen the cardiovascular and other toxic effects of this drug. MDMA also interferes with the metabolism of other drugs, including some of the adulterants that may be found in MDMA tablets.

In the hours after taking the drug, MDMA produces significant reductions in mental abilities. These changes, particularly those affecting memory, can last for up to a week, and possibly longer in regular users. The fact that MDMA markedly impairs information processing emphasizes the potential dangers of performing complex or skilled activities, such as driving a car, while under the influence of this drug.

Over the course of a week following moderate use of the drug, many MDMA users report feeling a range of emotions, including anxiety, restlessness, irritability, and sadness that in some individuals can be as severe as true clinical depression. Similarly, elevated anxiety, impulsiveness, and aggression, as well as sleep disturbances, lack of appetite, and reduced interest in and pleasure from sex have been observed in regular MDMA users. Some of these disturbances may not be directly attributable to MDMA, but may be related to some of the other drugs often used in combination with MDMA, such as cocaine or marijuana, or to adulterants commonly found in MDMA tablets.

What does MDMA do to the brain?

MDMA affects the brain by increasing the activity of at least three neurotransmitters (the chemical messengers of brain cells): serotonin, dopamine, and norepinephrine. Like other amphetamines, MDMA causes these neurotransmitters to be released from their storage sites in neurons, resulting in increased neurotransmitter activity. Compared to the very potent stimulant methamphetamine, MDMA causes greater serotonin release and somewhat lesser dopamine release. Serotonin is a neurotransmitter that plays an important role in the regulation of mood, sleep, pain, appetite, and other behaviors. The excess release of serotonin by MDMA likely causes the mood elevating effects experienced by MDMA users. However, by releasing large amounts of serotonin, MDMA causes the brain to become significantly depleted of this important neurotransmitter, contributing to the negative behavioral aftereffects that users often experience for several days after taking MDMA.

It is also important to keep in mind that many users of ecstasy may unknowingly be taking other drugs that are sold as ecstasy, and/or they may intentionally use other drugs, such as marijuana, which could contribute to these behavioral effects. Additionally, most studies in people do not have behavioral measures from before the users began taking drugs, making it difficult to rule out pre-existing conditions. Factors such as gender, dosage, frequency and intensity of use, age at which use began, the use of other drugs, as well as genetic and environmental factors all may play a role in some of the cognitive deficits that result from MDMA use and should be taken into consideration when studying the effects of MDMA in humans.

Given that most MDMA users are young and in their reproductive years, it is possible that some female users may be pregnant when they take MDMA, either inadvertently or intentionally, because of the misperception that it is a safe drug. The potential adverse effects of MDMA on the developing fetus are of great concern.

Is MDMA addictive?

For some people, MDMA can be addictive. A survey of young adult and adolescent MDMA users found that 43% of those who reported ecstasy use met the accepted diagnostic criteria for dependence, as evidenced by continued use despite knowledge of physical or psychological harm, withdrawal effects, and tolerance (or diminished response), and 34% met the criteria for drug abuse. Almost 60% of people who use MDMA report withdrawal symptoms, including fatigue, loss of appetite, depressed feelings, and trouble concentrating.

MDMA affects many of the same neurotransmitter systems in the brain that are targeted by other addictive drugs. Experiments have shown that animals prefer MDMA, much like they do cocaine, over other pleasurable stimuli, another hallmark of most addictive drugs.

What do we know about preventing MDMA abuse?

Because social context and networks seem to be an important component of MDMA use, the use of peer-led advocacy and drug prevention programs may be a promising approach to reduce MDMA use among adolescents and young adults. High schools and colleges can serve as important venues for delivering messages about the effects of MDMA use. Providing accurate scientific information regarding the effects of MDMA is important if we hope to reduce the damaging effects of this drug. Education is one of the most important tools for use in preventing MDMA abuse.

Are there effective treatments for MDMA abuse?

There are no specific treatments for MDMA abuse. The most effective treatments for drug abuse and addiction are cognitive behavioral interventions that are designed to help modify the patient's thinking, expectancies, and behaviors, and to increase skills in coping with life's stressors. Drug abuse recovery support groups may be effective in combination with behavioral interventions to support long-term, drug-free recovery. There are currently no pharmacological treatments for dependence on MDMA.

Chapter 27

Fentanyl

Drug name: Fentanyl

Trade names: Actiq®, Fentora®, Duragesic®

Street names: Apache, china girl, china white, dance fever, friend, goodfella, jackpot, murder 8, TNT, perc-o-pop, lollipop, tango, and cash

Introduction: Fentanyl is a potent synthetic opioid. It was introduced into medical practice as an intravenous anesthetic under the trade name of Sublimaze in the 1960s.

Licit uses: The clinical use of fentanyl has increased during the past decade. For example, fentanyl prescriptions increased from about 0.5 million in 1994 to 7.04 million in 2006 (IMS Health). Fentanyl pharmaceuticals are currently available in the dosage forms of oral transmucosal lozenges, commonly referred to as the fentanyl lollipops (Actiq®), effervescent buccal tablets (Fentora®), transdermal patches (Duragesic®), and injectable formulations. Oral transmucosal lozenges and effervescent buccal tablets are used for the management of breakthrough cancer pain in patients who are already receiving opioid medication for their underlying persistent pain. Transdermal patches are used in the management of chronic pain in patients who require

---

Text in this chapter is from "Fentanyl," Drug Enforcement Administration (DEA), September 2007.

continuous opioid analgesia for pain. Fentanyl citrate injections are administered intravenously, intramuscularly, spinally, or epidurally for potent analgesia and anesthesia. Fentanyl is frequently used in anesthetic practice for patients undergoing heart surgery or for patients with poor heart function. Because of a concern about deaths and overdoses resulting from fentanyl transdermal patches (Duragesic® and generic version), on July 15, 2005, the Food and Drug Administration issued safety warnings and reiterated the importance of strict adherence to the guidelines for the proper use of these products.

Chemistry and pharmacology: Fentanyl is 100 times more potent than morphine as an analgesic. It is a μ opioid receptor agonist with high lipid solubility and a rapid onset and short duration of effects. Fentanyl rapidly crosses the blood-brain barrier. It is similar to other μ agonists (like morphine or oxycodone) in its pharmacological effects and produces analgesia, sedation, respiratory depression, nausea, and vomiting. Fentanyl appears to produce muscle rigidity with greater frequency than other opioids. Unlike some μ opioid receptor agonists, fentanyl does not cause histamine release and has minimal depressant effects on the heart.

Illicit uses: Fentanyl is abused for its intense euphoric effects. Fentanyl can serve as a direct substitute for heroin in opioid dependent individuals. However, fentanyl is a very dangerous substitute for heroin because it is much more potent than heroin which results in frequent overdoses that can lead to respiratory depression and death.

Fentanyl patches are abused by removing the liquid contents from the patches and then injecting or ingesting these contents. Patches have also been frozen, cut into pieces and placed under the tongue or in the cheek cavity for drug absorption through the oral mucosa. Used patches are attractive to abusers as a large percentage of fentanyl remains in these patches even after a three-day use. Fentanyl oral transmucosal lozenges and fentanyl injectables are also diverted and abused.

Abuse of fentanyl initially appeared in mid-1970s and has increased in recent years. There have been reports of deaths associated with abuse of fentanyl products.

Illicit distribution: Fentanyl is diverted via pharmacy theft, fraudulent prescriptions, and illicit distribution by patients and registrants (physicians and pharmacists). Theft has also been identified at nursing homes and other long-term care facilities. Fentanyl oral transmucosal lozenges (Actiq®) are typically sold illicitly (street names:

perc-o-pop or lollipop) at $20 to $25 per unit or $450 per carton (contains 24 units) while transdermal patches (Duragesic®) are sold at prices ranging from $10 to $100 per patch depending upon the dose of the unit and geographical area. According to the National Forensic Laboratory Information System, state and local cases involving fentanyl expressed as a percent of the total of all drug cases increased by eighteen-fold from 0.0078 percent in 2001 (37 cases) to 0.144 percent in 2006 (1,472 cases involving 1,643 drug items).

Clandestine manufacture: In 2006, the distribution of clandestinely manufactured fentanyl has caused an unprecedented outbreak of hundreds of suspected fentanyl-related overdoses and over 972 confirmed and 162 suspected fentanyl-related deaths among the heroin user population. Most of these deaths have occurred in Delaware, Illinois, Maryland, Michigan, Missouri, New Jersey, and Pennsylvania. Drug Enforcement Administration (DEA) immediately undertook the development of regulations to control the precursor chemicals used by the clandestine laboratories to illicitly manufacture fentanyl. Recently, one of the precursors was designated as a List 1 chemical. DEA is now in the process of designating a second chemical as a schedule II immediate precursor.

Control status: Fentanyl is a schedule II substance under the federal Controlled Substances Act of 1970.

Chapter 28

Foxy

Drug name: 5-methoxy-N,N-diisopropyltryptamine (5-MeO-DIPT)

Street names: Foxy, or Foxy methoxy

Introduction: 5-methoxy-N,N-diisopropyltryptamine (5-MeO-DIPT) is a tryptamine derivative and shares many similarities with schedule I tryptamine hallucinogens such as alpha-ethyltryptamine, N,N-dimethyltryptamine, N,N-diethyltryptamine, bufotenine, psilocybin, and psilocin. Since 1999, there has been a growing popularity of 5-MeO-DIPT among drug abusers. This substance is abused for its hallucinogenic effects.

Licit uses: 5-MeO-DIPT has no approved medical uses in the United States.

Chemistry and pharmacology: 5-MeO-DIPT is a tryptamine derivative. The hydrochloride salt of 5-MeO-DIPT is a white crystalline powder. In animal behavioral studies, 5-MeO-DIPT has been shown to produce behavioral effects that are substantially similar to those of 1-(2,5-dimethoxy-4-methylphenyl)-2-aminopropane (DOM) and lysergic acid diethylamide (LSD), both schedule I hallucinogens.

"5-Methoxy-N,N-Diisopropyltryptamine," Drug Enforcement Administration (DEA), June 2009.

In humans, 5-MeO-DIPT elicits subjective effects including hallucinations similar to those produced by several schedule I hallucinogens such as 2C-B and 4-ethyl-2,5-dimethoxyphenyl-isopropylamine (DOET). The threshold dose of 5-MeO-DIPT to produce psychoactive effects is four milligrams (mg), while effective doses range from 6–20 mg. 5-MeO-DIPT produces effects with an onset of 20–30 minutes and with peak effects occurring between 1–1.5 hours after administration. Effects last about 3–6 hours. Initial effects include mild nausea, muscular hyperreflexia, and dilation of pupils. Other effects include relaxation associated with emotional enhancement, talkativeness, and behavioral disinhibition. High doses of 5-MeO-DIPT produce abstract eyes-closed imagery. 5-MeO-DIPT alters sensory perception and judgment and can pose serious health risks to the user and the general public. Abuse of 5-MeO-DIPT led to at least one emergency department admission.

Illicit uses: 5-MeO-DIPT is abused for its hallucinogenic-like effects and is used as a substitute for MDMA. It is often administered orally as either powder, tablets or capsules at doses ranging from 6–20 milligrams. Other routes of administration include smoking and snorting. Tablets often bear imprints commonly seen on MDMA tablets (spider and alien head logos) and vary in color. Powder in capsules was found to vary in colors.

User population: Youth and young adults are the main abusers of 5-MeO-DIPT.

Illicit distribution: According to National Forensic Laboratory Information System (NFLIS), law enforcement agents submitted thirty-five 5-MeO-DIPT items to federal laboratories for analysis between 2004 and 2008. Most of the items (19) were submitted in 2008. State and local labs received 214 drug items during that same time period. The number of 5-MeO-DIPT drug item seizures increased from 61 in 2007 to 135 in 2008.

5-MeO-DIPT has been illicitly available from United States and foreign chemical companies and from individuals through the internet. There is some evidence of the attempted clandestine production of 5-MeO-DIPT.

Control status: The Drug Enforcement Administration (DEA) placed 5-MeO-DIPT temporarily in schedule I of the Controlled Substances Act (CSA) on April 4, 2003, pursuant to the temporary scheduling provisions of the CSA (68 FR 16427). On September 29, 2004, 5-MeO-DIPT was controlled as schedule I substance under the CSA (69 FR 58050).

Chapter 29

Gamma Hydroxybutyrate (GHB)

Drug name: Gamma hydroxybutyric acid

Street names: GHB, liquid ecstasy, liquid X, goop, Georgia home boy, easy lay

Introduction: Gamma hydroxybutyric acid (GHB) is a schedule I depressant while the GHB-containing product, Xyrem, is a schedule III drug. GHB has been encountered in nearly every region of the country. It is used for the same reason as recreational drugs; for their euphoric and sedative effects. GHB abuse became popular among teens and young adults at dance clubs and raves in the 1990s, and gained notoriety as a date rape drug.

Licit uses: On July 17, 2002, the Food and Drug Administration (FDA) approved Xyrem (sodium oxybate) with orphan drug status and limited distribution through a central pharmacy. Xyrem oral solution is approved as a treatment to reduce the incidence of cataplexy and to improve daytime sleepiness in patients with narcolepsy

Chemistry and pharmacology: GHB is a solid substance but is generally dissolved in liquid. In liquid form, GHB is clear and colorless, and slightly salty in taste. GHB occurs naturally in the central nervous system in very small amounts. Scientific data suggest

---

This chapter includes text from "Gamma Hydroxybutyric Acid," Drug Enforcement Administration (DEA), September 2007.

that GHB can function as a neurotransmitter or neuromodulator in the brain. It produces dose-dependent depressant effects similar to those of the barbiturates and methaqualone. Low doses of GHB produce drowsiness, nausea, and visual distortion. At high doses, GHB overdose can result in unconsciousness, seizures, slowed heart rate, severe respiratory depression, decreased body temperature, vomiting, nausea, coma, or death. Sustained use of GHB can lead to addiction. Chronic abuse of GHB produces a withdrawal syndrome characterized by insomnia, anxiety, tremors, marked autonomic activation (for example, increased heart rate and blood pressure), and occasional psychotic thoughts. Currently, there is no antidote available for GHB intoxication.

Illicit uses: GHB is abused for its euphoric and sedative effects. GHB is mainly self-ingested orally in a liquid mixture. It is sometimes mixed with alcohol to intensify its effects resulting in respiratory depression and coma. The average oral dose range from 1–5 grams (depending on the purity of the compound this can be 1–2 teaspoons mixed in a beverage). The saturation and concentrations of these home-brews have varied so that the user is not usually aware of the actual dose they are drinking. The onset of action after oral ingestion is 15–30 minutes and the effects last 3–6 hours.

The most recent data from poison control centers, a high school survey, and forensic laboratory analyses of seized samples from System to Retrieve Information on Drug Evidence (STRIDE) and National Forensic Laboratory Information System (NFLIS) all suggest illicit activities with GHB and its analogues are declining although remaining a significant threat to the public safety. GHB analogues are often abused in place of GHB. Both gamma butyrolactone (GBL) and 1,4 butanediol (BD) metabolize to GHB upon ingestion. The ingestion of analogs produces physiological effects similar to GHB.

User population: GHB is abused by teens and young adults at all-night parties and raves. Monitoring the Future Survey indicated that in 2005, 0.5% of 8th graders, 0.8% of 10th graders, and 1.1% of 12th graders reported past year use of GHB.

Illicit distribution: GHB is produced illegally in both domestic and foreign clandestine laboratories. The major source of GHB on the street is through clandestine synthesis by local operators. GHB is sold usually as a white powder or as a clear liquid. GHB is packaged in vials or small bottles. At bars or rave parties, GHB is sold in liquid form by the capful or swig for $5 to $25 per cap. There has been almost no diversion or abuse of the pharmaceutical product, Xyrem.

Control status: On March 13, 2000, GHB, including its salts, isomers, and salts of isomers, were made a schedule I controlled substance (65 FR 13235-13238). On March 20, 2001, GHB was added in schedule IV of the 1971 Convention of Psychotropic Substances.

GBL became a list I chemical, subject to the criminal, civil, and administrative sanctions of the Controlled Substances Act, on February 18, 2000 under the provisions of the "Hillary Farias and Samantha Reid Date-Rape Prohibition Act."

Xyrem is a schedule III controlled substance. However, trafficking of Xyrem is subject to schedule I penalties.

Chapter 30

Heroin

Drug name: Heroin

Street names: Dope, dragon, brown sugar

Heroin is an opiate drug that is synthesized from morphine, a naturally occurring substance extracted from the seed pod of the Asian opium poppy plant. Heroin usually appears as a white or brown powder or as a black sticky substance, known as black tar heroin.

How is heroin abused?

Heroin can be injected, snorted (sniffed), or smoked—routes of administration that rapidly deliver the drug to the brain. Injecting is the use of a needle to administer the drug directly into the bloodstream. Snorting is the process of inhaling heroin powder through the nose, where it is absorbed into the bloodstream through the nasal tissues. Smoking involves inhaling heroin smoke into the lungs. All three methods of administering heroin can lead to addiction and other severe health problems.

How does heroin affect the brain?

Heroin enters the brain, where it is converted to morphine and binds to receptors known as opioid receptors. These receptors are located in

Text in this chapter is from "Heroin," National Institute on Drug Abuse (NIDA), September 2009.

many areas of the brain (and in the body), especially those involved in the perception of pain and in reward. Opioid receptors are also located in the brain stem—important for automatic processes critical for life, such as breathing (respiration), blood pressure, and arousal. Heroin overdoses frequently involve a suppression of respiration.

After an intravenous injection of heroin, users report feeling a surge of euphoria (rush) accompanied by dry mouth, a warm flushing of the skin, heaviness of the extremities, and clouded mental functioning. Following this initial euphoria, the user goes on the nod, an alternately wakeful and drowsy state. Users who do not inject the drug may not experience the initial rush, but other effects are the same.

With regular heroin use, tolerance develops, in which the user's physiological (and psychological) response to the drug decreases, and more heroin is needed to achieve the same intensity of effect. Heroin users are at high risk for addiction—it is estimated that about 23% of individuals who use heroin become dependent on it.

What other adverse effects does heroin have on health?

Heroin abuse is associated with serious health conditions, including fatal overdose, spontaneous abortion, and—particularly in users who inject the drug—infectious diseases, including human immunodeficiency virus (HIV)/acquired immunodeficiency syndrome (AIDS), and hepatitis. Chronic users may develop collapsed veins, infection of the heart lining and valves, abscesses, and liver or kidney disease. Pulmonary complications, including various types of pneumonia, may result from the poor health of the abuser as well as from heroin's depressing effects on respiration. In addition to the effects of the drug itself, street heroin often contains toxic contaminants or additives that can clog the blood vessels leading to the lungs, liver, kidneys, or brain, causing permanent damage to vital organs.

Chronic use of heroin leads to physical dependence, a state in which the body has adapted to the presence of the drug. If a dependent user reduces or stops use of the drug abruptly, he or she may experience severe symptoms of withdrawal. These symptoms—which can begin as early as a few hours after the last drug administration—can include restlessness, muscle and bone pain, insomnia, diarrhea and vomiting, cold flashes with goose bumps (cold turkey), and kicking movements (kicking the habit). Users also experience severe craving for the drug during withdrawal, which can precipitate continued abuse and/or relapse. Major withdrawal symptoms peak between 48 and 72 hours after the last dose of the drug and typically subside after about one week. Some individuals, however, may show persistent withdrawal symptoms for months. Although heroin withdrawal is considered less dangerous than alcohol or barbiturate withdrawal, sudden withdrawal by heavily dependent users who are in poor health is occasionally fatal. In addition, heroin craving can persist years after drug cessation, particularly upon exposure to triggers such as stress or people, places, and things associated with drug use.

Heroin abuse during pregnancy, together with related factors like poor nutrition and inadequate prenatal care, has been associated with adverse consequences including low birthweight, an important risk factor for later developmental delay. If the mother is regularly abusing the drug, the infant may be born physically dependent on heroin and could suffer from serious medical complications requiring hospitalization.

What treatment options exist?

A range of treatments exist for heroin addiction, including medications and behavioral therapies. Science has taught us that when medication treatment is combined with other supportive services, patients are often able to stop using heroin (or other opiates) and return to stable and productive lives.

Treatment usually begins with medically assisted detoxification to help patients withdraw from the drug safely. Medications such as clonidine, and now buprenorphine, can be used to help minimize symptoms of withdrawal. However, detoxification alone is not treatment and has not been shown to be effective in preventing relapse—it is merely the first step.

Medications to help prevent relapse include the following:

- **Methadone** has been used for more than 30 years to treat heroin addiction. It is a synthetic opiate medication that binds to the same receptors as heroin; but when taken orally, it has a gradual onset of action and sustained effects, reducing the desire for other opioid drugs while preventing withdrawal symptoms. Properly administered, methadone is not intoxicating or sedating, and its effects do not interfere with ordinary daily activities. Methadone maintenance treatment is usually conducted in specialized opiate treatment programs. The most effective methadone maintenance programs include individual and/or group counseling, as well as provision of or referral to other needed medical, psychological, and social services.

- **Buprenorphine** is a more recently approved treatment for heroin addiction (and other opiates). Compared with methadone, buprenorphine produces less risk for overdose and withdrawal effects and produces a lower level of physical dependence, so patients who discontinue the medication generally have fewer withdrawal symptoms than those who stop taking methadone. The development of buprenorphine and its authorized use in physicians' offices gives opiate-addicted patients more medical options and extends the reach of addiction medication. Its accessibility may even prompt attempts to obtain treatment earlier. However, not all patients respond to buprenorphine—some continue to require treatment with methadone.

- **Naltrexone** is approved for treating heroin addiction but has not been widely utilized due to poor patient compliance. This medication blocks opioids from binding to their receptors and thus prevents an addicted individual from feeling the effects of the drug. Naltrexone as a treatment for opioid addiction is usually prescribed in outpatient medical settings, although initiation of the treatment often begins after medical detoxification in a residential setting. To prevent withdrawal symptoms, individuals must be medically detoxified and opioid-free for several days before taking naltrexone. Naloxone is a shorter acting opioid receptor blocker, used to treat cases of overdose.

For pregnant heroin abusers, methadone maintenance combined with prenatal care and a comprehensive drug treatment program can improve many of the detrimental maternal and neonatal outcomes associated with untreated heroin abuse. Preliminary evidence suggests that buprenorphine may also be a safe and effective treatment during pregnancy, although infants exposed to either methadone or buprenorphine prenatally may still require treatment for withdrawal symptoms. For women who do not want or are not able to receive pharmacotherapy for their heroin addiction, detoxification from opiates during pregnancy can be accomplished with medical supervision, although potential risks to the fetus and the likelihood of relapse to heroin use should be considered.

There are many effective behavioral treatments available for heroin addiction—usually in combination with medication. These can be delivered in residential or outpatient settings. Examples are individual or group counseling; contingency management which uses a voucher-based system where patients earn points based on negative drug tests—the points can be exchanged for items that encourage healthy living; and cognitive-behavioral therapy designed to help modify a patient's expectations and behaviors related to drug abuse and to increase skills in coping with various life stressors.

How widespread is heroin abuse?

According to the Monitoring the Future survey, there were no significant changes between 2007 and 2008 in the proportions of students in 8th and 12th grades reporting lifetime, past-year, and past-month use of heroin. There also were no significant changes in past-year and past-month use for the 10th grade; however, lifetime use decreased significantly from 1.5% in 2007 to 1.2% in 2008.

Heroin use has been steadily declining since the mid-1990s. Recent peaks in heroin use were observed in 1996 for 8th-graders, 1997–2000 for 10th-graders, and 2000 for 12th-graders. Annual prevalence of heroin use in 2008 dropped significantly, by between 40% and 51%, from these recent peak use years for each grade surveyed.

According to the 2007 National Survey on Drug Use and Health, the number of current (past-month) heroin users in the United States decreased from 338,000 in 2006 to 153,000 in 2007. There were 106,000 first-time users of heroin aged 12 or older in 2007; the average age at first use of heroin was 21.8 years.

Chapter 31

Human Growth Hormone

Drug name: Human growth hormone

Trade names: Genotropin®, Humatrope®, Norditropin®, Nutropin®, Saizen®, Serostim®

Introduction: Human growth hormone (hGH) is a naturally occurring polypeptide hormone secreted by the pituitary gland and is essential for body growth. Daily secretion of hGH increases throughout childhood, peaking during adolescence, and steadily declining thereafter. In 1985, synthetic hGH was developed and approved by the U.S. Food and Drug Administration (FDA) for specific uses. However, it is commonly abused by athletes, bodybuilders, and aging adults for its ability increase muscle mass and decrease body fat, as well as its purported potential to improve athletic performance and reverse the effects of aging.

Licit uses: Several FDA-approved injectable hGH preparations are available by prescription from a supervising physician for clearly and narrowly defined indications. In children, hGH is approved for the treatment of poor growth due to Turner syndrome, Prader-Willi syndrome, and chronic renal insufficiency, hGH insufficiency/deficiency, for children born small for gestational age, and for idiopathic short

---

"Human Growth Hormone," Drug Enforcement Administration (DEA), August 2009.

stature. Accepted medical uses in adults include but are not limited to the treatment of the wasting syndrome of human immunodeficiency (HIV)/acquired immunodeficiency syndrome (AIDS), and hGH deficiency. Depending on the clinical presentation, pediatric dosages range from 24–100 microgram/kilogram/day to adult dosages from 0.9–25 microgram/kilogram/day, dependent on product. The FDA-approved injectable formulations are available as liquid preparations, or as powder with a diluent for reconstitution.

Chemistry and pharmacology: Using recombinant deoxyribonucleic acid (DNA) technology, two forms of synthetic hGH were developed, somatropin and somatrem. Somatropin is identical to the endogenous pituitary-derived hGH, whereas somatrem has an extra amino acid on the N-terminus. Both synthetic forms have similar biological actions and potencies as the endogenous hGH polypeptide. Synthetic hGH also is chemically indistinguishable from the naturally occurring hormone in blood and urine tests. hGH binds to growth hormone receptors present on cells throughout the body. hGH functions to regulate body composition, fluid homeostasis, glucose and lipid metabolism, skeletal muscle and bone growth, and possibly cardiac functioning. Sleep, exercise, and stress all increase the secretion of hGH.

The use of hGH is associated with several adverse effects including edema, carpal tunnel syndrome, joint pain, muscle pain, and abnormal skin sensations (for example, numbness and tingling). It may also increase the growth of pre-existing malignant cells, and increase the possibility of developing diabetes. hGH is administered by subcutaneous or intramuscular injection. The circulating half-life of hGH is relatively short half-life (20–30 minutes), while its biological half-life is much longer (9–17 hours) due to its indirect effects.

Illicit uses: Human growth hormone is illicitly used as an anti-aging agent, to improve athletic performance, and for bodybuilding purposes. It is marketed, distributed, and illegally prescribed off-label to aging adults to replenish declining hGH levels and reverse age-related bodily deterioration. It is also abused for its ability to alter body composition by reducing body fat and increasing skeletal muscle mass. It is often used in combination with other performance enhancing drugs, such as anabolic steroids. Athletes also use it to improve their athletic performance, although the ability of hGH to increase athletic performance is debatable.

Abuser population: Athletes, bodybuilders, and aging adults are the primary abusers of hGH. Because the illicit use of synthetic hGH is difficult to detect, its use in sports is believed to be widespread. Over the past few years, numerous professional athletes have admitted to using hGH. Bodybuilders, as well as celebrities also purportedly use it for its ability to alter body composition. Aging adults looking to reverse the effects of aging are increasingly using synthetic hGH.

Illicit distribution: The illicit distribution of hGH occurs as the result of physicians illegally prescribing it for off-label uses, and for the treatment of FDA-approved medical conditions without examination and supervision. Illicit distribution also involves diverted hGH obtained through theft, smuggled hGH illegally imported from other countries, and counterfeit hGH.

The illicit distribution of injectable synthetic hGH formulations is thought to be primarily through internet pharmacies, as well as wellness and anti-aging clinics and websites. Internet pharmacies are often partnered with a physician willing to write prescriptions for a fee without a physical examination. Individuals may also obtain hGH without a prescription through the black market. hGH is often marketed with other performance enhancing drugs (such as anabolic steroids).

According to the National Forensic Laboratory Information System, law enforcement officials submitted 27 hGH items/exhibits to state and local forensic laboratories between 2004 and 2008. There were no hGH items submitted to federal laboratories during the same time period. The number of seized hGH items have increased recently; in 2006, three items were submitted to state and local laboratories; in 2007, seven items were submitted; and ten items were submitted in 2008.

Various oral preparations (sprays and pills) purported to contain hGH are also marketed and distributed. However, hGH is only bioavailable in the injectable form. The hGH molecule is too large for absorption across the lining of the oral mucosa and the hormone is digested by the stomach before absorption can occur.

Control status: Human growth hormone is not controlled under the Controlled Substances Act (CSA). However, as part of the 1990 Anabolic Steroid Control Act, the distribution and possession, with the intent to distribute, of hGH "for any use...other than the treatment of a disease or other recognized medical condition, where such

179

use has been authorized by the Secretary of Health and Human Services...and pursuant to the order of a physician..." was criminalized as a five-year felony under the penalties chapter of the Food, Drug, and Cosmetics Act of the FDA.

Also, hGH is listed by the World Anti-Doping Agency and the International Olympic Committee as a performance enhancing drug barring athletes from using it.

Chapter 32

Kava

Drug name: Kava

Other names: Ava, intoxicating pepper, kawa kawa, kew, sakau, tonga, yangona

Introduction: Kava, also known as *Piper methysticum* (intoxicating pepper), is a perennial shrub native to the South Pacific Islands, including Hawaii. This relatively slow growing plant is harvested for its rootstock, which contains the pharmacologically active compounds kavalactones.

The term kava also refers to the non-fermented, psychoactive beverage prepared from the rootstock. For many centuries, Pacific Island societies have consumed kava beverages for social, ceremonial, and medical purposes. Traditionally, kava beverages are prepared by chewing or pounding the rootstock to produce a cloudy, milky pulp that is then soaked in water before the liquid is filtered to drink.

Kava-containing dietary supplements are marketed in the United States (U.S.) for the treatment of anxiety and insomnia. There is also an increasing use of kava for recreational purposes. The reinforcing effects of kava include mild euphoria, muscle relaxation, sedation, and analgesia. Currently, kava is not controlled under the federal Controlled Substances Act (CSA).

"Kava," Drug Enforcement Administration (DEA), May 2008.

Licit uses: In the U.S., kava is sold as dietary supplements promoted as natural alternatives to anti-anxiety drugs and sleeping pills. A meta-analysis of six randomized, placebo-controlled, double-blind kava clinical trials found that kava (60–200 milligrams [mg] of kavalactones/day) produced a significant reduction in anxiety compared to placebo. However, the U.S. Food and Drug Administration (FDA) has not made a determination about the ability of dietary supplements containing kava to provide such benefits.

Kava dietary supplements are commonly formulated as tablets and capsules (30–90 percent kavalactones; 50–250 mg per capsule). Kava is also available as whole root, powdered root, extracts (powder, paste, and liquid), tea bags, and instant powdered drink mix. Kava is frequently found in products containing a variety of herbs or vitamins, or both.

A number of cases of liver damage (hepatitis and cirrhosis), and liver failure have been associated with commercial extract preparations of kava. In 2002, the FDA issued an advisory alerting consumers and health care providers to the potential risk of liver related injuries associated with the use a kava dietary supplements.

Chemistry and pharmacology: The pharmacologically active kavalactones are found in the lipid soluble resin of the kava rootstock. Of the 18 isolated and identified, yangonin, methysticin, dihydromethysticin, dihydrokawain, kawain, and desmethoxyyangoin are the six major kavalactones. Different varieties of kava plants possess varying concentrations of the kavalactones. The pharmacokinetics of the kavalactones has not been extensively studied. Kavalactones are thought to be relatively quickly absorbed in the gut. There may be differences in the bioavailability between the different kavalactones. The limbic structures, amygdala complex, and reticular formation of the brain appear to be the preferential sites of action of kavalactones. However, the exact molecular mechanisms of action are not clear.

Kava has the potential for causing drug interactions through the inhibition of CYP450 enzymes that are responsible for the metabolism of many pharmaceutical agents and other herbal remedies. Chronic use of kava in large quantities may cause a dry scaly skin or yellow skin discoloration known as kava dermopathy. It may also cause liver toxicity, and extrapyramidal effects (for example, tremor and abnormal body movement). The National Toxicology Program is currently conducting toxicology studies of the kava extract.

Individuals may experience a numbing or tingling of the mouth upon drinking kava due to its local anesthetic action. High doses of kavalactones can also produce central nervous system depressant effects (such as sedation and muscle weakness) that appear to be transient.

Illicit uses: Information on the illicit use of kava in the U.S. is anecdotal. Based on information on the internet, kava is being used recreationally to relax the body and achieve a mild euphoria. It is typically consumed as a beverage made from dried kava root powder, flavored and unflavored powdered extracts, and liquid extract dissolved in pure grain alcohol and vegetable glycerin. Individuals may consume 25 grams of kavalactones, which is about 125 times the daily dose in kava dietary supplements.

Intoxicated individuals typically have sensible thought processes and comprehensive conversations, but have difficulty coordinating movement and often fall asleep. Kava users do not exhibit the generalized confusion and delirium that occurs with high levels of alcohol intoxication. However, while kava alone does not produce the motor and cognitive impairments caused by alcohol, kava does potentiate both the perceived and measured impairment produced by alcohol alone.

User population: Information on user population in the U.S. is very limited. Kava use is not monitored by any national drug abuse surveys. In the 1980s, kava was introduced to Australian Aboriginal communities where it quickly became a drug of abuse. It has become a serious social problem in regions of Northern Australia.

Distribution: Kava is widely available on the internet. Some websites promoting and selling kava products also sell other uncontrolled psychoactive products such as Salvia divinorum and kratom. Several kava bars and lounges in the U.S. sell kava drinks.

Control status: Kava is not a controlled substance in the U.S. Due to concerns of liver toxicity, many countries including Australia, Canada, France, Germany, Malaysia, Singapore, Switzerland, and the United Kingdom have placed regulatory controls on kava. These controls range from warning consumers of the dangers of taking kava to removing kava products from the marketplace.

Chapter 33

Ketamine

Drug name: Ketamine

Trade names: Ketalar, Ketaset, Ketajet, Ketavet, Vetamine, Vetaket, and Ketamine Hydrochloride Injection

Street names: Special K, "K", kit kat, cat valium, super acid, purple

Introduction: Ketamine is a dissociative anesthetic that has gained popularity as a drug of abuse. On the street, it is commonly known as "K" or "special K." Other street names include cat valium, super acid, special la coke, purple, jet (Texas), and vitamin K. Slang for experiences related to ketamine or effects of ketamine include: "k-land" (refers to a mellow and colorful experience), "K-hole" (refers to the out-of-body, near death experience), "baby food" (users sink into blissful, infantile inertia), and "God" (users are convinced that they have met their maker).

Licit uses: Since the 1970s, ketamine has been marketed in the United States as an injectable short-acting anesthetic for use in humans and animals. It is imported into the United States and formulated into dosage forms for distribution under the trade names Ketalar, Ketaset, Ketajet, Ketavet, Vetamine, Vetaket, and Ketamine Hydrochloride Injection.

"Ketamine," Drug Enforcement Administration (DEA), August 2007.

Chemistry and pharmacology: Ketamine hydrochloride, 2-(2-chlorophenyl)-2-(methylamino)-cyclohexanone hydrochloride, is a white crystalline powder, which is soluble in water. It is a rapid-acting non-barbiturate dissociative anesthetic, structurally and pharmacologically similar to phencyclidine (PCP). It produces sedation, immobility, amnesia, and marked analgesia. At low doses and upon emergence from anesthesia, it produces changes in mood, body image, and hallucination. Relative to PCP, ketamine is less potent as an anesthetic, has a faster onset and shorter duration of action.

Illicit uses: Ketamine distorts perceptions of sight and sound and makes the user feel disconnected and not in control. A "special K" trip is touted as better than that of lysergic acid diethylamide (LSD) or phencyclidine (PCP) because its hallucinatory effects are relatively short in duration, lasting approximately 30 to 60 minutes as opposed to several hours.

Ketamine powder is usually snorted , mixed in drinks, or smoked. Liquid ketamine is injected, applied on a smokeable material or consumed in drinks. Most abusers of ketamine take small lines or "bumps" for a mild, dreamy effect. A dose of 100 milligrams (mg) is usually enough to enter a "k-hole" experience. A dose is referred to as a bump.

User population: Ketamine is abused by teenagers and young adults.

Illicit distribution: Drug Enforcement Administration (DEA) reports indicate that a major source of illicit ketamine in the United States is Mexico. Despite DEA and Mexican law enforcement dismantling the major drug ring of illicit ketamine in the United States in September 2002, Mexico continues to be a major supplier of ketamine into the United States. In November 2005, DEA successfully dismantled a large ketamine distribution organization operating throughout Los Angeles, Riverside, and Orange counties in California. At that time approximately 35,000 dosage units of ketamine smuggled from Mexico were seized.

Law enforcement information indicated that another source was an international pharmaceutical drug organization. This organization was smuggling ketamine from India into the United States. In April 2005, that organization was taken down and 108 kilograms of Indian ketamine seized with an estimated street value of approximately $1.62 million.

Ketamine is distributed as a dried powder or as a liquid in small vials or bottles. It is snorted, smoked, ingested orally, or injected. Powdered ketamine is formed from pharmaceutical ketamine by evaporating the liquid off. The national average price for ketamine is $20 to $40 per dosage unit and $65 to $100 per 10 milliliter (ml) vial containing one gram of ketamine.

Ketamine is mainly found by itself. However, it has also been found in combination with MDMA, amphetamine, methamphetamine, cocaine, or carisoprodol. Occasionally, ketamine is found in polydrug MDMA (ecstasy) tablets.

According to the System to Retrieve Information from Drug Evidence (STRIDE), a federal database for drug seizures analyzed by DEA laboratories, there were 185 cases involving 408 exhibits in 2001 and 166 cases involving 330 exhibits in 2002. Recent seizure data indicate that ketamine availability is decreasing. Since 2003, the number of STRIDE cases involving ketamine showed small decline: 2003: 144 cases involving 236 exhibits; 2004: 111 cases involving 233 exhibits; 2005: 79 cases involving 152 exhibits; 2006: 140 cases involving 294 exhibits. According to the National Forensic Laboratory Information System (NFLIS), state and local forensic laboratories analyzed 1,153 drug items (925 cases), 1,526 drug items (1,222 cases), 762 drug items (643 cases), 535 drug items (456 cases), 498 drug items (414 cases), and 1,171 drug items (942 cases) in 2001, 2002, 2003, 2004, 2005, and 2006 respectively.

Control status: On August 12, 1999, ketamine including its salts, isomers, and salts of isomers, became a schedule III nonnarcotic substance under the federal Controlled Substances Act (CSA).

Chapter 34

Khat

Drug name: Khat

Street names: Abyssinian tea, African salad, bushman's tea, chat, gat, Graba, kat, miraa, oat, qat, Somali tea, tohai, tschat

What is khat?

Khat (Catha edulis) is a flowering shrub native to East Africa and the Arabian Peninsula. The term khat refers to the leaves and young shoots of Catha edulis. The plant has been widely used since the thirteenth century as a recreational drug by the indigenous people of East Africa, the Arabian Peninsula, and the Middle East. Individuals chew khat leaves because of their stimulant and euphoric effects, which are similar to, but less intense than, those resulting from the abuse of cocaine or methamphetamine.

What does khat look like?

When fresh, khat leaves are glossy and crimson-brown in color, resembling withered basil. Khat leaves typically begin to deteriorate 48 hours after being harvested from the shrub on which they grow. Deteriorating khat leaves are leathery and turn yellow-green.

"Khat Fast Facts," U.S. Department of Justice, November 2008.

How is khat used?

Fresh khat typically is chewed and then retained in the cheek and chewed intermittently until the juices are extracted. Dried khat can be brewed into tea or made into a chewable paste. Less common methods of administering khat are smoking or sprinkling on food. Immediate effects of khat use include increased heart and breathing rates, elevated body temperature and blood pressure, and increased alertness, excitement, energy, and talkativeness. The effects of khat usually last between 90 minutes and three hours. After-effects of khat use include lack of concentration, numbness, and insomnia.

Who uses khat?

The use of khat is accepted within Somali, Ethiopian, and Yemeni cultures; in the United States, khat use is most prevalent among immigrants from those countries. Abuse levels are highest in cities with sizable immigrant populations from Somalia, Ethiopia, and Yemen, such as Boston, Columbus, Dallas, Detroit, Kansas City, Los Angeles, Minneapolis, Nashville, New York City, and Washington, DC.

What are the risks?

Khat abuse causes psychological dependence, and chronic abuse can lead to behavioral changes and mental health impairment. Clinical symptoms include manic behavior with grandiose delusions, violence, suicidal depression, and schizophreniform psychosis characterized by paranoid delusions. Chronic abuse can also produce physical exhaustion, anorexia, periodontal disease, and gastrointestinal illness.

Is khat illegal?

There is no licit use for khat in the United States. Khat contains two central nervous system stimulants: cathinone—a schedule I drug[1] under the federal Controlled Substances Act—and cathine—a schedule IV drug.[2] Cathinone is the principal active stimulant; its levels are highest in fresh khat. Once the plant is harvested, cathinone levels begin to decline; cooling the cut plant material reduces the rate of decline. In dried or dehydrated khat, also known as Graba, cathinone may be detected for many months or even years. Cathine, which is about ten times less potent than cathinone, remains stable in khat after the plant has been harvested. Khat samples in which any level of cathinone is found by chemical analysis are treated as schedule I plant material. Khat samples in which only cathine is detectable by chemical analysis are treated as schedule IV plant material.

End Notes

1. Schedule I drugs under the Controlled Substances Act (CSA) are classified as having a high potential for abuse, no currently accepted medical use in the United States, and a lack of accepted safety for use of the drug under medical supervision.

2. Schedule IV drugs under the CSA are classified as having a low potential for abuse relative to the drugs or other substances in schedule III, a currently accepted medical use in the United States, and abuse of the drug may lead to limited physical dependence or psychological dependence relative to the drugs or other substances in schedule III.

Chapter 35

Kratom

Drug name: Kratom (*Mitragyna speciosa Korth*)

Street names: Thang, kakuam, thom, ketum, biak

Introduction: Kratom, botanically known as *Mitragyna speciosa Korth*, is a tropical tree indigenous to Thailand, Malaysia, Myanmar, and other areas of Southeast Asia. Kratom is in the same family as the coffee tree (*Rubiaceae*). The tree reaches heights of 50 feet with a spread of over 15 feet.

Kratom has been used by natives of Thailand and other regions of Southeast Asia as an herbal drug for decades. Traditionally, kratom was mostly used as a stimulant by Thai peasants, laborers, and farmers to overcome the burdens of hard work. Thai natives chewed the leaves to make them work harder and feel good. Kratom was also used in Southeast Asia and by Thai natives to alleviate opium withdrawal. In 1943, the Thai government passed the Kratom Act 2486 that made planting of the tree illegal. In 1979, the Thai government enacted the Narcotics Act B.E. 2522, placing kratom along with marijuana in category V of a five category classification of narcotics.

Kratom remains a popular drug in Thailand. As of December 2006, kratom is the third most popular drug within southern Thailand, after methamphetamine and marijuana. In a November 2005 article in

---

"Kratom (*Mitragyna speciosa Korth*)," Drug Enforcement Administration (DEA), August 2007.

the *Bangkok Post*, it was reported that young Thai militants were offered to drink a "4x100" kratom formula to make them "more bold and fearless and easy to control." The two "4x100" kratom formulas are described as a mixture of a boiled kratom leaves and mosquito coils and cola, or a mixture of boiled cough syrup, kratom leaves, and cola served with ice. In this report it was also mentioned that the "4x100" formula was gaining popularity among Muslim youngsters in several districts of Yala (Southern Thailand) and was available in local coffee and tea shops.

Kratom is promoted as a legal psychoactive product on numerous websites in the United States (U.S.). On those websites, topics range from vendors listings, preparation of tea, and recommended doses, to alleged medicinal uses, and user reports of drug experiences.

Licit uses: There is no legitimate medical use for kratom in the U. S.

Chemistry and pharmacology: Over 25 alkaloids have been isolated from kratom, of which the indole alkaloid, mitragynine, is the most important. Mitragynine, chemically known as 9-methoxy-corynantheidine, is the primary active alkaloid in the plant.

Pharmacology studies show that mitragynine has opioid-like activity in animals. It inhibits electrically stimulated ileum and vas deferens smooth muscle contraction. Through actions on centrally located opioid receptor, it inhibits gastric secretion and reduces pain response.

Kratom has been described as producing both stimulant and sedative effects. At low doses, it produces stimulant effects, with users reporting increased alertness, physical energy, talkativeness, and sociable behavior. At high doses, it produces sedative and euphoric effects, and possibly an aphrodisiac effect. Effects occur within 5–10 minutes after ingestion and last for 2–5 hours. Acute side effects include nausea, itching, sweating, dry mouth, constipation, increased urination, and loss of appetite.

Kratom consumption can lead to addiction. In a study of Thai kratom addicts, it was observed that some addicts chewed kratom daily for 3–30 years (mean of 18.6 years). Long-term use of kratom produced anorexia, weight loss, insomnia, skin darkening, dry mouth, frequent urination, and constipation. A withdrawal syndrome was observed, consisting of symptoms of hostility, aggression, emotional lability, wet nose, achy muscles and bones, and jerky movement of the limbs. Furthermore, several cases of kratom psychosis were observed, where kratom addicts exhibited psychotic symptoms that included hallucinations, delusion, and confusion.

Illicit uses: Information on the illicit use of kratom in the U.S. is anecdotal. Based on information posted on the internet, kratom is mainly being abused orally as a tea. Chewing kratom leaves is another method of consumption. Doses in the range of 2–10 grams are recommended to achieve the desired effects. Users report that the dominant effects are similar to those of psychostimulant drugs.

Other countries are reporting emerging new trends in the use of kratom. In the United Kingdom, kratom is promoted as an herbal speedball. In Malaysia, kratom (known as ketum) juice preparations are illegally available.

User population: Information on user population in the U.S. is very limited. Kratom abuse is not monitored by any national drug abuse surveys.

Illicit distribution: Kratom is widely available on the internet. There are numerous vendors within and outside of the U.S. selling kratom, many of which sell other uncontrolled psychoactive products such as *Salvia divinorum*. Forms of kratom available through the internet, includes leaves (whole or crushed), powder, extract, encapsulated powder, and extract resin "pies" (40 gram pellets made from reduced extract). The kratom available from these vendors through the internet is allegedly imported from Thailand, Bali, New Guinea, and Hawaii. Seeds and whole trees are also available from some vendors through the internet, suggesting the possibility of domestic cultivation.

Control status: Kratom is not a controlled substance in the U.S. It is illegal to possess kratom in Thailand, Australia, Malaysia, and Myanmar.

Chapter 36

Lysergic Acid Diethylamide (LSD)

Drug name: D-lysergic acid diethylamide

Street names: LSD, acid, blotter acid, window pane

Introduction: Lysergic acid diethylamide (LSD), commonly referred to as acid, is a synthetic schedule I hallucinogen. LSD is the most potent hallucinogen known; with only microgram amounts required to produce overt hallucinations. LSD has been abused for its hallucinogenic properties since the 1960s. While LSD is available throughout the United States (U.S.), its availability has declined significantly since 2001.

Chemistry and pharmacology: LSD is manufactured from lysergic acid, which is found in ergot, a fungus that grows on rye and other grains. LSD's physiological effects are mediated primarily through the serotonergic neuronal system. It increases heart rate, blood pressure, and body temperature, and causes pupil dilation and sweating.

LSD induces a heightened awareness of sensory input that is accompanied by an enhanced sense of clarity, but reduced ability to control what is experienced. The LSD trip is made up of perceptual and psychic effects. A user may experience the following perceptual effects:

"D-Lysergic Acid Diethylamide," Drug Enforcement Administration (DEA), August 2007.

visual distortion in the size and shape of objects, movements, color, sound, touch, and the user's own body image. The user may report hearing colors or seeing sounds. The psychic effects experienced by the user may include feelings of obtaining true insight; intensified emotions; sudden and dramatic mood swings; impairment of attention, concentration, and motivation; distortion of time, and depersonalization.

High doses of LSD can induce a bad trip characterized by intense anxiety or panic, confusion, and combative behaviors. After a LSD trip, a user may also experience fatigue, acute anxiety, or depression for 12–24 hours.

Illicit uses: LSD is abused for its hallucinogenic effects. LSD is mainly ingested in a variety of forms. The average effective oral dose is from 20–80 micrograms. Following ingestion, effects occur within 30–60 minutes and last 10–12 hours.

User population: LSD is abused by teenagers and young adults in connection with raves, nightclubs, and concert settings.

Illicit distribution: According to the National Forensic Laboratory Information System (NFLIS), state and local forensic laboratories analyzed 1,435 and 1,325 exhibits of LSD in 2000 and 2001, respectively. In 2002, the number of LSD items dropped dramatically to 249 due to the seizure of a large LSD lab in Kansas City. With the arrest of clandestine chemists and with the dismantling of their laboratory, within two years, the availability of LSD in the U.S. was reduced by 95%. The number of LSD samples analyzed by state and local forensic laboratories remained low for 2003, 2004, 2005, and 2006, with 310, 312, 502, and 533 exhibits reported, respectively.

According to the System to Retrieve Information from Drug Evidence (STRIDE) database, the number of LSD drug items analyzed by the Drug Enforcement Administration (DEA) forensic laboratories substantially reduced in 2002. Moreover, similar to the NFLIS database, since 2002, the number of LSD drug exhibits analyzed by DEA forensic laboratories has remained comparatively low since 2002 with a small increase in 2006: 20 exhibits in 2005 and 36 exhibits in 2006.

LSD is odorless, colorless and tasteless. It is sold in a variety of formulations. Some of the streets names include acid, battery acid, blotter, window pane, microdots, loony toons, sunshine, and zen. Prices range from $2 to $5 per unit or hit.

LSD is most commonly found in the form of small squares of paper called blotter; that is generally decorated with artwork or designs, perforated, soaked in liquid LSD solution, and dried. Each square represents one dose of LSD. There have been some instances of blotter paper being found impregnated with hallucinogens other than LSD. For example, the hallucinogens 2,5-dimethoxyamphetamine (DMA) and 4-bromo-2,5-dimethoxyamphetamine (DOB) have been found on blotter paper passed off as LSD.

Other forms of LSD include tablets (known as microdots), gelatin squares (known as window pane), and impregnated sugar cubes. LSD has also been available in gel wraps which look like bubble-wrap packing material, and is blue in color. LSD is also distributed in liquid form which often is packaged in small bottles typically sold as breath drops. Additionally, LSD has been embedded in candy such as Gummy Worms®, Sweet Tarts®, Smartie®, and Pez®. The most common venues for retail LSD distribution are raves, dance clubs, and concerts.

Control status: Lysergic acid diethylamide acid is in schedule I of the Controlled Substances Act (CSA). Its two precursor's lysergic acid and lysergic acid amide are both in schedule III of the CSA. The LSD precursor's ergotamine and ergonovine are list I chemicals.

Chapter 37

Marijuana, Hashish, and Hash Oil

Drug name: Marijuana, hashish, hash oil

Street names: Pot, herb, weed, grass, boom, Mary Jane, gangster, chronic

Marijuana is a green, brown, or gray mixture of dried, shredded leaves, stems, seeds, and flowers of the hemp plant. You may hear marijuana called by street names such as pot, herb, weed, grass, boom, Mary Jane, gangster, or chronic. There are more than 200 slang terms for marijuana. Sinsemilla (sin-seh-me-yah; it's a Spanish word), hashish (hash for short), and hash oil are stronger forms of marijuana.

All forms of marijuana are mind-altering (psychoactive). In other words, they change how the brain works. They all contain THC (delta-9-tetrahydrocannabinol), the main active chemical in marijuana. They also contain more than 400 other chemicals. Marijuana's effects on the user depend on its strength or potency, which is related to the amount of THC it contains. The THC content of marijuana has been increasing since the 1970s. For the year 2006, most marijuana contained, on average, seven percent THC.

Most users roll loose marijuana into a cigarette (called a joint or a nail) or smoke it in a pipe or water pipe, sometimes referred to as a bong. Some users mix marijuana into foods or use it to brew a tea.

Text in this chapter is from "Marijuana: Facts for Teens," National Institute on Drug Abuse (NIDA), NIH Publication No. 04-4037, revised March 2008.

Another method is to slice open a cigar and replace the tobacco with marijuana, making what's called a blunt. Marijuana cigarettes or blunts sometimes contain other substances as well including crack cocaine.

THC in marijuana is rapidly absorbed by fatty tissues in various organs. Generally, traces (metabolites) of THC can be detected by standard urine testing methods several days after a smoking session. In heavy users, however, traces can sometimes be detected for weeks after they have stopped using marijuana.

Contrary to popular belief, most teenagers do not use marijuana. Among students surveyed in a yearly national survey, only about one in seven 10th graders report they are current marijuana users (that is, used marijuana within the past month). Fewer than one in five high school seniors is a current marijuana user.

There are many reasons why some children and young teens start smoking marijuana. Many young people smoke marijuana because they see their brothers, sisters, friends, or even older family members using it. Some use marijuana because of peer pressure. Others may think it's cool to use marijuana because they hear songs about it and see it on television and in movies. Some teens may feel they need marijuana and other drugs to help them escape from problems at home, at school, or with friends.

What happens if you smoke marijuana?

The way the drug affects each person depends on many factors, including:

- the user's previous experience with the drug;
- how strong the marijuana is (how much THC it has);
- what the user expects to happen;
- where the drug is used;
- how it is taken; and
- whether the user is drinking alcohol or using other drugs.

Some people feel nothing at all when they smoke marijuana. Others may feel relaxed or high. Sometimes marijuana makes users feel thirsty and very hungry—an effect called the munchies. Some users can suffer bad reactions from abusing marijuana. They may experience sudden feelings of anxiety and have paranoid thoughts. This is more likely to happen when a more potent variety of marijuana is used.

Short-term effects of marijuana use include:

- problems with memory and learning;
- distorted perception (sights, sounds, time, touch);
- trouble with thinking and problem solving;
- loss of motor coordination; and
- increased heart rate.

Effects can be unpredictable, especially when other drugs are mixed with marijuana.

Marijuana can affect school, sports, or other activities. Marijuana affects memory, judgment, and perception. The drug can make you mess up in school, in sports or clubs, or with your friends. If you're high on marijuana, you are more likely to make mistakes that could embarrass or even hurt you. If you use marijuana a lot, you could start to lose interest in how you look and how you're getting along at school or work.

Athletes could find their performance is off; timing, movements, and coordination are all affected by THC. Also, since marijuana can affect judgment and decision making, its use can lead to risky sexual behavior, resulting in exposure to sexually transmitted diseases like human immunodeficiency virus (HIV), the virus that causes acquired immunodeficiency syndrome (AIDS).

Long term effects: Findings so far show that regular use of marijuana or THC may play a role in some kinds of cancer and in problems with the respiratory and immune systems.

- **Cancer:** It's hard to know for sure whether marijuana use alone causes cancer, because many people who smoke marijuana also smoke cigarettes and use other drugs. But it is known that marijuana smoke contains some of the same, and sometimes even more, of the cancer-causing chemicals found in tobacco smoke. Studies show that someone who smokes five joints per day may be taking in as many cancer-causing chemicals as someone who smokes a full pack of cigarettes every day.

- **Lungs and airways:** People who smoke marijuana often develop the same kinds of breathing problems that cigarette smokers have: coughing and wheezing. They tend to have more chest colds than nonusers. They are also at greater risk of getting lung infections like pneumonia.

- **Immune system:** Our immune system protects the body from many agents that cause disease. It is not certain whether marijuana damages the immune system of people, but both animal and human studies have shown that marijuana impairs the ability of T-cells in the lungs' immune system to fight off some infections.

Marijuana and other drug use: Long-term studies of high school students and their patterns of drug use show that very few young people use other illegal drugs without first trying marijuana. For example, the risk of using cocaine is much greater for those who have tried marijuana than for those who have never tried it. Using marijuana puts children and teens in contact with people who are users and sellers of other drugs. So there is more of a risk that a marijuana user will be exposed to and urged to try more drugs. Although many young people who use marijuana do not go on to use other drugs, further research is needed to determine who will be at greatest risk.

How can you tell if someone has been using marijuana?

If someone is high on marijuana, he or she might seem dizzy and have trouble walking; seem silly and giggly for no reason; have very red, bloodshot eyes; and have a hard time remembering things that just happened. When the early effects fade, over a few hours, the user can become very sleepy.

Is marijuana sometimes used as a medicine?

There has been much talk about the possible medical use of marijuana. Under United States law since 1970, marijuana has been a Schedule I controlled substance. This means that the drug, at least in its smoked form, has no commonly accepted medical use. However, THC, the active chemical in marijuana, is manufactured into a pill available by prescription that can be used to treat the nausea and vomiting that occur with certain cancer treatments and to help AIDS patients eat more to keep up their weight. Scientists are studying whether THC, and related chemicals in marijuana (called cannabinoids) may have other medical uses. Because of the adverse effects of smoking marijuana, research on other cannabinoids appears more promising for the development of new medications.

How does marijuana affect driving?

Marijuana affects many skills required for safe driving: alertness, concentration, coordination, and reaction time. Marijuana use can make it difficult to judge distances and react to signals and sounds on the road. Marijuana may play a role in car accidents. In one study conducted in Memphis, Tennessee, researchers found that, of 150 reckless drivers who were tested for drugs at the arrest scene, 33 percent tested positive for marijuana, and 12 percent tested positive for both marijuana and cocaine. Data have also shown that while smoking marijuana, people show the same lack of coordination on standard drunk driver tests as do people who have had too much to drink.

If a woman is pregnant and smokes marijuana, will it hurt the baby?

Doctors advise pregnant women not to use any drugs because they could harm the growing fetus. Studies in children born to mothers who used marijuana have shown increased behavioral problems during infancy and preschool years. In school, these children are more likely to have problems with decision making, memory, and the ability to remain attentive.

Researchers are not certain whether health problems that may be caused by early exposure to marijuana will remain as the child grows into adulthood. However, since some parts of the brain continue to develop throughout adolescence, it is also possible that certain kinds of problems may appear as the child matures.

What does marijuana do to the brain?

Some studies show that when people have smoked large amounts of marijuana for years, the drug takes its toll on mental functions. Heavy or daily use of marijuana affects the parts of the brain that control memory, attention, and learning. A working short-term memory is needed to learn and perform tasks that call for more than one or two steps. Smoking marijuana causes some changes in the brain that are like those caused by cocaine, heroin, and alcohol. Scientists are still learning about the many ways that marijuana can affect the brain.

Can people become addicted to marijuana?

Yes. Long-term marijuana use leads to addiction in some people. That is, they cannot control their urges to seek out and use marijuana, even though it negatively affects their family relationships, school performance, and recreational activities. According to one study, marijuana use by teenagers who have prior antisocial problems can quickly lead to addiction. In addition, some frequent, heavy marijuana users develop tolerance to its effects. This means they need larger and larger amounts of marijuana to get the same desired effects as they used to get from smaller amounts.

What if a person wants to quit using the drug?

In 2004, over 298,000 people entering drug treatment programs reported marijuana as their primary drug of abuse. However, up until a few years ago, it was hard to find treatment programs specifically for marijuana users.

Now researchers are testing different ways to help marijuana users abstain from drug use. There are currently no medications for treating marijuana addiction. Treatment programs focus on counseling and group support systems. There are also a number of programs designed especially to help teenagers who are abusers. Family doctors can be a good source for information and help when dealing with marijuana problems.

Chapter 38

Methadone

Drug name: Methadone

Trade names: Methadose®, Dolophine®

Street names: Fizzies, amidone, chocolate chip cookies

Introduction: Methadone, a pharmaceutical opioid, is currently marketed as oral concentrate (10 milligrams per milliliter [mg/ml]), oral solution (5 mg, and 10 mg/5 ml), tablet (5, 10, and 40 mg), injectable (10 mg/ml) and powder (50, 100, and 500 mg/bottle for prescription compounding). Recently there have been increasing concerns about the marked escalation of diversion and abuse of methadone and its adverse health consequences. According to the Centers for Disease Control and Prevention (CDC), methadone-related deaths increased about four-fold from 786 (4% of all poisoning deaths) in 1999 to 3,849 (13% of all poisoning deaths) in 2004. According to the National Poison Data System, American Poison Control Centers reported 4,558 methadone-related toxic exposures in 2006. Florida Department of Law Enforcement reported that methadone-related deaths increased about five-fold from 209 in 2000 to 1,095 in 2007. On November 27,

---

This chapter includes "Methadone," Drug Enforcement Administration (DEA), August 2008; and excerpts from "Methadone Diversion, Abuse, and Misuse: Deaths Increasing at Alarming Rate," U.S. Department of Justice, Document ID 2007-Q0317-001, November 16, 2007.

2006, the Food and Drug Administration (FDA) issued a public health advisory stating that methadone use in pain control may result in life-threatening cardiac and respiratory changes and deaths. FDA further advised that methadone doses for pain should be carefully selected, slowly titrated and carefully monitored by the prescribing physician. As of January 1, 2008, manufacturers of 40 mg methadone hydrochloride dispersible tablets have voluntarily agreed to restrict distribution of this formulation to only those facilities authorized for detoxification and maintenance treatment of opioid addiction, and hospitals. The 40 mg product is not FDA approved for use in the management of pain.

Licit uses: Methadone has been used for over forty years primarily as a detoxification and maintenance treatment of opioid addiction. In recent years, methadone is also increasingly being prescribed for the relief of moderate to severe pain. The prescriptions for methadone products have increased by about eight-fold from about 0.5 million in 1998 to about four million in 2007 (IMS National Prescription Audit Plus™). Aggregate production quota for methadone as established by the Drug Enforcement Administration (DEA) for legitimate national needs increased from 5,975 kilograms in 1998 to 25,000 kilograms in 2007. Methadone products when used for treatment of narcotic addiction in detoxification or maintenance programs shall be dispensed only by pharmacies approved by appropriate regulatory authorities. These products when used as analgesics may be dispensed in any licensed pharmacy.

Chemistry and pharmacology: Methadone, [3-heptanone, 6-(dimethyl-amino)-4,4-diphenyl-, hydrochloride] is a synthetic drug with m-opioid receptor agonist activity. Pharmacological and toxic effects, abuse and dependence liabilities of methadone are qualitatively similar to those of other schedule II opioid analgesics such as morphine and oxycodone. Analgesic activity of racemic methadone is entirely due to its l-isomer which is 8–50 times more potent than d-isomer. D-isomer lacks significant respiratory depressant action and addiction liability, but possesses antitussive activity. Analgesic effect of 8–10 mg of methadone is approximately equivalent to that of ten milligrams of morphine. With respect to total analgesic effects, methadone given orally is one-half as effective as its parenteral administration. Pain relief from a dose of methadone lasts about 4–8 hours, but the drug may stay in the body for longer period (8–59 hours).

Methadone binds strongly to proteins in various tissues, including brain tissue. Upon discontinuation of its administration, slow release from tissue binding sites maintains low concentrations of methadone. Notable features of methadone are its efficacy by the oral route, its prolonged duration of action in suppressing withdrawal symptoms in physically dependent individuals, and its tendency to produce persistent effects with repeated administration. Acute overdose of methadone, similar to morphine, can produce severe respiratory depression, somnolence, coma, skeletal muscle flaccidity, cool clammy skin, constricted pupils, reduction in blood pressure and heart rate, pulmonary edema, and death. Pure opioid antagonists such as naloxone are specific antidotes against respiratory depression from methadone overdose.

Illicit uses: Methadone, similar to other schedule II opioids, has abuse potential and may produce psychic and physical dependence and tolerance. Methadone abuse has escalated markedly in recent years in the United States. According to the National Survey on Drug Use and Health, about 1.5 million individuals age 12 and older have used it for non-medical purpose at least once in their lifetime in 2006.

Illicit distribution: DEA field offices reported that the street prices for methadone ranged from $2 to $30 per tablet and $10 to $40 per diskette in 2005. The majority of the diversion involves methadone tablets. According to the National Forensic Laboratory Information System, methadone drug items analyzed by the state, local, and DEA laboratories increased about 14-fold from 511 in 2000 to 7,425 in 2007.

Control status: Methadone products are in schedule II of the Controlled Substances Act of 1970.

Methadone Deaths Increasing at Alarming Rate

From 1999 through 2006 the number of methadone-related deaths increased significantly. Most deaths are attributed to the abuse of methadone diverted from hospitals, pharmacies, practitioners, and pain management physicians. Some deaths result from misuse of legitimately prescribed methadone or methadone obtained from narcotic treatment programs, including use in combination with other drugs and/or alcohol. Methadone is a safe and effective drug when used as prescribed; however, when it is misused or abused—particularly in combination with other prescription drugs, illicit drugs, or alcohol—death or nonfatal overdose is likely to occur. This assessment analyzes increases in methadone diversion, abuse, and misuse that have occurred since 1999.

Methadone poisoning deaths increased 390% from 1999 through 2004. Additionally, selected state health department data indicate methadone poisoning deaths increased through 2006. The percentage increase in methadone deaths exceeds the percentage increase in other opioid (including oxycodone, morphine, hydromorphone, and hydrocodone) deaths during the same period. Other opioid deaths increased 90% during that time and accounted for a much larger percentage of total opioid-related deaths. Methadone deaths receive more media attention than do oxycodone- or hydrocodone-related deaths, very likely because of the drug's association with narcotic treatment programs (NTP). A 2004 Substance Abuse and Mental Health Services Administration (SAMHSA) study reported that most methadone deaths involve abuse or misuse of methadone diverted in ways other than from NTP and taken in combination with other drugs and/or alcohol.

Various methods are used to divert methadone. Wholesale-level quantities of methadone are stolen from delivery trucks and reverse distributors, and midlevel quantities are stolen from businesses such as hospitals and pharmacies. Retail-level quantities frequently are obtained through traditional prescription drug diversion methods such as doctor-shopping, prescription fraud, and to a much lesser extent, rogue internet pharmacies. Methadone can be misused by patients being treated for chronic or cancer pain who obtain the drug using legitimate prescriptions. Following increases in OxyContin (oxycodone) addiction and death rates, many practitioners began using methadone to manage chronic pain and pain associated with cancer. Methadone is a safe and effective drug when used as prescribed; however, patients who are prescribed methadone need to be monitored by a physician well trained in the pharmacodynamic and pharmacokinetic properties of the drug, particularly if the patients have no prior history of opioid use for pain management.

Key Judgments

- The total amount of methadone legitimately distributed to businesses increased from 2001 through 2006; the greatest percentage change occurred at the practitioner level, indicating that pain management and general practitioners are dispensing the drug more frequently in the management of pain.

- Theft of methadone during transit from the manufacturers to businesses and theft from businesses and reverse distributors increased the availability of methadone at the midlevel and retail level.

- Diversion from pain management facilities, hospitals, pharmacies, general practitioners, family and friends, and to a lesser extent, narcotic treatment programs increased availability, primarily at the retail level.

- Retail-level distribution of diverted methadone may be occurring more frequently than law enforcement reporting indicates.

- Methadone poisoning deaths rose at a higher rate than such deaths involving any other prescription opioid from 1999 through 2004, although the total number of methadone deaths was far fewer than the number of deaths involving other prescription opioids (morphine, oxycodone, hydrocodone, and hydromorphone).

- Most methadone deaths are the result of methadone diverted from hospitals, pharmacies, practitioners, pain management physicians, and to a much lesser extent, NTP and used in combination with other drugs and/or alcohol.

- Some methadone deaths and nonfatal overdoses are the result of misuse of legitimately prescribed methadone by individuals who may not have been properly counseled by their physicians about the dangers of taking the drug in ways other than those prescribed, including in combination with other drugs and/or alcohol.

Chapter 39

Methamphetamine

Drug name: Methamphetamine

Street name: Meth

Methamphetamine is a central nervous system stimulant drug that is similar in structure to amphetamine. Due to its high potential for abuse, methamphetamine is classified as a schedule II drug and is available only through a prescription that cannot be refilled. Although methamphetamine can be prescribed by a doctor, its medical uses are limited, and the doses that are prescribed are much lower than those typically abused. Most of the methamphetamine abused in this country comes from foreign or domestic super labs, although it can also be made in small, illegal laboratories, where its production endangers the people in the labs, neighbors, and the environment.

Methamphetamine is a white, odorless, bitter-tasting crystalline powder that easily dissolves in water or alcohol and is taken orally, intranasally (snorting the powder), by needle injection, or by smoking.

Methamphetamine Affects the Brain

Methamphetamine increases the release and blocks the reuptake of the brain chemical (or neurotransmitter) dopamine, leading to high

Text in this chapter is from "NIDA InfoFacts: Methamphetamine," National Institute on Drug Abuse (NIDA), July 2009.

levels of the chemical in the brain, a common mechanism of action for most drugs of abuse. Dopamine is involved in reward, motivation, the experience of pleasure, and motor function. Methamphetamine's ability to rapidly release dopamine in reward regions of the brain produces the intense euphoria, or rush, that many users feel after snorting, smoking, or injecting the drug.

Chronic methamphetamine abuse significantly changes how the brain functions. Noninvasive human brain imaging studies have shown alterations in the activity of the dopamine system that are associated with reduced motor skills and impaired verbal learning.[1] Recent studies in chronic methamphetamine abusers have also revealed severe structural and functional changes in areas of the brain associated with emotion and memory,[2,3] which may account for many of the emotional and cognitive problems observed in chronic methamphetamine abusers.

Repeated methamphetamine abuse can also lead to addiction—a chronic, relapsing disease, characterized by compulsive drug seeking and use, which is accompanied by chemical and molecular changes in the brain. Some of these changes persist long after methamphetamine abuse is stopped. Reversal of some of the changes, however, may be observed after sustained periods of abstinence (more than one year).[4]

Other Adverse Health Effects from Methamphetamine Use

Taking even small amounts of methamphetamine can result in many of the same physical effects of other stimulants, such as cocaine or amphetamines, including increased wakefulness, increased physical activity, decreased appetite, increased respiration, rapid heart rate, irregular heartbeat, increased blood pressure, and hyperthermia.

Long-term methamphetamine abuse has many negative health consequences, including extreme weight loss, severe dental problems (meth mouth), anxiety, confusion, insomnia, mood disturbances, and violent behavior. Chronic methamphetamine abusers can also display a number of psychotic features, including paranoia, visual and auditory hallucinations, and delusions (for example, the sensation of insects crawling under the skin).

Transmission of human immunodeficiency (HIV) and hepatitis B and C can be consequences of methamphetamine abuse. The intoxicating effects of methamphetamine, regardless of how it is taken, can also alter judgment and inhibition and lead people to engage in unsafe behaviors, including risky sexual behavior. Among abusers who inject the drug, HIV and other infectious diseases can be spread through contaminated needles, syringes, and other injection equipment that is used by more than one person. Methamphetamine abuse may also worsen the progression of HIV and its consequences. Studies of methamphetamine abusers who are HIV-positive indicate that HIV causes greater neuronal injury and cognitive impairment for individuals in this group compared with HIV-positive people who do not use the drug.[5,6]

Treatment Options

Currently, the most effective treatments for methamphetamine addiction are comprehensive cognitive-behavioral interventions. For example, the Matrix Model—a behavioral treatment approach that combines behavioral therapy, family education, individual counseling, 12-step support, drug testing, and encouragement for non-drug-related activities—has been shown to be effective in reducing methamphetamine abuse.[7] Contingency management interventions, which provide tangible incentives in exchange for engaging in treatment and maintaining abstinence, have also been shown to be effective.[8] There are no medications at this time approved to treat methamphetamine addiction.

Prevalence of Methamphetamine Abuse

According to the 2008 Monitoring the Future survey*—a national survey of 8th-, 10th-, and 12th- graders—methamphetamine abuse among students has shown a general decline in recent years; however, it remains a concern. Survey results show that 2.3% of 8th-graders, 2.4% of 10th-graders, and 2.8% of 12th-graders have used methamphetamine in their lifetime. In addition, 0.7% of 8th-graders, 0.7% of 10th-graders, and 0.6% of 12th-graders were current (past-month) methamphetamine abusers. Past-year use of methamphetamine remained steady across all grades surveyed from 2007 to 2008.

The number of individuals aged 12 years or older reporting past-year methamphetamine use declined from 1.9 million in 2006 to 1.3 million in 2007. An estimated 529,000 Americans were current (past-month) users of methamphetamine (0.2% of the population). Of the 157,000 people who used methamphetamine for the first time in 2007, the mean age at first use was 19.1 years, which is down from the mean age of 22.2 in 2006.

* These data are from the 2008 Monitoring the Future survey, funded by the National Institute on Drug Abuse, National Institutes of Health, Department of Health and Human Services, and conducted by the University of Michigan's Institute for Social Research. The study has tracked 12th-graders' illicit drug abuse and related attitudes since 1975; in 1991, 8th- and 10th-graders were added to the study. The latest data are online at www.drugabuse.gov.

End Notes

1. Volkow ND, Chang L, Wang GJ, et al. Association of dopamine transporter reduction with psychomotor impairment in methamphetamine abusers. *Am J Psychiatry* 158:377–382, 2001.

2. London ED, Simon SL, Berman SM, et al.. Mood disturbances and regional cerebral metabolic abnormalities in recently abstinent methamphetamine abusers. *Arch Gen Psychiatry* 61:73–84, 2004.

3. Thompson PM, Hayashi KM, Simon SL, et al. Structural abnormalities in the brains of human subjects who use methamphetamine. *J Neurosci* 24:6028–6036, 2004.

4. Wang GJ, Volkow ND, Chang L, et al. Partial recovery of brain metabolism in methamphetamine abusers after protracted abstinence. *Am J Psychiatry* 161:242–248, 2004.

5. Chang L, Ernst T, Speck O, Grob CS. Additive effects of HIV and chronic methamphetamine use on brain metabolite abnormalities. *Am J Psychiatry* 162:361–369, 2005.

6. Rippeth JD, Heaton RK, Carey CL, et al. Methamphetamine dependence increases risk of neuropsychological impairment in HIV infected persons. *J Int Neuropsychol Soc* 10:1–14, 2004.

7. Rawson RA, Marinelli-Casey P, Anglin MD, et al. A multi-site comparison of psychosocial approaches for the treatment of methamphetamine dependence. *Addiction* 99:708–717, 2004.

8. Roll JM, Petry NM, Stitzer ML, et al. Contingency management for the treatment of methamphetamine use disorders. *Am J Psychiatry* 163:1993–1999, 2006.

Chapter 40

Oxycodone

Drug name: Oxycodone

Trade names: Tylox®, Percodan®, OxyContin®

Street names: OC, oxy, oxycotton, hillbilly heroin, kicker

Introduction: Oxycodone is a schedule II narcotic analgesic and is widely used in clinical medicine. It is marketed either alone as controlled release (OxyContin®) and immediate release formulations (OxyIR®, OxyFast®), or in combination with other nonnarcotic analgesics such as aspirin (Percodan®) or acetaminophen (Percocet®). The introduction in 1996 of OxyContin®, commonly known on the street as OC, OX, oxy, oxycotton, hillbilly heroin, and kicker, led to a marked escalation of its abuse as reported by drug abuse treatment centers, law enforcement personnel, and health care professionals. Although the diversion and abuse of OxyContin® appeared initially in the eastern United States (U.S.), it has now spread to the western U.S. including Alaska and Hawaii. Oxycodone-related adverse health effects increased markedly in recent years. In 2004, Food and Drug Administration (FDA) approved generic forms of controlled release oxycodone products for marketing.

"Oxycodone," Drug Enforcement Administration (DEA), September 2007.

Licit uses: Products containing oxycodone in combination with aspirin or acetaminophen are used for the relief of moderate to moderately severe pain. Oxycodone controlled-release tablets are prescribed for the management of moderate to severe pain when a continuous, around-the-clock analgesic is needed for an extended period of time. Oxycodone is a widely prescribed in the U.S. Prescriptions for OxyContin® (1.57 million) and similar controlled release products accounted for 7.6 million of the 42.3 million total prescriptions for oxycodone in 2006 (IMS Health™).

Chemistry and pharmacology: Oxycodone, [4,5-epoxy-14-hydroxy-3-methoxy-17-methyl-morphinan-6-one, dihydrohydroxycodeinone] is a semi-synthetic opioid agonist derived from thebaine, a constituent of opium. Oxycodone will test positive for an opiate in the available field test kits. Pharmacology of oxycodone is essentially similar to that of morphine, in all respects, including its abuse and dependence liabilities. Pharmacological effects include analgesia, sedation, euphoria, feelings of relaxation, respiratory depression, constipation, papillary constriction, and cough suppression. A ten milligram (mg) dose of orally-administered oxycodone is equivalent to a ten mg dose of subcutaneously administered morphine as an analgesic in the normal population. Oxycodone's behavioral effects can last up to five hours. The drug is most often administered orally. The controlled-release product, OxyContin®, has a longer duration of action (8–12 hours). As with most opiates, oxycodone abuse may lead to dependence and tolerance. Acute overdose of oxycodone can produce severe respiratory depression, skeletal muscle flaccidity, cold and clammy skin, reduction in blood pressure and heart rate, coma, respiratory arrest, and death.

Illicit uses: Oxycodone abuse has been a continuing problem in the U.S. since the early 1960s. Oxycodone is abused for its euphoric effects. It is equipotent to morphine in relieving abstinence symptoms from chronic opiate (heroin, morphine) administration. For this reason, it is often used to alleviate or prevent the onset of opiate withdrawal by street users of heroin and methadone. The large amount of oxycodone (10–80 mg) present in controlled release formulations (OxyContin®) renders these products highly attractive to opioid abusers and doctor-shoppers. They are abused either as intact tablets or by crushing or chewing the tablet and then swallowing, snorting, or injecting. Products containing oxycodone in combination with acetaminophen or aspirin are abused orally. Acetaminophen present in the combination products poses an additional risk of liver toxicity upon chronic abuse. According to the Florida Department of Law Enforcement, oxycodone was found in 5.6% (716) of the total drug-related deaths in Florida in 2005. Based on the toxicology reports, oxycodone was cited as a causative drug in 340 deaths. The manner of oxycodone deaths cited included accidental (65%), suicide (16%), natural (13%), and undetermined (4%).

User population: Every age-group has been affected by the relative prevalence of oxycodone availability and the perceived safety of oxycodone products by professionals. Sometimes seen as a white-collar addiction, oxycodone abuse has increased among all ethnic and economic groups.

Illicit distribution: Oxycodone-containing products are in tablet, capsule, and liquid forms. A variety of colors, markings, and packaging are available. The main sources of oxycodone on the street have been through forged prescriptions, professional diversion through unscrupulous pharmacists, doctors, and dentists, doctor-shopping, armed robberies, and night break-ins of pharmacies and nursing homes. The diversion and abuse of OxyContin® has become a major public health problem in recent years. In 2006, 4.1 million people aged 12 or older used OxyContin® for nonmedical use at least once during their life time (National Survey on Drug Use and Health, 2006). According to reports from Drug Enforcement Administration (DEA) field offices, oxycodone products sell at an average price of $1 per milligram, the 40 mg OxyContin® tablet being the most popular. According to the System to Retrieve Information from Drug Evidence, DEA forensic laboratories analyzed 51 items (38 cases) and 607 items (237 cases) of oxycodone in 1998 and 2006, respectively. According to the National Forensic Laboratory Information System, state and local forensic laboratories analyzed 19,056 oxycodone drug items in 2006.

Control status: Oxycodone products are in schedule II of the federal Controlled Substances Act of 1970.

Chapter 41

PCP

Drug name: Phencyclidine

Street names: PCP, angel dust, supergrass, boat, tic tac, zoom, shermans

Introduction: After a decline in abuse during the late 1980s and 1990s, phencyclidine (PCP) has re-emerged as a drug of abuse. PCP is considered a club drug and is abused by young adults involved in the rave culture. Street names include angel dust, hog, ozone, rocket fuel, shermans, wack, crystal, and embalming fluid. Street names for PCP combined with marijuana include killer joints, super grass, fry, lovelies, wets, and waters.

Licit uses: Once marketed as an anesthetic in the United States under the trade names, Sernyl and Sernylan, PCP is no longer produced or used for medical purposes in the United States.

Chemistry and pharmacology: Phencyclidine, 1-(1-phencyclohexyl) piperidine, is a white crystalline powder that is readily soluble in water. PCP is clandestinely manufactured for purposes of abuse.

PCP is known as a dissociative anesthetic because it distorts sight and sound and produces feelings of detachment from one's environment

---

"Phencyclidine (Street Names: PCP, Angel Dust, Supergrass, Boat, Tic Tac, Zoom, Shermans)," Drug Enforcement Administration (DEA), August 2007.

and self. Its pharmacological effects include the ability to produce sedation, immobility, amnesia, and marked analgesia. The drug effects of PCP vary by the route of administration and dose. The effects can be felt within 2–5 minutes after smoking and 30–60 minutes after oral ingestion. PCP intoxication may last between 4–8 hours when consumed as recreational dose, although some users report subjective effects lasting between 24–48 hours. Low to moderate doses (1–5 milligrams [mg]) of PCP often cause the user to feel detached, distant, and estranged from his surroundings. Numbness, slurred speech, and loss of coordination may be accompanied by a sense of strength and invulnerability. A blank stare, rapid and involuntary eye movements, and an exaggerated gait are among the more observable effects. High doses (ten milligrams or more) of PCP produce illusions and hallucination (auditory). Physiological effects include increased blood pressure, rapid and shallow breathing, elevated heart rate, and elevated temperature.

Chronic use of PCP can result in dependency with a withdrawal syndrome upon cessation of the drug. Chronic abuse of PCP can impair memory and thinking. The user can have persistent speech difficulties such as slurred speech, stuttering, inability to articulate, and inability to speak. Other symptoms from long-term use include suicidal ideation, anxiety, depression, social withdrawal, and social isolation

Illicit uses: PCP is abused for its mind altering effects. It is abused in one of three ways: snorted, smoked, or swallowed. Smoking is the most common method of abusing PCP. Leafy material such as mint, parsley, oregano, tobacco, or marijuana are saturated with powdered PCP which is than rolled into a cigarette, called a joint, and smoked. A marijuana joint or cigarette dipped in liquid PCP is known as a dipper. PCP is typically used in small quantities with 5–10 milligrams being considered an average dose.

User population: PCP is abused by young adults and high school students. According to the 2005 National Survey on Drug Use and Health, 2.7% (6.6 millions) and 0.1% (164,000) of Americans aged 12 and older surveyed reported PCP use in their lifetime and past year, respectively. The 2004, 2005, and 2006 Monitoring the Future survey reported that 0.7%, 1.3%, and 0.7% of high school seniors acknowledged using PCP within the past year, respectively.

Illicit distribution: PCP is available in powder, crystal, tablet, capsule, and liquid forms. It is most commonly sold in powder and liquid forms. Tablets sold as MDMA (ecstasy) occasionally are found to contain PCP. Prices for PCP range from $5–$15 for tablets, $20–$30 for a gram of powder PCP, and $200–$300 for an ounce of liquid PCP. The dipper sells for $10–$20 each.

The Los Angeles area is the primary source of the majority of PCP found in the United States. According to the El Paso Intelligence Center National Clandestine Laboratory Seizure System (EPIC) data, six PCP laboratories seized in 2004 were in the Los Angeles County. Several major PCP producers operating in Southern California were arrested in 2005 and 2006. It is typically produced in liquid form and subsequently distributed to mid-level distributors in Chicago, Houston, Los Angeles, Milwaukee, New Orleans, Newark, New York City, Philadelphia, and Washington DC. PCP is available throughout the country; however, primarily it's found in metropolitan areas such as Philadelphia and Washington DC.

According to the System to Retrieve Information from Drug Evidence, Drug Enforcement Administration (DEA) forensic laboratories analyzed 494 PCP exhibits from 271 cases in 2003. PCP exhibits declined to 207 (121 cases) and 266 (152 cases) in 2004 and 2005, respectively. In 2006, there were 400 PCP exhibits (222 cases). According to the National Forensic Laboratory Information System, state and local forensic laboratories analyzed 3,386 (3,044 cases), 2,765 (2,501 cases), 2,827 (2,580 cases), and 2,990 (2,634 cases) PCP drug items in 2003, 2004, 2005, and 2006, respectively.

Control status: On January 25, 1978, PCP was transferred from schedule III to schedule II under the federal Controlled Substances Act.

Chapter 42

Ritalin and Other ADHD Medications: Methylphenidate and Amphetamines

Methylphenidate

Drug name: Methylphenidate

Trade names: Ritalin®, Concerta®, Metadate®, Methylin®, and Focalin®

Introduction: Methylphenidate (d,l-threo-methyl-I-phenyl-2-pip-eridine-acetate hydrochloride) is a central nervous system (CNS) stimulant that has been marketed in the United States since the 1950s. For many years, Ritalin® (immediate release [IR] product), was the only brand-name product available. In recent years, other IR, extended release [ER], and long acting [LA] methylphenidate products have entered the market. These products are primarily prescribed to children for the treatment of attention deficit hyperactivity disorder (ADHD).

Domestic and worldwide use of methylphenidate has increased dramatically since 1990. According to the 2004 United Nations International Narcotic Control Board (INCB) report, the United States is the main consumer of methylphenidate accounting for about 70% of the global medical use of methylphenidate.

This chapter includes text from "Methylphenidate," Drug Enforcement Administration (DEA), June 2009; and text from "NIDA InfoFacts: Stimulant ADHD Medications—Methylphenidate and Amphetamines," National Institute on Drug Abuse (NIDA), June 2009.

Licit use: Methylphenidate is used almost exclusively for the treatment of ADHD. There is a considerable body of literature on the short-term efficacy of methylphenidate pharmaceutical-therapy for the treatment of ADHD. However, attentional improvement is not diagnostic of ADHD. There is no diagnostic test that can confirm an ADHD diagnosis.

Recent data suggests that some children may continue to have significant ADHD-symptoms into adulthood. As a consequence, the prescription of methylphenidate for individuals 18 and older is the most rapidly growing market. Longer acting products, primarily Concerta®, have gained a significant share of the total methylphenidate market. The IMS Health National Prescription Audit Plus™ reported 14.8 million methylphenidate prescriptions dispensed in 2008.

Illicit use: Like other potent stimulants, methylphenidate is abused for its feel good stimulant effects. The occasional abuser may use methylphenidate as a study aid to increase attention and stay awake. Others may use methylphenidate recreationally and combine it with alcohol or some other depressant to feel more alert or less drunk. Serious methylphenidate abusers often snort or inject methylphenidate for its intense euphoric effects or to alleviate the severe depression and craving associated with a stimulant withdrawal syndrome.

Monitoring the Future (MTF) is a National Institute on Drug Abuse (NIDA) funded study conducted by the University of Michigan. In 2008, the MTF survey indicated that 3.4% of 12th grade students, 2.9% of 10th grade students and 1.6% of 8th grade students reported non-medical use of Ritalin® in the past year.

The National Survey on Drug Use and Health (NSDUH) is a database that measures drug use by people living in households. In 2007, the highest non-medical use of methylphenidate among youth was in the 18–25 year old age group with 4.8% reporting lifetime non-medical use. It is estimated that 1.61 million people misused methylphenidate in their lifetime, according to the 2007 NSDUH report.

The American Association of Poison Control Centers (AAPCC) report indicates 8,766 methylphenidate case mentions and 6,062 single exposures in 2006. In 2007, 8,994 case mentions and 6,355 single exposures reported to AAPCC were associated with methylphenidate. Nonmedical use of methylphenidate accounted for 2,192 visits to the emergency department in 2006 according to the Drug Abuse Warning Network (New DAWN ED).

The National Forensic Laboratory Information System (NFLIS) is a database that collects data on analyzed drug seizures from federal, state and local forensic laboratories. In 2008, the NFLIS reported law enforcement submitted 1,382 exhibits of methylphenidate to state and local labs and 81 exhibits to federal labs to be analyzed.

User population: While a wide spectrum of the population has abused methylphenidate products, the primary abusers are individuals less than 25 years of age who often obtain methylphenidate from a friend or classmate and use this drug as a study aid or to party.

Illicit distribution: Unlike other potent stimulants, there is no clandestine production of methylphenidate and diverted pharmaceutical products are the only source for abuse purposes. Methylphenidate is obtained from fraudulent prescriptions, doctor shopping, pharmacy theft, and from friends or associates who have obtained the drug through a prescription.

Control status: Methylphenidate is a schedule II substance under the Controlled Substances Act.

Stimulant ADHD Medications: Methylphenidate and Amphetamines

Stimulant medications (for example, methylphenidate and amphetamines) are often prescribed to treat individuals diagnosed with attention deficit/hyperactivity disorder (ADHD). ADHD is characterized by a persistent pattern of inattention and/or hyperactivity-impulsivity that is more frequently displayed and more severe than is typically observed in individuals at a comparable level of development. This pattern of behavior usually becomes evident in the preschool or early elementary years with the median age of onset of ADHD symptoms is seven years. For many individuals, ADHD symptoms improve during adolescence or as age increases, but the disorder can persist into adulthood. In the United States, ADHD is diagnosed in an estimated eight percent of children ages 4–17 and in 2.9–4.4% of adults.[1,2,3]

How do prescription stimulants affect the brain?

All stimulants work by increasing dopamine levels in the brain—dopamine is a brain chemical (or neurotransmitter) associated with pleasure, movement, and attention. The therapeutic effect of stimulants is achieved by slow and steady increases of dopamine, which are similar to the natural production of the chemical by the brain. The doses prescribed by physicians start low and increase gradually until a therapeutic effect is reached. However, when taken in doses and routes other than those prescribed, stimulants can increase brain dopamine in a rapid and highly amplified manner—as do most other drugs of abuse—disrupting normal communication between brain cells, producing euphoria, and increasing the risk of addiction.

What is the role of stimulants in the treatment of ADHD?

Treatment of ADHD with stimulants, often in conjunction with psychotherapy, helps to improve the symptoms of ADHD, as well as the self-esteem, cognition, and social and family interactions of the patient. The most commonly prescribed medications include amphetamines (for example, Adderall®, a mix of amphetamine salts) and methylphenidate (such as, Ritalin® and Concerta®—a formulation that releases medication in the body over a period of time). These medications have a paradoxically calming and focusing effect on individuals with ADHD. Researchers speculate that because methylphenidate amplifies the release of dopamine, it can improve attention and focus in individuals who have dopamine signals that are weak.[4]

One of the most controversial issues in child psychiatry is whether the use of stimulant medications to treat ADHD increases the risk of substance abuse in adulthood. Research thus far suggests that individuals with ADHD do not become addicted to their stimulant medications when taken in the form and dosage prescribed by their doctors. Furthermore, several studies report that stimulant therapy in childhood does not increase the risk for subsequent drug and alcohol abuse disorders later in life.[5,6,7] More research is needed, however, particularly in adolescents treated with stimulant medications.

Why and how are prescription stimulants abused?

Stimulants have been abused for both performance enhancement and recreational purposes (to get high). For the former, they suppress appetite (to facilitate weight loss), increase wakefulness, and increase focus and attention. The euphoric effects of stimulants usually occur when they are crushed and then snorted or injected. Some abusers dissolve the tablets in water and inject the mixture. Complications from this method of use can arise because insoluble fillers in the tablets can block small blood vessels.

What adverse effect does prescription stimulant abuse have on health?

Stimulants can increase blood pressure, heart rate, body temperature, and decrease sleep and appetite, which can lead to malnutrition and its consequences. Repeated use of stimulants can lead to feelings of hostility and paranoia. At high doses, they can lead to serious cardiovascular complications, including stroke.

Addiction to stimulants is also a very real consideration for anyone taking them without medical supervision. This most likely occurs because stimulants, when taken in doses and routes other than those prescribed by a doctor, can induce a rapid rise in dopamine in the brain. Furthermore, if stimulants are used chronically, withdrawal symptoms—including fatigue, depression, and disturbed sleep patterns—can emerge when the drugs are discontinued.

End Notes

1. Centers for Disease Control and Prevention. Mental health in the United States. Prevalence of diagnosis and medication treatment for attention-deficit/hyperactivity disorder–United States, 2003. *Morb Mortal Wkly Rep* 54:842–847, 2005.

2. Kessler RC, Adler L, Barkley R, et al. The prevalence and correlates of adult ADHD in the United States: results from the National Comorbidity Survey Replication. *Am J Psychiatry* 163:716–723, 2006.

3. Faraone SV, Biederman J. *Prevalence of adult ADHD in the United States*. Paper presented at the American Psychiatric Association annual meeting, New York, 2008.

4. Volkow ND, Fowler JS, Wang G, Ding Y, Gatley SJ. Mechanism of action of methylphenidate: insights from PET imaging studies. *J Attention Disorders* 6(Suppl. 1):S31–S43, 2002.

5. Wilens TE, Faraone SV, Biederman J, Gunawardene S. Does stimulant therapy of attention-deficit/hyperactivity disorder beget later substance abuse? A meta-analytic review of the literature. *Pediatrics* 111:179–185, 2003.

6. Mannuzza S, Klein RG, Truong NL, et al. Age of methylphenidate treatment initiation in children with ADHD and later substance abuse: prospective follow-up into adulthood.

Am J Psychiatry 165(5):604–609, 2008. Epub April 1, 2008. Available at: http://www.ncbi.nlm.nih.gov/pubmed/18381904?dopt=Abstract.

7. Biederman J, Monuteaux MC, Spencer T, Wilens TE, MacPherson HA, Faraone SV. Stimulant therapy and risk for subsequent substance use disorders in male adults with ADHD: a naturalistic controlled 10-year follow-up study. *Am J Psychiatry* 165(5):597-603, 2008. Epub March 3, 2008. Available at: http://ajp.psychiatryonline.org/cgi/content/abstract/appi.ajp.2007.07091486v1.

Chapter 43

Salvia Divinorum *and*
Salvinorin A

Drug name: *Salvia divinorum* and salvinorin A

Street names: Maria Pastora, sage of the seers, diviner's sage, salvia, Sally-D, magic mint

Introduction: *Salvia divinorum* is a perennial herb in the mint family native to certain areas of the Sierra Mazateca region of Oaxaca, Mexico. The plant, which can grow to over three feet in height, has large green leaves, hollow square stems, and white flowers with purple calyces, can also be grown successfully outside of this region. *Salvia divinorum* has been used by the Mazatec Indians for its ritual divination and healing. The active constituent of *Salvia divinorum* has been identified as salvinorin A. Currently, neither *Salvia divinorum* nor any of its constituents, including salvinorin A, are controlled under the federal Controlled Substances Act (CSA).

Licit uses: Neither *Salvia divinorum* nor its active constituent salvinorin A has an approved medical use in the United States (U.S.).

Chemistry and pharmacology: Salvinorin A, also called divinorin A, is believed to be the ingredient responsible for the hallucinogenic effects of *Salvia divinorum*. Chemically, it is a neoclerodane

"*Salvia Divinorum* and Salvinorin A," Drug Enforcement Administration (DEA), November 2008.

diterpene found primarily in the leaves, and to a lesser extent in the stems. Although several other substances have been isolated from the plant, none have been shown to be psychoactive.

In the U.S., plant material is typically either chewed or smoked. When chewed, the leaf mass and juice are maintained within the cheek area with absorption occurring across the lining of the oral mucosa (buccal). Effects first appear within 5–10 minutes. Dried leaves, as well as extract-enhanced leaves purported to be enriched with salvinorin A, are also smoked. Smoking pure salvinorin A, at a dose of 200–500 micrograms, results in effects within 30 seconds and lasts about 30 minutes.

A limited number of studies have reported the effects of using either plant material or salvinorin A. Psychic effects include perceptions of bright lights, vivid colors and shapes, as well as body movements, and body or object distortions. Other effects include dysphoria, uncontrolled laughter, a sense of loss of body, overlapping realities, and hallucinations (seeing objects that are not present). Adverse physical effects may include incoordination, dizziness, and slurred speech.

Scientific studies show that salvinorin A is a potent and selective kappa opioid receptor agonist. Other drugs that act at the kappa opioid receptor also produce hallucinogenic effects and dysphoria similar to that produced by salvinorin A. Salvinorin A does not activate the serotonin 2A receptor, which mediates the effects of other schedule I hallucinogens.

Illicit uses: Salvinorin A and *Salvia divinorum* products are abused for their ability to evoke hallucinogenic effects, which, in general, are similar to those of other scheduled hallucinogenic substances.

User population: According to a National Survey on Drug Use and Health Report published by Substance Abuse and Mental Health Services Administration (SAMHSA) in February 2008, it is estimated that 1.8 million persons aged 12 or older used *Salvia divinorum* in their lifetime, and approximately 750,000 did so in the past year. Use was more common among young adults (18 to 25 years old) as opposed to older adults (those over 26 years of age). Young adults were three times more likely than youths aged 12–17 to have used *Salvia divinorum* in the past year. Use is more common in males than females.

Illicit distribution: *Salvia divinorum* is grown domestically and imported from Mexico and Central and South America. The internet is used for the promotion and distribution of *Salvia divinorum*. It is sold as seeds, plant cuttings, whole plants, fresh and dried leaves, extract-enhanced leaves of various strengths (for example, 5 times [x], 10x, 20x, 30x), and liquid extracts purported to contain salvinorin A. These products are also sold at local shops (such as head shops and tobacco shops).

Control status: *Salvia divinorum* and salvinorin A are not currently controlled under the CSA. However, a number of states have placed controls on *Salvia divinorum* and/or salvinorin A. As of November 2008, thirteen states have enacted legislation placing regulatory controls on *Salvia divinorum* and/or salvinorin A. Delaware, Florida, Illinois, Kansas, Mississippi, Missouri, North Dakota, Oklahoma, and Virginia have placed *Salvia divinorum* and/or salvinorin A into schedule I of state law. California, Louisiana, Maine and Tennessee enacted other forms of legislation restricting the distribution of the plant. States in which legislative bills proposing regulatory controls died are Alabama, Alaska, Hawaii, Indiana, Iowa, Minnesota, Nebraska, Oregon, South Carolina, and Utah. Legislative bills proposing regulatory controls are pending in Michigan, New Jersey, New York, Ohio, Pennsylvania, Texas and Wisconsin.

Salvinorin A and/or *Salvia divinorum* have been placed under regulatory controls in Australia, Belgium, Denmark, Estonia, Finland, Italy, Japan, Spain, and Sweden.

Chapter 44

Spirals

Drug name: Alpha-methyltryptamine (AMT)

Street name: Spirals

Introduction: Alpha-methyltryptamine (AMT) is a tryptamine derivative and shares many pharmacological similarities with those of schedule I hallucinogens such as alpha-ethyltryptamine, N,N-dimethyltryptamine, psilocybin, and lysergic acid diethylamide (LSD). Since 1999, there has been a growing popularity of AMT among drug abusers for its hallucinogenic-like effects. In the 1960s, following extensive clinical studies on AMT as a possible antidepressant drug, the Upjohn Company concluded that AMT was a toxic substance that produces psychosis.

Licit uses: AMT has no approved medical uses in the United States.

Chemistry and pharmacology: AMT is a tryptamine (indolethylamine) derivative. The hydrochloride salt of AMT is a white crystalline powder. AMT, similar to several schedule I hallucinogens, binds with moderate affinities to serotonin (5-HT) receptors (5-HT1 and 5-HT2). AMT inhibits the uptake of monoamines especially 5-HT and is a potent inhibitor of monoamine oxidase (MAO) (especially MAO-A),

---

"Alpha-Methyltryptamine," Drug Enforcement Administration (DEA), June 2009.

an enzyme critical for the metabolic degradation of monoamines, the brain chemicals important for sensory, emotional, and other behavioral functions. AMT has been shown to produce locomotor stimulant effects in animals. It has been hypothesized that both 5-HT and dopamine systems mediate the stimulant effects of AMT. In animals, AMT produces behavioral effects that are substantially similar to those of 1-(2,5-dimethoxy-4-methylphenyl)-2-aminopropane (DOM) and methylene-dioxymethamphetamine (MDMA), both schedule I hallucinogens, in animals.

In humans, AMT elicits subjective effects including hallucinations. It has an onset of action of about 3–4 hours and duration of about 12–24 hours, but may produce an extended duration of two days in some subjects. Subjects report uncomfortable feelings, muscular tension, nervous tension, irritability, restlessness, unsettled feeling in stomach, and the inability to relax and sleep. AMT can alter sensory perception and judgment and can pose serious health risks to the user and the general public. Abuse of AMT led to two emergency department admissions and one death. AMT increases blood pressure and heart rate and dilates pupils, causes deep tendon reflexes, and impairs coordination.

Illicit uses: AMT is abused for its hallucinogenic effects and is used as substitute for MDMA. It is often administered orally as either powder or capsules at doses ranging from 15–40 milligrams. Other routes of administration include smoking and snorting.

User population: Youth and young adults are the main abusers of AMT. Internet websites are a source that high school students and United States soldiers have used to obtain and abuse AMT.

Illicit distribution: According to the System to Retrieve Information from Drug Evidence (STRIDE) data, first recorded submission by law enforcement to Drug Enforcement Administration (DEA) laboratories of a drug exhibit containing AMT occurred in 1999. Following federal control of AMT as a schedule I substance in 2003, number of AMT encounters by law enforcement as reported in STRIDE decreased.

According to the National Forensic Laboratory Information System (NFLIS), law enforcement officials seized and submitted six AMT drug items in 2004 and one item in 2005 to federal laboratories. There were no recorded submissions from 2006 to 2008 for federal laboratories. In the past five years, there were four AMT drug items submitted to state and local laboratories. Two items were submitted in

2007 and no AMT items were submitted in 2008. AMT has been illicitly available from United States and foreign chemical companies and from internet websites. Additionally, there is evidence of attempted clandestine production of AMT.

Control status: The Drug Enforcement Administration (DEA) placed AMT temporarily in schedule I of the Controlled Substances Act (CSA) on April 4, 2003, pursuant to the temporary scheduling provisions of the CSA (68 FR 16427). On September 29, 2004, AMT was controlled as a schedule I substance under the CSA (69 FR 58050).

Chapter 45

Toonies (Nexus)

Drug name: 4-bromo-2,5-dimethoxyphenethylamine

Street names: 2C-B, Nexus, 2's, toonies, bromo, spectrum, venus

Introduction: 4-bromo-2,5-dimethoxyphenethylamine (2C-B, 4-bromo-2,5-DMPEA) is a synthetic schedule I hallucinogen. It is abused for its hallucinogenic effects primarily as a club drug in the rave culture and circuit party scene.

Licit uses: 2C-B has no approved medical uses in the United States.

Chemistry and pharmacology: 4-Bromo-2,5-dimethoxyphenethylamine is closely related to the phenylisopropylamine hallucinogen 1-(4-bromo-2, 5-dimethoxyphenyl)-2-aminopropane (DOB) and is referred to as alpha-desmethyl DOB. 2C-B produces effects similar to 2,5-dimethoxy-4-methylamphetamine (DOM) and DOB. 2C-B displays high affinity for central serotonin receptors. 2C-B produces dose dependent psychoactive effects. Threshold effects are noted at approximately four milligrams (mg) of an oral dose; the user becomes passive and relaxed and is aware of an integration of sensory perception with emotional states. There is euphoria with increased body awareness and enhanced receptiveness of visual,

---

"4-Bromo-2,5-Dimethoxyphenethylamine" Drug Enforcement Administration (DEA), June 2009.

auditory, olfactory, and tactile sensation. Oral doses of 8–10 mg produce stimulant effects and cause a full intoxicated state. Doses in the range of 20–40 mg produce lysergic acid diethylamide (LSD)-like hallucinations. Doses greater than 50 mg have produced extremely fearful hallucinations and morbid delusions. Onset of subjective effects following 2C-B ingestion is between 20–30 minutes with peak effects occurring at 1.5–2 hours. Effects of 2C-B can last up to eight hours.

Radioimmunoassay detection system that is commonly used for testing amphetamine and hallucinogens does not detect 2C-B. In the Marquis Reagent Field Test-902, 2C-B produces a bright green color. 2C-B is the only known drug to produce a bright green color when using this test.

Illicit uses: 2C-B is abused for its hallucinogenic effects. 2C-B is abused orally in tablet or capsule forms or snorted in its powder form. The drug has been misrepresented by distributors and sold as other hallucinogens such as MDMA and LSD. Some user's abuse 2C-B in combination with LSD (referred to as a banana split) or MDMA (called a party pack).

User population: 2C-B is used by the same population as those using Ecstasy and other club drugs, high school and college students, and other young adults who frequent rave or techno parties.

Illicit distribution: 2C-B is distributed as tablets, capsules or in powder form. Usually sold as MDMA, a single dosage unit of 2C-B typically sells for $10 to $30 per tablet. The illicit source of 2C-B currently available on the street has not been identified by Drug Enforcement Administration (DEA). Prior to its control, DEA seized both clandestine laboratories and illicit repacking shops. As the name implies, these shops would repackage and reformulate the doses of the tablets prior to illicit sales.

According to the System to Retrieve Information from Drug Evidence (STRIDE) data, the first recorded submission by law enforcement to DEA forensic laboratories of a drug exhibit containing 2C-B occurred in 1986.

The National Forensic Laboratory Information System (NFLIS) database reports an increase of 2C-B items/exhibits submitted to federal, state, and local forensic laboratories, from nine in 2004 to 49 in 2008. According to NFLIS, 2C-B has been seized in a number of states including Arkansas, Alabama, California, Florida, Iowa, Illinois, Kansas,

Kentucky, Minnesota, Missouri, Nevada, New York, North Carolina, Ohio, Oregon, Pennsylvania, South Carolina, South Dakota, Texas, Virginia, Washington, and Wyoming.

Control status: The Drug Enforcement Administration placed 2C-B in schedule I of the Controlled Substances Act (CSA).

Part Three

The Causes and
Consequences of
Drug Abuse and Addiction

Chapter 46

Understanding Drug Abuse and Addiction

Many people do not understand why individuals become addicted to drugs or how drugs change the brain to foster compulsive drug abuse. They mistakenly view drug abuse and addiction as strictly a social problem and may characterize those who take drugs as morally weak. One very common belief is that drug abusers should be able to just stop taking drugs if they are only willing to change their behavior. What people often underestimate is the complexity of drug addiction—that it is a disease that impacts the brain and because of that, stopping drug abuse is not simply a matter of willpower. Through scientific advances we now know much more about how exactly drugs work in the brain, and we also know that drug addiction can be successfully treated to help people stop abusing drugs and resume their productive lives.

Drug abuse and addiction are a major burden to society. Estimates of the total overall costs of substance abuse in the United States—including health- and crime-related costs as well as losses in productivity—exceed half a trillion dollars annually. This includes approximately $181 billion for illicit drugs, $168 billion for tobacco, and $185 billion for alcohol. Staggering as these numbers are, however, they do not fully describe the breadth of deleterious public health—and safety—implications, which include family disintegration, loss of employment, failure in school, domestic violence, child abuse, and other crimes.

This chapter includes text from "Understanding Drug Abuse and Addiction," National Institute on Drug Abuse (NIDA), July 27, 2009; and excerpts from "NIDA Frequently Asked Questions," NIDA, July 31, 2009.

What is drug addiction?

Addiction is a chronic, often relapsing brain disease that causes compulsive drug seeking and use despite harmful consequences to the individual who is addicted and to those around them. Drug addiction is a brain disease because the abuse of drugs leads to changes in the structure and function of the brain. Although it is true that for most people the initial decision to take drugs is voluntary, over time the changes in the brain caused by repeated drug abuse can affect a person's self control and ability to make sound decisions, and at the same time send intense impulses to take drugs.

It is because of these changes in the brain that it is so challenging for a person who is addicted to stop abusing drugs. Fortunately, there are treatments that help people to counteract addiction's powerful disruptive effects and regain control. Research shows that combining addiction treatment medications, if available, with behavioral therapy is the best way to ensure success for most patients. Treatment approaches that are tailored to each patient's drug abuse patterns and any co-occurring medical, psychiatric, and social problems can lead to sustained recovery and a life without drug abuse.

Similar to other chronic, relapsing diseases, such as diabetes, asthma, or heart disease, drug addiction can be managed successfully. And, as with other chronic diseases, it is not uncommon for a person to relapse and begin abusing drugs again. Relapse, however, does not signal failure—rather, it indicates that treatment should be reinstated, adjusted, or that alternate treatment is needed to help the individual regain control and recover.

What happens to your brain when you take drugs?

Drugs are chemicals that tap into the brain's communication system and disrupt the way nerve cells normally send, receive, and process information. There are at least two ways that drugs are able to do this: (1) by imitating the brain's natural chemical messengers, and/or (2) by overstimulating the reward circuit of the brain. Some drugs, such as marijuana and heroin, have a similar structure to chemical messengers, called neurotransmitters, which are naturally produced by the brain. Because of this similarity, these drugs are able to fool the brain's receptors and activate nerve cells to send abnormal messages. Other drugs, such as cocaine or methamphetamine, can cause the nerve cells to release abnormally large amounts of natural neurotransmitters, or prevent the normal recycling of these brain chemicals, which is needed to shut off the signal between neurons. This disruption produces a greatly amplified message that ultimately disrupts normal communication patterns.

Nearly all drugs, directly or indirectly, target the brain's reward system by flooding the circuit with dopamine. Dopamine is a neurotransmitter present in regions of the brain that control movement, emotion, motivation, and feelings of pleasure. The overstimulation of this system which normally responds to natural behaviors that are linked to survival (eating, spending time with loved ones, and so forth) produces euphoric effects in response to the drugs. This reaction sets in motion a pattern that teaches people to repeat the behavior of abusing drugs. As a person continues to abuse drugs, the brain adapts to the overwhelming surges in dopamine by producing less dopamine or by reducing the number of dopamine receptors in the reward circuit. As a result, dopamine's impact on the reward circuit is lessened, reducing the abuser's ability to enjoy the drugs and the things that previously brought pleasure. This decrease compels those addicted to drugs to keep abusing drugs in order to attempt to bring their dopamine function back to normal. And, they may now require larger amounts of the drug than they first did to achieve the dopamine high—an effect known as tolerance.

Long-term abuse causes changes in other brain chemical systems and circuits as well. Glutamate is a neurotransmitter that influences the reward circuit and the ability to learn. When the optimal concentration of glutamate is altered by drug abuse, the brain attempts to compensate, which can impair cognitive function. Drugs of abuse facilitate unconscious (conditioned) learning, which leads the user to experience uncontrollable cravings when they see a place or person they associate with the drug experience, even when the drug itself is not available. Brain imaging studies of drug-addicted individuals show changes in areas of the brain that are critical to judgment, decision making, learning and memory, and behavior control. Together, these changes can drive an abuser to seek out and take drugs compulsively despite adverse consequences—in other words, to become addicted to drugs.

Why do some people become addicted, while others do not?

No single factor can predict whether or not a person will become addicted to drugs. Risk for addiction is influenced by a person's biology, social environment, and age or stage of development. The more risk factors an individual has, the greater the chance that taking drugs can lead to addiction. For example:

- **Biology:** The genes that people are born with—in combination with environmental influences—account for about half of their addiction vulnerability. Additionally, gender, ethnicity, and the presence of other mental disorders may influence risk for drug abuse and addiction.

- **Environment:** A person's environment includes many different influences—from family and friends to socioeconomic status and quality of life in general. Factors such as peer pressure, physical and sexual abuse, stress, and parental involvement can greatly influence the course of drug abuse and addiction in a person's life.

- **Development:** Genetic and environmental factors interact with critical developmental stages in a person's life to affect addiction vulnerability, and adolescents experience a double challenge. Although taking drugs at any age can lead to addiction, the earlier that drug use begins, the more likely it is to progress to more serious abuse. And because adolescents' brains are still developing in the areas that govern decision making, judgment, and self-control, they are especially prone to risk-taking behaviors, including trying drugs of abuse.

Prevention Is the Key

Drug addiction is a preventable disease. Results from National Institute on Drug Abuse (NIDA)-funded research have shown that prevention programs that involve families, schools, communities, and the media are effective in reducing drug abuse. Although many events and cultural factors affect drug abuse trends, when youths perceive drug abuse as harmful, they reduce their drug taking. It is necessary, therefore, to help youth and the general public to understand the risks of drug abuse, and for teachers, parents, and healthcare professionals to keep sending the message that drug addiction can be prevented if a person never abuses drugs.

Frequently Asked Questions

How quickly can I become addicted to a drug?

There is no easy answer to this. If and how quickly you might become addicted to a drug depends on many factors including the biology of your body. All drugs are potentially harmful and may have life-threatening consequences associated with their abuse. There are also vast differences among individuals in sensitivity to various drugs. While one person may use a drug one or many times and suffer no ill effects, another person may be particularly vulnerable and overdose with first use. There is no way of knowing in advance how someone may react.

How do I know if someone is addicted to drugs?

If a person is compulsively seeking and using a drug despite negative consequences, such as loss of job, debt, physical problems brought on by drug abuse, or family problems, then he or she probably is addicted. Seek professional help to determine if this is the case and, if so, the appropriate treatment.

What are the physical signs of abuse or addiction?

The physical signs of abuse or addiction can vary depending on the person and the drug being abused. For example, someone who abuses marijuana may have a chronic cough or worsening of asthmatic symptoms. Each drug has short-term and long-term physical effects. Stimulants like cocaine increase heart rate and blood pressure, whereas opioids like heroin may slow the heart rate and reduce respiration.

Are there effective treatments for drug addiction?

Drug addiction can be effectively treated with behavioral-based therapies and, for addiction to some drugs such as heroin or nicotine, medications. Treatment will vary for each person depending on the type of drug(s) being used, and multiple courses of treatment may be needed to achieve success. For referrals to treatment programs:

Substance Abuse and Mental Health Services Administration (SAMHSA)
Toll-Free: 800-662-HELP (4357)
Website: http://findtreatment.samhsa.gov

Chapter 47

Factors That Impact Drug Abuse and Addiction

Drugs, Brains, and Behavior

In general, people begin taking drugs for a variety of reasons:

- **To feel good:** Most abused drugs produce intense feelings of pleasure. This initial sensation of euphoria is followed by other effects, which differ with the type of drug used. For example, with stimulants such as cocaine, the high is followed by feelings of power, self-confidence, and increased energy. In contrast, the euphoria caused by opiates such as heroin is followed by feelings of relaxation and satisfaction.

- **To feel better:** Some people who suffer from social anxiety, stress-related disorders, and depression begin abusing drugs in an attempt to lessen feelings of distress. Stress can play a major role in beginning drug use, continuing drug abuse, or relapse in patients recovering from addiction.

- **To do better:** The increasing pressure that some individuals feel to chemically enhance or improve their athletic or cognitive performance can similarly play a role in initial experimentation and continued drug abuse.

This chapter includes text from "Drugs, Brains, and Behavior: The Science of Addiction (Part I)," National Institute on Drug Abuse (NIDA), April 2007; excerpts from "Genetics of Addiction," NIDA, April 2008; and text from "Stress and Substance Abuse," NIDA, February 2006.

- **Curiosity and because others are doing it:** In this respect adolescents are particularly vulnerable because of the strong influence of peer pressure; they are more likely, for example, to engage in thrilling and daring behaviors.

The initial decision to take drugs is mostly voluntary. However, when drug abuse takes over, a person's ability to exert self control can become seriously impaired. Brain imaging studies from drug-addicted individuals show physical changes in areas of the brain that are critical to judgment, decision making, learning and memory, and behavior control. Scientists believe that these changes alter the way the brain works, and may help explain the compulsive and destructive behaviors of addiction.

Table 47.1. Examples of Risk and Protective Factors

Risk Factors	Domain	Protective Factors
Early aggressive behavior	Individual	Self-control
Poor social skills	Individual	Positive relationships
Lack of parental supervision	Family	Parental monitoring and support
Substance abuse	Peer	Academic competence
Drug availability	School	Anti-drug use policies
Poverty	Community	Strong neighborhood attachment

Why do some people become addicted to drugs, while others do not?

As with any other disease, vulnerability to addiction differs from person to person. In general, the more risk factors an individual has, the greater the chance that taking drugs will lead to abuse and addiction. Protective factors reduce a person's risk of developing addiction.

No single factor determines whether a person will become addicted to drugs. The overall risk for addiction is impacted by the biological makeup of the individual—it can even be influenced by gender or ethnicity, his or her developmental stage, and the surrounding social environment (for example, conditions at home, at school, and in the neighborhood).

Scientists estimate that genetic factors account for between 40 and 60% of a person's vulnerability to addiction, including the effects of environment on gene expression and function. Adolescents and individuals with mental disorders are at greater risk of drug abuse and addiction than the general population.

Environment factors that increase the risk of addiction include the following:

- **Home and family:** The influence of the home environment is usually most important in childhood. Parents or older family members who abuse alcohol or drugs, or who engage in criminal behavior, can increase children's risks of developing their own drug problems.

- **Peers and school:** Friends and acquaintances have the greatest influence during adolescence. Drug-abusing peers can sway even those without risk factors to try drugs for the first time. Academic failure or poor social skills can put a child further at risk for drug abuse.

What other factors increase the risk of addiction?

Early use: Although taking drugs at any age can lead to addiction, research shows that the earlier a person begins to use drugs the more likely they are to progress to more serious abuse. This may reflect the harmful effect that drugs can have on the developing brain; it also may result from a constellation of early biological and social vulnerability factors, including genetic susceptibility, mental illness, unstable family relationships, and exposure to physical or sexual abuse. Still, the fact remains that early use is a strong indicator of problems ahead, among them, substance abuse and addiction.

Method of administration: Smoking a drug or injecting it into a vein increases its addictive potential. Both smoked and injected drugs enter the brain within seconds, producing a powerful rush of pleasure. However, this intense high can fade within a few minutes, taking the abuser down to lower, more normal levels. It is a starkly felt contrast, and scientists believe that this low feeling drives individuals to repeated drug abuse in an attempt to recapture the high pleasurable state.

Brain development: The brain continues to develop into adulthood and undergoes dramatic changes during adolescence. One of the brain areas still maturing during adolescence is the prefrontal cortex—the part of the brain that enables us to assess situations, make sound decisions, and keep our emotions and desires under control. The fact that this critical part of an adolescent's brain is still a work-in-progress puts them at increased risk for poor decisions (such as trying drugs or continued abuse). Thus, introducing drugs while the brain is still developing may have profound and long-lasting consequences.

Genetics: The Blueprint of Health and Disease

Why do some people become addicted, while others do not? Studies of identical twins indicate that as much as half of an individual's risk of becoming addicted to nicotine, alcohol, or other drugs depends on his or her genes. Pinning down the biological basis for this risk is an important avenue of research for scientists trying to solve the problem of drug abuse.

Genes—functional units that make up our deoxyribonucleic acid (DNA)—provide the information that directs our bodies' basic cellular activities. Research on the human genome has shown that the DNA sequences of any two individuals are 99.9% identical. However, that 0.1% variation is profoundly important, contributing to visible differences, like height and hair color, and to invisible differences, such as increased risks for, or protection from, heart attack, stroke, diabetes, and addiction.

What role does the environment play in a disease like addiction?

That old saying "nature or nurture" might be better phrased "nature and nurture," because research shows that individual health is the result of dynamic interactions between genes and environmental conditions. For example, susceptibility to high blood pressure is influenced by both genetics and lifestyle, including diet, stress, and exercise. Environmental influences, such as exposure to drugs or stress, can alter both gene expression and gene function. In some cases, these effects may persist throughout a person's life. Research suggests that genes can also influence how a person responds to his or her environment, placing some individuals at higher risk than others.

Research advance: A recent study highlights the complex interactions between genetics, drug exposure, and age of use in the risk of developing a mental disorder. The COMT gene produces an enzyme that regulates dopamine, a brain chemical involved in schizophrenia.

COMT comes in two forms: Met and Val. Individuals with one or two copies of the Val variant have a higher risk of developing symptoms of psychosis and schizophrenic-type disorders if they used cannabis during adolescence.

The promise of personalized medicine: The emerging science of pharmacogenomics promises to harness the power of genomic information to improve treatments for addiction. Clinicians often find substantial variability in how individual patients respond to treatment. Part of that variability is due to genetics. Genes influence the numbers and types of receptors in our brains, how quickly our bodies metabolize drugs, and how well we respond to different medications.

A National Institute on Drug Abuse (NIDA)-sponsored study of alcohol dependent patients treated with naltrexone found that patients with a specific variant in an opioid receptor gene, Asp40, had a significantly lower rate of relapse (26.1%) than patients with the Asn40 variant (47.9%). In the future, identifying which mu-opioid receptor gene variant a patient possesses may help predict the most effective choice of medication for alcohol addiction.

Stress and Substance Abuse

Stress is a term that is hard to define because it means different things to different people. Stress is a normal occurrence in life for people of all ages. The body responds to stress in order to protect itself from emotional or physical distress or, in extreme situations, from danger. What is stressful for one person may or may not be stressful for another, and each of us responds to stress in different ways. How a person copes with stress—by reaching for a beer or cigarette or by heading to the gym—also plays an important role in the impact that stress will have on our bodies. By using their own support systems, some people are able to cope effectively with the emotional and physical demands brought on by stressful and traumatic experiences. However, individuals who experience prolonged reactions to stress that disrupt their daily functioning may require treatment by a trained and experienced mental health professional.

The Body's Response to Stress

The stress response is mediated by a highly complex, integrated network that involves the central nervous system, the adrenal system, the immune system, and the cardiovascular system. Stress activates adaptive responses. It releases the neurotransmitter norepinephrine, which is involved in memory. Stress also increases the release of a hormone known as corticotropin-releasing factor (CRF). CRF is found throughout the brain and initiates our biological response to stressors. During all stressful experiences, certain regions of the brain show increased levels of CRF. Interestingly, almost all drugs of abuse have also been found to increase CRF levels, suggesting a neurobiological connection between stress and drug abuse.

Stress and Substance Abuse

Stressful events can profoundly influence the abuse of alcohol or other drugs. Stress is a major contributor to the initiation and continuation of alcohol or other drug abuse, as well as to substance abuse relapse after periods of abstinence. Children exposed to severe stress may be more vulnerable to drug abuse. A number of clinical and epidemiological studies show a strong association between psychosocial stressors early in life (for example, parental loss or child abuse) and an increased risk for depression, anxiety, impulsive behavior, and substance abuse in adulthood.

Stress, Drugs, and Vulnerable Populations

Stressful experiences increase the vulnerability of an individual to relapse to drug use, even after prolonged abstinence. Individuals who have achieved abstinence from drugs must continue to sustain their abstinence by avoiding environmental triggers, recognizing their psychosocial and emotional triggers, and developing healthy behaviors to handle life's stresses. A number of relapse prevention approaches have been developed to help clinicians address relapse. Treatment techniques that foster coping skills, problem solving skills, and social support play a role in successful treatment. Physicians should be aware of which medications their patients are taking. Some people may need medications for stress-related symptoms or for treatment of depression and anxiety.

Post-Traumatic Stress Disorder (PTSD) and Substance Abuse

Post-traumatic stress disorder (PTSD) is an anxiety disorder that can develop in some people after exposure to a terrifying event or ordeal in which grave physical harm occurred or was threatened. Emerging research has documented a strong association between PTSD and substance abuse. In some cases, substance use begins after the exposure to trauma and the development of PTSD, thus making PTSD a risk factor for drug abuse.

Early intervention to help children and adolescents who have suffered trauma from violence or a disaster is critical. Children who witness or are exposed to a traumatic event and are clinically diagnosed with PTSD have a greater likelihood for developing later drug and/or alcohol use disorders. Among individuals with substance use disorders, 30 to 60% meet the criteria for comorbid PTSD. Patients with substance use disorders tend to suffer from more severe PTSD symptoms than do PTSD patients without substance use disorders.

Helping Those Who Suffer from PTSD and Drug Abuse

Healthcare professionals must be alert to the fact that PTSD frequently co-occurs with depression, other anxiety disorders, and alcohol and other substance abuse. Patients who are experiencing the symptoms of PTSD need support from physicians and healthcare providers to develop coping skills and reduce substance abuse risk. The likelihood of treatment success increases when these concurrent disorders are appropriately identified and treated. For substance abuse there are effective medications and behavioral therapies. For symptoms of PTSD, some antianxiety and antidepressant medications may be useful.

Several behavioral treatments can help individuals who suffer from PTSD. Improvements have been shown with some forms of group therapy and with cognitive-behavioral therapy, especially when it includes an exposure component for trauma victims. Exposure therapy allows patients to gradually and repeatedly re-experience the frightening event(s) under controlled conditions to help them work through the trauma. Exposure therapy is thought to be one of the most effective ways to manage PTSD, when it is conducted by a trained therapist. Treatment of patients with comorbid PTSD and addictions will vary, and for some patients, successful treatment may require initial inpatient hospitalization. Finally, support from family and friends can play an important role in recovery from both disorders.

Chapter 48

How Drugs Affect the Brain

The human brain is the most complex organ in the body. This three-pound mass of gray and white matter sits at the center of all human activity—you need it to drive a car, to enjoy a meal, to breathe, to create an artistic masterpiece, and to enjoy everyday activities. In brief, the brain regulates your basic body functions; enables you to interpret and respond to everything you experience; and shapes your thoughts, emotions, and behavior. The brain is made up of many parts that all work together as a team. Different parts of the brain are responsible for coordinating and performing specific functions. Drugs can alter important brain areas that are necessary for life-sustaining functions and can drive the compulsive drug abuse that marks addiction. Brain areas affected by drug abuse include the following:

- The brain stem controls basic functions critical to life, such as heart rate, breathing, and sleeping.

- The limbic system contains the brain's reward circuit—it links together a number of brain structures that control and regulate our ability to feel pleasure. Feeling pleasure motivates us to repeat behaviors such as eating—actions that are critical to our existence. The limbic system is activated when we perform these activities— and also by drugs of abuse. In addition, the limbic system is responsible for our perception of other emotions, both

Text in this chapter is from "Drugs, Brains, and Behavior: The Science of Addiction (Part III)," National Institute on Drug Abuse (NIDA), April 2007.

positive and negative, which explains the mood-altering properties of many drugs.

- The cerebral cortex is divided into areas that control specific functions. Different areas process information from our senses, enabling us to see, feel, hear, and taste. The front part of the cortex, the frontal cortex or forebrain, is the thinking center of the brain; it powers our ability to think, plan, solve problems, and make decisions.

How do drugs work in the brain?

Drugs are chemicals. They work in the brain by tapping into the brain's communication system and interfering with the way nerve cells normally send, receive, and process information. Some drugs, such as marijuana and heroin, can activate neurons because their chemical structure mimics that of a natural neurotransmitter. This similarity in structure fools receptors and allows the drugs to lock onto and activate the nerve cells. Although these drugs mimic brain chemicals, they don't activate nerve cells in the same way as a natural neurotransmitter, and they lead to abnormal messages being transmitted through the network.

Other drugs, such as amphetamine or cocaine, can cause the nerve cells to release abnormally large amounts of natural neurotransmitters or prevent the normal recycling of these brain chemicals. This disruption produces a greatly amplified message, ultimately disrupting communication channels. The difference in effect can be described as the difference between someone whispering into your ear and someone shouting into a microphone.

How do drugs work in the brain to produce pleasure?

All drugs of abuse directly or indirectly target the brain's reward system by flooding the circuit with dopamine. Dopamine is a neurotransmitter present in regions of the brain that regulate movement, emotion, cognition, motivation, and feelings of pleasure. The overstimulation of this system, which rewards our natural behaviors, produces the euphoric effects sought by people who abuse drugs and teaches them to repeat the behavior.

Our brains are wired to ensure that we will repeat life-sustaining activities by associating those activities with pleasure or reward. Whenever this reward circuit is activated, the brain notes that something important is happening that needs to be remembered, and teaches us to do it again and again, without thinking about it. Because drugs of abuse stimulate the same circuit, we learn to abuse drugs in the same way.

Why are drugs more addictive than natural rewards?

When some drugs of abuse are taken, they can release 2–10 times the amount of dopamine that natural rewards do. In some cases, this occurs almost immediately (as when drugs are smoked or injected), and the effects can last much longer than those produced by natural rewards. The resulting effects on the brain's pleasure circuit dwarfs those produced by naturally rewarding behaviors such as eating and sex. The effect of such a powerful reward strongly motivates people to take drugs again and again. This is why scientists sometimes say that drug abuse is something we learn to do very, very well.

Just as we turn down the volume on a radio that is too loud, the brain adjusts to the overwhelming surges in dopamine (and other neurotransmitters) by producing less dopamine or by reducing the number of receptors that can receive and transmit signals. As a result, dopamine's impact on the reward circuit of a drug abuser's brain can become abnormally low, and the ability to experience any pleasure is reduced. This is why the abuser eventually feels flat, lifeless, and depressed, and is unable to enjoy things that previously brought them pleasure. Now, they need to take drugs just to bring their dopamine function back up to normal. And, they must take larger amounts of the drug than they first did to create the dopamine high—an effect known as tolerance.

How does long-term drug taking affect brain circuits?

We know that the same sort of mechanisms involved in the development of tolerance can eventually lead to profound changes in neurons and brain circuits, with the potential to severely compromise the long-term health of the brain. For example, glutamate is another neurotransmitter that influences the reward circuit and the ability to learn. When the optimal concentration of glutamate is altered by drug abuse, the brain attempts to compensate for this change, which can cause impairment in cognitive function. Similarly, long-term drug abuse can trigger adaptations in habit or unconscious memory systems. Conditioning is one example of this type of learning, whereby environmental cues become associated with the drug experience and can trigger uncontrollable cravings if the individual is later exposed to these cues, even without the drug itself being available. This learned reflex is extremely robust and can emerge even after many years of abstinence.

Chronic exposure to drugs of abuse disrupts the way critical brain structures interact to control behavior—behavior specifically related to drug abuse. Just as continued abuse may lead to tolerance or the need for higher drug dosages to produce an effect, it may also lead to addiction, which can drive an abuser to seek out and take drugs compulsively. Drug addiction erodes a person's self-control and ability to make sound decisions, while sending intense impulses to take drugs.

Chapter 49

Uses and Effects of Drugs That Are Abused

The Controlled Substances Act (CSA) regulates five classes of drugs: narcotics, depressants, stimulants, hallucinogens, and anabolic steroids. Each class has distinguishing properties, and drugs within each class often produce similar effects. However, all controlled substances, regardless of class, share a number of common features.

All controlled substances have abuse potential or are immediate precursors to substances with abuse potential. With the exception of anabolic steroids, controlled substances are abused to alter mood, thought, and feeling through their actions on the central nervous system (brain and spinal cord). Some of these drugs alleviate pain, anxiety, or depression. Some induce sleep and others energize. Though therapeutically useful, the feel good effects of these drugs contribute to their abuse. The extent to which a substance is reliably capable of producing intensely pleasurable feelings (euphoria) increases the likelihood of that substance being abused.

When drugs are used in a manner or amount inconsistent with the medical or social patterns of a culture, it is called drug abuse. In legal terms, the non-sanctioned use of substances controlled in schedules I through V of the CSA is considered drug abuse. While legal pharmaceuticals placed under control in the CSA are prescribed and used by patients for medical treatment, the use of these same pharmaceuticals outside the scope of sound medical practice is drug abuse.

Excerpted from "Drugs of Abuse/Uses and Effects," U.S. Department of Justice, 2005.

Table 49.1. Drugs of Abuse/Uses and Effects

Drugs	Medical Uses	Physical Dependence	Psychological Dependence	Tolerance	Possible Effects	Effects of Overdose
Narcotics						
Heroin	None in U.S., analgesic, antitussive	High	High	Yes	Euphoria, drowsiness, respiratory depression, constricted pupils, nausea	Slow and shallow breathing, clammy skin, convulsions, coma, possible death
Morphine	Analgesic	High	High	Yes		
Hydrocodone	Analgesic, antitussive	High	High	Yes		
Hydromorphone	Analgesic	High	High	Yes		
Oxycodone	Analgesic	High	High	Yes		
Codeine	Analgesic, antitussive	Moderate	Moderate	Yes		
Depressants						
gamma Hydroxybutyric acid	None in U.S., anesthetic	Moderate	Moderate	Yes	Slurred speech, disorientation, drunken behavior without odor of alcohol, impaired memory of events, interacts with alcohol	Shallow respiration, clammy skin, dilated pupils, weak and rapid pulse, coma, possible death
Benzodiazepines	Antianxiety, sedative, anticonvulsant, hypnotic, muscle relaxant	Moderate	Moderate	Yes		
Stimulants						
Cocaine	Local anesthetic	Possible	High	Yes	Increased alertness, excitation, euphoria, increased pulse rate and blood pressure, insomnia, loss of appetite	Agitation, increased body temperature, hallucinations, convulsions, possible death

Uses and Effects of Drugs That Are Abused

	Medical Uses	Physical Dependence	Psychological Dependence	Tolerance	Possible Effects	Effects of Overdose
Amphetamine/methamphetamine	ADHD disorder, narcolepsy, weight control	Possible	High	Yes		
Methylphenidate	ADHD disorder	Possible	High	Yes		
Hallucinogens						
MDMA and analogs	None	None	Moderate	Yes	Heightened senses, teeth grinding and dehydration	Increased body temperature, electrolyte imbalance, cardiac arrest
LSD	None	None	Unknown	Yes	Illusions and hallucinations, altered perception of time and distance	Longer more intense trip episodes
PCP and analogs	Anesthetic (ketamine)	Possible	High	Yes		Unable to direct movement, feel pain, or remember
Cannabis						
Marijuana	None	Unknown	Moderate	Yes	Euphoria, relaxed inhibitions, creased appetite, disorientation	Fatigue, paranoia, possible in psychosis
Tetrahydrocannabinol	Antinauseant, appetite stimulant	Yes	Moderate	Yes		
Hashish and hashish oil	None	Unknown	Moderate	Yes		
Anabolic steroids						
Testosterone	Hypogonadism	Unknown	Unknown	Unknown	Virilization, edema, testicular atrophy, gynecomastia, acne, aggressive behavior	Unknown
Inhalants						
Amyl and butyl nitrite	Angina (amyl)	Unknown	Unknown	No	Flushing, hypotension, headache	Methemoglobinemia
Nitrous oxide	Anesthetic	Unknown	Low	No	Impaired memory, slurred speech, drunken behavior, slow onset vitamin deficiency, organ damage	Vomiting, respiratory depression, loss of consciousness, possible death

In addition to having abuse potential, most controlled substances are capable of producing dependence, either physical or psychological. Physical dependence refers to the changes that have occurred in the body after repeated use of a drug that necessitates the continued administration of the drug to prevent a withdrawal syndrome. This withdrawal syndrome can range from mildly unpleasant to life-threatening and is dependent on a number of factors. The type of withdrawal experienced is related to: the drug being used; the dose and route of administration; concurrent use of other drugs; frequency and duration of drug use; and the age, sex, health, and genetic makeup of the user. Psychological dependence refers to the perceived need or craving for a drug. Individuals who are psychologically dependent on a particular substance often feel that they cannot function without continued use of that substance. While physical dependence disappears within days or weeks after drug use stops, psychological dependence can last much longer and is one of the primary reasons for relapse (initiation of drug use after a period of abstinence).

Contrary to common belief, physical dependence is not addiction. While addicts are usually physically dependent on the drug they are abusing, physical dependence can exist without addiction. For example, patients who take narcotics for chronic pain management or benzodiazepines to treat anxiety are likely to be physically dependent on that medication. Addiction is defined as compulsive drug-seeking behavior where acquiring and using a drug becomes the most important activity in the user's life. This definition implies a loss of control regarding drug use, and the addict will continue to use a drug despite serious medical and/or social consequences. The National Institute on Drug Abuse (NIDA) estimates that about five million Americans suffer from drug addiction.

Individuals that abuse drugs often have a preferred drug that they use, but may substitute other drugs that produce similar effects (often found in the same drug class) when they have difficulty obtaining their drug of choice. Drugs within a class are often compared with each other with terms like potency and efficacy. Potency refers to the amount of a drug that must be taken to produce a certain effect, while efficacy refers to whether or not a drug is capable of producing a given effect regardless of dose. Both the strength and the ability of a substance to produce certain effects play a role in whether that drug is selected by the drug abuser.

It is important to keep in mind that the effect produced by any drug can vary significantly and is largely dependent on the dose and route of administration. Concurrent use of other drugs can enhance or block an effect and substance abusers often take more than one drug to boost the desired effects or counter unwanted side effects. The risks associated with drug abuse cannot be accurately predicted because each user has his or her own unique sensitivity to a drug. There are a number of theories that attempt to explain these differences, and it is clear that a genetic component may predispose an individual to certain toxicities or even addictive behavior.

Youths are especially vulnerable to drug abuse. According to NIDA, young Americans engaged in extraordinary levels of illicit drug use in the last third of the twentieth century. Today, the majority of young people (about 53%) have used an illicit drug by the time they leave high school and about 25% of all seniors are current (within the past month) users. The behaviors associated with teen and preteen drug use often result in tragic consequences with untold harm to others, themselves, and their families. For example, an analysis of data from the National Household Survey on Drug Abuse indicates that youngsters between the ages of 12 and 17 who have smoked marijuana within the past year are more than twice as likely to cut class, steal, commit assault, and destroy property than are those who did not smoke marijuana. The more frequently a youth smokes marijuana, the more likely he or she is to engage in these antisocial behaviors.

Chapter 50

Misuse of Over-the-Counter Cough and Cold Medication

The cough suppressant dextromethorphan (DXM) is found in more than 140 cough and cold medications that are available without a prescription (over-the-counter or OTC) in the United States and is generally safe when taken at the recommended doses. When taken in large amounts, however, DXM can produce hallucinations or dissociative, out-of-body experiences similar to those caused by the hallucinogens phencyclidine (PCP) and ketamine and can cause other adverse health effects. Abuse of DXM among American youths aged 12 to 17 and young adults aged 18 to 25 has become a matter of concern in a number of states and metropolitan areas due to increased poison control calls involving DXM. The 2006 National Survey on Drug Use and Health (NSDUH) asks persons aged 12 or older questions related to their use of OTC cough or cold medications during their lifetime (lifetime or ever used) and the past 12 months (past year use) for the purpose of getting high (misuse).

Persons who reported that they used OTC cough or cold medications to get high in the past year were asked to specify the names of up to five OTC medications that they had used for this purpose. The report examines the prevalence and patterns of the use of OTC cough and cold medications to get high among persons aged 12 to 25, the

This chapter includes text from "The NSDUH Report: Misuse of Over-the-Counter Cough and Cold Medications among Persons Aged 12 to 25," Substance Abuse and Mental Health Services Administration (SAMHSA), January 10, 2008.

269

age group with the highest rates of such use. The report also examines the specific OTC cough and cold medications that were most commonly misused in the past year and the use of selected illicit drugs among persons who misused OTC cough and cold medications in their lifetime. Findings presented are based on 2006 NSDUH data.

Lifetime Misuse of OTC Cough and Cold Medications

About 3.1 million persons aged 12 to 25 (5.3%) had misused OTC cough and cold medications at least once in their lifetime (Table 50.1). Young adults aged 18 to 25 were more likely than youths aged 12 to 17 to have misused OTC cough and cold medications in their lifetime (6.5% versus 3.7%).

Among persons aged 12 to 25 who had ever misused OTC cough and cold medications, 81.9% also were lifetime users of marijuana. Slightly less than half were lifetime users of the hallucinogens lysergic acid diethylamide (LSD), PCP, or ecstasy (44.2%) or were lifetime users of inhalants (49.3%). Youths and young adults who had ever misused OTC cough and cold medications had comparable lifetime rates of inhalant use. However, young adults who had ever misused OTC cough and cold medications were more likely than the corresponding youths to have ever used marijuana or the hallucinogens LSD, PCP, or ecstasy. Males aged 12 to 25 who had ever misused OTC cough and cold medications were more likely than their female counterparts to have used LSD, PCP, or ecstasy. Males and females who had ever misused these medications had similar rates of lifetime use of marijuana and inhalants.

Past Year Misuse of OTC Cough and Cold Medications

Nearly one million persons aged 12 to 25 (1.7%) misused OTC cough and cold medications in the past year (Table 50.1). Unlike the pattern for lifetime misuse, youths aged 12 to 17 were more likely than young adults aged 18 to 25 to have misused OTC cough and cold medications in the past year (1.9% versus 1.6%). Males and females aged 12 to 25 had the same rate of past year misuse of these medications (1.7%). When examined separately for adolescents and young adults, however, the patterns varied by gender. Among youths aged 12 to 17, females were more likely than males to have misused OTC cough and cold medications in the past year (2.3% versus 1.5%). Among young adults aged 18 to 25, however, males were more likely than females to have misused these medications (1.8% versus 1.3%).

The rate of past year misuse of OTC cough and cold medications among whites aged 12 to 25 (2.1%) was about three times higher than the rate among Blacks (0.6%) and was also higher than the rate among Hispanics (1.4%). In this age group, Hispanics also were more likely than Blacks to be past year abusers. Rates of past year misuse among persons aged 12 to 25 did not differ significantly by county type or region.

Among persons aged 12 to 25 who had misused an OTC cough and cold medication in the past year, 30.5% misused a NyQuil® product, 18.1% misused a Coricidin® product, and 17.8% misused a Robitussin® product. More than 40% of the abusers in this age group misused any of a wide variety of other OTC medications.

Table 50.1. Misuse of Over-the-Counter (OTC) Cough or Cold Medications in the Lifetime and the Past Year among Persons Aged 12 to 25, by Demographic Characteristics: 2006

Demographic Characteristic	Lifetime (%)	Past Year (%)
Total Aged 12 to 25	5.3	1.7
Age Group		
12 to 17	3.7	1.9
18 to 25	6.5	1.6
Gender		
Male	5.6	1.7
Female	4.9	1.7
Age Group, by Gender		
12 to 17, Male	3.0	1.5
12 to 17, Female	4.3	2.3
18 to 25 Male	7.7	1.8
18 to 25, Female	5.4	1.3
Race/Ethnicity		
White	6.2	2.1
Black or African American	2.5	0.6
Hispanic or Latino	4.7	1.4

Source: SAMHSA, 2006 NSDUH

Chapter 51

Nonmedical Use and Abuse of Prescription Drugs

Chapter Contents

Section 51.1—Scientific Research on
            Prescription Drug Abuse 274

Section 51.2—Pain Reliever Abuse 278

Section 51.3—Tranquilizer Abuse 282

Section 51.4—Stimulant Abuse 285

Section 51.5—Sedative Abuse 288

Section 51.1

Scientific Research on Prescription Drug Abuse

Excerpted from "Scientific Research on Prescription Drug Abuse, Before the Subcommittee on the Judiciary and Caucus on International Narcotics Control," National Institute on Drug Abuse (NIDA), March 12, 2008.

Several factors have recently contributed to the severity of prescription drug abuse, including drastic increases in the number of prescriptions written, greater social acceptance of using medications, and aggressive marketing by pharmaceutical companies. These factors together have helped create the broad environmental availability of prescription drugs. To illustrate, the total number of stimulant prescriptions in the United States (U.S.) has soared from around five million in 1991 to nearly 35 million in 2007. Prescriptions for opiates (hydrocodone and oxycodone products) have escalated from around 40 million in 1991 to nearly 180 million in 2007, with the U.S. their biggest consumer. The U.S. is supplied 99% of the world total for hydrocodone (Vicodin®) and 71% of oxycodone (OxyContin®).

This greater availability of prescription drugs has been accompanied by increases in their abuse. Unlike illicit drug use, which shows a continuing downward trend, prescription drug abuse, particularly of opioid pain medications, has seen a continual rise through the 1990s and has remained stubbornly steady among persons 12 or older during recent years.[1] Because prescription drugs act directly or indirectly on the same brain systems affected by illicit drugs, their abuse carries substantial abuse and addiction liabilities. They are most dangerous when taken to get high via methods that increase their addictive potential (for example, crushing the pills, then snorting or injecting their contents, or combining them with alcohol or illicit drugs). Some people also take prescription drugs for their intended purpose, though not as prescribed, thus heightening the risk of dangerous adverse reactions; and still others may become addicted even when they take them as prescribed. Given that more than 30 million people suffer from chronic pain in this country, even if a fraction of this group takes prescription drugs for their pain and becomes addicted, it could affect a large number of people.

What is the scope of the prescription drug problem in this country?

Several indicators show that prescription drug abuse is a significant problem in the United States. According to the National Survey on Drug Use and Health (NSDUH), conducted by the Substance Abuse and Mental Health Services Administration (SAMHSA), in 2006 approximately seven million persons 12 and older took a psychotherapeutic drug for nonmedical purposes in the 30 days before the survey. Most reported abusing opiate pain relievers in particular. In fact, 2.2 million persons aged 12 and over initiated abuse of pain relievers in the past year. Young adults (ages 18–25) by far showed the greatest use overall and the largest increases in past month, past year, and lifetime use between 2002 and 2006, compared to all other age groups (NSDUH, 2007). Still, even by the time they graduate from high school, roughly a quarter of 12th graders report having abused a prescription drug (Monitoring the Future [MTF], 2007). Other significant indicators of the prescription drug problem include the following:

- In 2006, more than half a million adolescents aged 12–17 used stimulants nonmedically in the past year (NSDUH, 2007).

- Although abuse of sedatives decreased among high school seniors between 2005 and 2007, it is still near peak levels, at over 6% among this group (MTF, 2007).

- Nearly 6% of 12th graders reported abusing cough medicine to get high in 2007 (MTF, 2007).

- Data on drug-related emergency department visits that involved prescription opioids show a 153% increase from 1995–2002, from 42,857 to 108,320 (SAMHSA's Drug Abuse Warning Network, 2004).

- Treatment admissions for opiates other than heroin surged from 16,121 in 1995 to 67,887 in 2005, a 321% increase (SAMHSA's Treatment Episode Data Set, 1995–2005).

- Prescribed pain medications are driving the upward trend in drug poisoning mortality. The number of deaths involving prescription opioid analgesics increased 160% in just five years from 1999 to 2004. By 2004, opioid painkiller abuse deaths outnumbered total deaths involving heroin and cocaine (Centers for Disease Control and Prevention, 2006).

What factors are driving abuse of prescription drugs?

The far-ranging scope of prescription drug abuse in this country stems not only from the greater prescribing of medications, but also from misperceptions of their safety. For example, many students, and even some parents, see nothing wrong in the abuse of stimulants to improve cognitive function and academic performance. In fact, being in college may even be a risk factor for greater use of amphetamines or Ritalin® nonmedically, with reports of students taking pills before tests and of those with prescribed medications being approached to divert them to others. Pain relievers show a similar link with regard to access. Evidence suggests that parents sometimes provide their children with prescription medications not prescribed by a physician for the child to relieve their discomfort.[3] According to the 2006 NSDUH, 55.7% of those 12 and older who misused pain relievers said they received their medications from a friend or family member, the vast majority of whom had gotten the drugs from just one doctor. Only 3.9% cited obtaining these drugs from a drug dealer or stranger, and only 0.1% cited an internet purchase. Notably, the leading reason for the abuse is to relieve pain, although other top motives include intent to get high and experimentation.

Similar motivations characterize younger groups, with high school students reporting that they primarily abuse prescription drugs for the medications' intended purpose, albeit without a prescription. Using these medications without a prescription, or in ways other than prescribed, poses multiple risks including dangerous interactions with other medications, accidental poisoning, and risk of addiction.

Nonmedical use among children and adolescents is particularly troublesome, given that adolescence is the period of greatest risk not only for drug experimentation but also for developing addiction. At this stage, the brain is still developing and exposure to drugs could interfere with these carefully orchestrated developmental changes. Today we know that the last part of the brain to fully mature is the prefrontal cortex, a region that governs judgment and decision-making functions. This may help explain why teens are prone to risk-taking and to experimentation with alcohol and other drugs.

Research also shows that adolescents who abuse prescription drugs are twice as likely to have engaged in delinquent behavior and nearly three times as likely to have experienced an episode of major depression compared to teens who did not abuse prescription medications over the past year. Finally, several studies link the illicit use of prescription drugs with increased rates of cigarette smoking, heavy drinking, and marijuana and other illicit drug use in adolescents and young adults in the U.S.

Older adults represent another area for particular concern. Although this group currently comprises just 13% of the U.S. population, they receive approximately one-third of all medications prescribed in the nation. In a culture in which medications are considered a quick fix for whatever ails you, combined with the greater rates of lifetime drug abuse among the baby boom generation as compared to those in the current older generation relative to its size, it is possible that the number of persons aged 50 or older abusing prescription drugs could increase 190% over the next two decades, from 911,000 in 2001 to almost 2.7 million in 2020.[4] Because older adults also experience higher rates of other illness as well as normal changes in drug metabolism, it makes sense that even moderate abuse or unintentional misuse of prescription drugs by elderly persons could lead to more severe health consequences. Therefore, physicians need to be aware of the possibility of abuse and to discuss the health implications with their patients.

End Notes

1. *The NSDUH Report: Patterns and Trends in Nonmedical Prescription Pain Reliever Use: 2002 to 2005*, Substance Abuse and Mental Health Services Administration, Department of Health and Human Services, 2007.

2. For purposes of this testimony, the focus will be only on psychotherapeutic drugs, so even though NIDA's prescription drug portfolio includes work on other prescribed drug categories, such as anabolic steroids, these will be excluded from this discussion.

3. Boyd et al. Medical and nonmedical use of prescription pain medication by youth in a Detroit-area public school district. *Drug and Alcohol Dependence* 81:37–45, 2006.

4. Colliver JD, Compton WM, Grroerer JC, Condon, T. Projecting drug use among aging baby boomers in 2020. *Ann Epidemiol.* 2006 Apr;16(4):257–65.

Section 51.2

Pain Reliever Abuse

This section includes text from "Trends in Nonmedical Use of Prescription Pain Relievers: 2002 to 2007," Substance Abuse and Mental Health Services Administration (SAMHSA), February 5, 2009; and "How Young Adults Obtain Prescription Pain Relievers for Nonmedical Use," SAMHSA, 2006.

Trends in Nonmedical Use of Prescription Pain Relievers

Use of prescription pain relievers without a doctor's prescription or only for the experience or feeling they caused (nonmedical use) is, after marijuana use, the second most common form of illicit drug use in the United States. When used appropriately under medical supervision, hydrocodone (Vicodin®), oxycodone (OxyContin®), morphine, and similar prescription pain relievers provide indispensable medical benefit by reducing pain and suffering, but when taken without a physician's direction and oversight, these medications can cause serious adverse consequences and produce dependence and abuse. According to the Drug Abuse Warning Network (DAWN), approximately 324,000 emergency department visits in 2006 involved the nonmedical use of pain relievers (including both prescription and over-the-counter pain medications).

In 2007, 2.1% of persons aged 12 or older (an estimated 5.2 million persons) reported using prescription pain relievers nonmedically in the past month; this rate does not differ significantly from that in 2002. Among youths aged 12 to 17, nonmedical use of pain relievers in the past month declined from 3.2% in 2002 to 2.7% in 2007. In contrast, use increased among young adults aged 18 to 25 and among adults aged 26 or older. Among young adults, the rate of nonmedical use of pain relievers in the past month increased from 4.1% in 2002 to 4.6% in 2007. Among adults aged 26 or older, use increased from 1.3% in 2002 to 1.6% in 2007. In 2007, 2.7% of youths, 4.6% of young adults, and 1.6% of adults aged 26 or older used prescription pain relievers nonmedically in the past month. These percentages represent an estimated 670,000 youths, 1.5 million young adults, and 3.0 million adults aged 26 or older.

Table 51.1 Nonmedical Use of Prescription Pain Relievers in the Past Month among Persons Aged 12 or Older: Percentages, 2002 to 2007

Year	Percent
2002	1.9%
2003	2.0%
2004	1.8%
2005	1.9%
2006	2.1%
2007	2.1%

Source: SAMHSA, 2002 to 2007 NSDUH

Among males aged 12 or older, the rates of nonmedical use of prescription pain relievers increased between 2002 (2.0%) and 2007 (2.6%). Among females, the rate of nonmedical use of pain relievers in the past month did not change significantly over the period from 2002 through 2007, remaining in the range of 1.7% to 1.9%. The 2.6% of males who used prescription pain relievers nonmedically in the past month in 2007 represent an estimated 3.1 million persons, and the 1.7% of females is equivalent to an estimated 2.1 million persons.

Although nonmedical use of prescription pain relievers in the past month was lower in 2007 than in 2002 among youths aged 12 to 17, the rates have been increasing over time for adults aged 18 or older. These increases for adults may place greater demands on the health care system due to adverse consequences such as overdoses, and additional resources may be needed to treat dependence and abuse involving these medications. To reduce rates of nonmedical use of pain relievers, physicians and other medical practitioners must not only continue to exercise care in prescribing and monitoring their patients or clients for signs of misuse, but also should counsel them about not sharing their prescription medications, preventing others from having access to their medications, and properly disposing of remaining dosage units once the need for the medication has passed. Policy makers at the national and state levels need to consider measures to reduce diversion of prescription pain relievers from legitimate medical use to nonmedical use.

How Young Adults Obtain Prescription Pain Relievers for Nonmedical Use

There has been a growing concern in both the law enforcement and public health arenas about the increase in the use of pharmaceutical drugs for nonmedical use, especially among young adults. The National Survey on Drug Use and Health (NSDUH) asks persons aged 12 or older questions related to their nonmedical use of prescription-type drugs, including prescription pain relievers, during the past year. The 2005 NSDUH also asks individuals who used prescription pain relievers nonmedically in the past year how they obtained prescription pain relievers the last time they used them.

Nonmedical Use of Prescription Pain Relievers in the Past Year

In 2005, 12.4% of young adults aged 18 to 25 (4.0 million persons) used prescription pain relievers nonmedically in the past year, and 1.7% met the criteria for past year prescription pain reliever dependence or abuse. In this age group, males were more likely than females to have used prescription pain relievers nonmedically in the past year (13.5% versus 11.3%). Unemployed persons aged 18 to 25 were more likely to have used prescription pain relievers nonmedically (15.5%) than those employed part time or full time or those in the other employment group (12.6%, 12.2%, and 11.3%, respectively). Among young adults aged 18 to 22, the prevalence of past year nonmedical prescription pain reliever use did not differ significantly between those enrolled and those not enrolled in college.

Method of Obtaining Prescription Pain Relievers for Nonmedical Purposes

Among young adults aged 18 to 25 who used prescription pain relievers nonmedically in the past year, over half (53.0%) obtained them from a friend or relative for free when they last used pain relievers nonmedically Young adult females were more likely than their male counterparts to have obtained the prescription pain relievers that they used most recently for nonmedical purposes for free from a friend or relative (58.9% versus 48.2%). Conversely, males were nearly twice as likely as females to have bought their most recently used prescription pain relievers from a friend or relative (13.4% versus 7.2%) and three times as likely to have bought them from a drug dealer or other stranger (6.9% versus 2.3%).

Among young adults aged 18 to 25 who used prescription pain relievers nonmedically in the past year and met the criteria for prescription pain reliever dependence or abuse, 37.5% obtained the prescription pain relievers that they used most recently for nonmedical purposes for free from a friend or relative, 19.9% bought them from a friend or relative, and 13.6% obtained them from one doctor. Young adult females who met the criteria for prescription pain reliever dependence or abuse were more likely than their male counterparts to have obtained their most recently used prescription pain relievers from a friend or relative for free (46.6% versus 30.6%) and were less likely to have bought them from a drug dealer or other stranger (8.1% versus 15.9%).

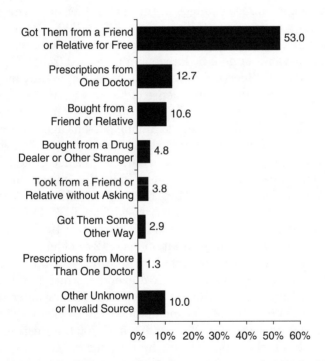

Figure 51.1. *Percentages of Reported Method* of Obtaining Prescription Pain Relievers for Their Most Recent Nonmedical Use in the Past Year among Persons Aged 18 to 25: 2005 NSDUH. (*The following response options were reported at less than 1% and, therefore, are not shown: "Wrote a fake prescription;" "Bought on the internet;" and "Stole them from a health facility.") (Source: SAMHSA, 2005 NSDUH).*

Section 51.3

Tranquilizer Abuse

Excerpted from "Patterns in Nonmedical Use of Specific Prescription
Drugs: Chapter 3," Substance Abuse and Mental Health Administration
(SAMHSA), June 3, 2008.

Recent Trends in Lifetime Nonmedical Use of Tranquilizer Prescription Drugs

This section examines changes in the rate of lifetime misuse of particular prescription-type tranquilizers from 2002 to 2004. Among persons aged 12 or older, the rate of lifetime nonmedical use of Xanax®, generic alprazolam, Ativan®, or generic lorazepam increased from 3.5% in 2002 to 3.9% in 2004. This increase appeared to be driven mainly by persons aged 18 to 25, for whom the prevalence of lifetime misuse of that group of drugs increased from 6.7% to 7.7%. Misuse of two muscle relaxants, Flexeril® and Soma®, also increased among persons aged 18 to 25; lifetime nonmedical use of Flexeril® increased from 0.9% to 1.4%, while the rate for Soma® increased from 2.3% to 3.0% in this age group. Two categories of tranquilizers showed decreases in lifetime misuse among persons aged 26 or older: the rate of Atarax® use declined from 0.2% to 0.1%, and the rate of Librium® misuse decreased from 0.8% to 0.5%. These changes among persons aged 26 or older drove statistically significant decreases among the overall population aged 12 or older.

The most frequently reported tranquilizer that was used nonmedically was Valium® or generic diazepam, which had been misused by an estimated 14.6 million persons aged 12 or older (6.1% of the population and 73.6% of lifetime nonmedical users of any tranquilizer). Based on averages for 2002, 2003, and 2004, an estimated 9.0 million (3.8% of the population) had misused Xanax®, generic alprazolam, Ativan®, or generic lorazepam at least once in their lifetime. Lifetime misuse of the major tranquilizers Klonopin® or clonazepam ranked a distant third with 2.7 million persons (1.1%).

Analysis by drug group indicates that an estimated 18.6 million persons aged 12 or older misused anxiolytic benzodiazepines in their lifetime; this is 93.9% of lifetime nonmedical tranquilizer users and

7.8% of the population. This group includes Klonopin® or clonazepam, Xanax® or alprazolam, Ativan® or lorazepam, Valium® or diazepam, Librium®, Limbitrol®, Rohypnol®, Serax®, and Tranxene®, plus responses to the "other-specify" tranquilizer item that fell into the benzodiazepine category; benzodiazepines that are prescribed for use as sedatives are not included in this group.

Table 51.2. Lifetime Nonmedical Use of Selected Tranquilizers among Persons Aged 12 or Older: Percentages, 2002–2004

Specific Tranquilizer[1]	Estimated Number (in 1,000s)	Percentage of Population	Percentage of Lifetime Nonmedical Users of Any Tranquilizer
Any Tranquilizer	19,780	8.3	100.0
Valium® or Diazepam	14,555	6.1	73.6
Xanax®, Alprazolam, Ativan®, or Lorazepam	9,025	3.8	45.6
Klonopin® or Clonazepam	2,657	1.1	13.4
Soma®	2,488	1.0	12.6
Flexeril®	1,914	0.8	9.7
Librium®	1,185	0.5	6.0
BuSpar®	661	0.3	3.3
Rohypnol®	376	0.2	1.9
Vistaril®	296	0.1	1.5
Atarax®	283	0.1	1.4
Tranxene®	182	0.1	0.9
Serax®	167	0.1	0.8
Meprobamate	153	0.1	0.8
Miltown®	113	0.0	0.6
Equanil®	94	0.0	0.5
Limbitrol®	84	0.0	0.4

[1]In descending order of prevalence.

Source: SAMHSA, Office of Applied Studies, National Survey on Drug Use and Health, 2002, 2003, and 2004.

Demographic Differences

Using the average for 2002 through 2004, the prevalence of lifetime nonmedical use of specific tranquilizers was examined among males and females and among adolescents aged 12 to 17, young adults aged 18 to 25, and adults aged 26 or older. Lifetime misuse of any tranquilizer was more prevalent for males (8.9%) than females (7.8%). Specific drugs for which this difference reached statistical significance between males and females included Valium® or diazepam (7.0% among males versus 5.3% among females), Klonopin® or clonazepam (1.2% versus 1.0%), Rohypnol® (0.2% versus 0.1%), and Soma® (1.2% versus 0.9%). There were no specific tranquilizers for which a statistically significant reversal of this pattern was found.

The lifetime prevalence of nonmedical use of any prescription-type tranquilizer was higher for young adults aged 25 (11.9%) than for older adults aged 26 or older (8.4%), who in turn had a higher rate than youths aged 12 to 17 (3.4%). Statistically significant differences following this pattern were observed for Klonopin® or clonazepam; Xanax®, alprazolam, Ativan®, or lorazepam; Valium® or diazepam; Flexeril®; and Soma®. Exceptions to this pattern were found for lifetime misuse of Librium®, which was more common among older adults (0.6%) than younger adults (0.2%), and Miltown® (0.1% versus 0.0%, respectively). However, these latter drugs have been on the market longer than drugs such as alprazolam (Xanax®).

Use of Tranquilizer Drugs among Past Year Initiates of Any Drug in Class

An estimated 1.1 million persons initiated nonmedical use of any tranquilizer in the year prior to the survey interview; this constitutes 5.8% of the estimated 19.8 million lifetime nonmedical users of any tranquilizer. Among the new initiates, the specific tranquilizers used most frequently were Xanax®, alprazolam, Ativan®, or lorazepam (used by 50.9% of new users), and the second-ranking tranquilizer was Valium® or diazepam (42.0%). Among all lifetime nonmedical users of tranquilizers, however, the relative rankings of these two drug groups was reversed, possibly reflecting the fact that Valium® (diazepam) has been on the market since 1962 whereas Xanax® (alprazolam) and Ativan® (lorazepam) were first approved for marketing in 1977. Lifetime misuse of Librium® was reported by 1.3% of new initiates compared with 6.0% of all lifetime nonmedical users of tranquilizers.

Section 51.4

Stimulant Abuse

Excerpted from "Patterns in Nonmedical Use of Specific Prescription Drugs: Chapter 3," Substance Abuse and Mental Health Administration (SAMHSA), June 3, 2008.

Recent Trends in Lifetime Nonmedical Use of Stimulant Prescription Drugs

This section examines changes in the rate of lifetime misuse of particular prescription-type stimulants from 2002 to 2004. Between 2002 and 2004, lifetime nonmedical use of stimulants overall declined from 9.0% to 8.3%. Among particular stimulants, significant decreases were observed for prescription diet pills (from 3.8% to 3.4%), Dexedrine® (from 1.4% to 1.1%), and Preludin® (from 0.4% to 0.2%). These decreases were driven primarily by declines among persons aged 26 or older. In addition, Preludin® is no longer approved for marketing in the United States. Among youths aged 12 to 17, decreases were seen in lifetime nonmedical use of methamphetamine, Desoxyn®, or Methedrine® (from 1.5% to 1.2%), and Ritalin® or methylphenidate (from 2.4% to 1.8%).

Basic Prevalence Information

The stimulant that had the highest lifetime prevalence of misuse was methamphetamine, with an estimated 12.1 million lifetime users (5.1% of the population and 58.9% of all lifetime stimulant users). This category includes both prescription-type methamphetamine (for example, Desoxyn®) and street methamphetamine (referred to as crank, crystal, ice, or speed in the survey instrument). Prescription diet pills ranked second, with 8.6 million lifetime nonmedical users (3.6% of the population), and Ritalin® or generic methylphenidate ranked third with 4.3 million users (1.8% of the population).

285

Table 51.3. Lifetime Nonmedical Use of Specific Stimulants among Persons Aged 12 or Older: Annual Averages Based on 2002–2004

Specific Stimulant[1]	Estimated Number (in 1,000s)	Percentage of Population	Percentage of Lifetime Nonmedical Users of Any Stimulant
Any Stimulant	20,617	8.7	100.0
Methamphetamine, Desoxyn®, or Methedrine®	12,138	5.1	58.9
Prescription diet pills	8,585	3.6	41.6
Ritalin® or Methylphenidate	4,293	1.8	20.8
Dexedrine®	2,803	1.2	13.6
Preludin®	697	0.3	3.4
Dextroamphetamine	575	0.2	2.8
Ionamin®	511	0.2	2.5
Eskatrol®	227	0.1	1.1
Tenuate®	214	0.1	1.0
Cylert®	209	0.1	1.0
Didrex®	186	0.1	0.9
Sanorex®	116	0.0	0.6
Mazanor®	54	0.0	0.3
Plegine®	46	0.0	0.2
Obedrin-LA®	33	0.0	0.2

[1]In descending order of prevalence.

Source: SAMHSA, Office of Applied Studies, National Survey on Drug Use and Health, 2002, 2003, and 2004.

Demographic Differences

Using the average for 2002 through 2004, the prevalence of lifetime nonmedical use of specific stimulants was examined among males and females and among adolescents aged 12 to 17, young adults aged 18 to 25, and adults aged 26 or older. Misuse of any stimulant in the lifetime was higher among males than females (9.9 versus 7.5%), and this pattern was apparent for most of the specific drugs in this category although the difference did not reach statistical significance in all cases. Lifetime misuse of methamphetamine, Desoxyn®, or Methedrine®, for example, was reported by 6.3% of males compared with 4.0% of females. There were no statistically significant reversals of this pattern.

Age group differences in lifetime misuse of any stimulant showed the same pattern as tranquilizers; the rate was higher for adults aged 18 to 25 (10.7%) than for adults aged 26 or older (9.0%), who in turn had a higher rate than youths aged 12 to 17 (3.9%). Compared with youths, young adults had higher lifetime rates of misuse of methamphetamine, Desoxyn®, or Methedrine®; prescription diet pills; Ritalin® or methylphenidate; Dexedrine®; dextroamphetamine; and Preludin®. Compared with young adults aged 18 to 25, older adults aged 26 or older had higher lifetime rates of nonmedical use of prescription diet pills, Dexedrine®, Eskatrol®, Ionamin®, Preludin®, and Tenuate®. Misuse of Ritalin® or methylphenidate, however, was more prevalent among young adults than older adults (5.5 versus 1.1%). An estimated 2.1% of youths aged 12 to 17 reported lifetime nonmedical use of Ritalin® or methylphenidate.

Use of Stimulant Drugs among Past Year Initiates of Any Drug in Class

Persons who initiated nonmedical use of stimulants in the year prior to the survey were estimated to number 764,000; this is 3.7% of the estimated 20.6 million lifetime nonmedical users of any stimulant. Ritalin® or methylphenidate was the most frequently used specific stimulant among new initiates (42.3%).

Methamphetamine, Desoxyn®, or Methedrine® ranked second (31.5%) in this therapeutic class. Among all lifetime nonmedical users of stimulants, methamphetamine, Desoxyn®, or Methedrine® ranked first, and Ritalin® or methylphenidate ranked third. The higher profile of Ritalin® or methylphenidate among new initiates may be associated with differential rates of use among young people because Ritalin® is typically prescribed to ameliorate the symptoms of attention deficit/hyperactivity disorder (ADHD). Consequently, misuse of this stimulant may differentially involve young people. Comparison of the age-specific rates among all lifetime nonmedical users (including new initiates, continuing users, and former users) indicates that Ritalin® or methylphenidate was the most frequently reported specific drug among those aged 12 to 17 (53.6%); it was roughly equal to methamphetamine among those aged 18 to 25 (51.0% for Ritalin® or methylphenidate versus 50.0% for methamphetamine) and ranked fourth among adults aged 26 or older (12.5%). Nonmedical use of Preludin® (phenmetrazine) was reported by 0.3% of past year stimulant initiates compared with 3.4% of lifetime users. As noted, Preludin® and its generic equivalent are no longer approved for marketing in the United States.

Section 51.5

Sedative Abuse

Excerpted from "Patterns in Nonmedical Use of Specific Prescription
Drugs: Chapter 3," Substance Abuse and Mental Health Administration
(SAMHSA), June 3, 2008.

Recent Trends in Lifetime Nonmedical Use of Sedative Prescription Drugs

This section examines changes in the rate of lifetime misuse of
particular prescription-type sedatives from 2002 to 2004. The rate of
lifetime nonmedical use of any barbiturate decreased from 1.7% in
2002 to 1.4% in 2004 among persons aged 12 or older, based largely
on a decline from 2.1% to 1.7% among persons aged 26 or older. Corresponding decreases were seen for the separate categories of generic
barbiturates, phenobarbital, and Tuinal®. Tuinal® is not currently
approved for marketing in the United States (U.S.). Among adults
aged 26 or older, there were small but statistically significant decreases in lifetime misuse of the sedative benzodiazepines Restoril®
or temazepam (from 0.5% to 0.3%) and Halcion® (from 0.5% to 0.3%);
these decreases appeared to drive decreases in the overall category
of temazepam, flurazepam, or triazolam and in the corresponding drug
categories among all persons aged 12 or older.

Basic Prevalence Information

Methaqualone, Sopor®, or Quaalude®, which is now a schedule I
drug and can no longer be manufactured, distributed, or used legally
in the United States, was the most commonly reported sedative that
was misused by persons aged 12 or older in their lifetime. An estimated 7.1 million (3.0% of the population) had used these methaqualone products nonmedically in their lifetime. Similarly, an estimated
3.1 million persons aged 12 or older (1.3%) had misused barbiturates,

based on a NSDUH question about nonmedical barbiturate use that provided selected examples of barbiturates but not an exhaustive list. In addition, an estimated 1.8 million persons (0.7%) had misused sedative benzodiazepines in their lifetime; these include drugs in the generic categories of temazepam, flurazepam, and triazolam and their corresponding brand names.

Table 51.4. Lifetime Nonmedical Use of Specific Sedatives among Persons Aged 12 or Older: Annual Averages Based on 2002–2004

Specific Sedative[1]	Estimated Number (in 1,000s)	Percentage of Population	Percentage of Lifetime Nonmedical Users of Any Sedative
Any Sedative	9,787	4.1	100.0
Methaqualone, Sopor®, or Quaalude®	7,144	3.0	73.0
Barbiturates[2]	3,093	1.3	31.6
Phenobarbital	1,333	0.6	13.6
Tuinal®	1,164	0.5	11.9
Placidyl®	905	0.4	9.2
Restoril® or Temazepam	901	0.4	9.2
Halcion®	760	0.3	7.8
Dalmane®	504	0.2	5.2
Amytal®	244	0.1	2.5
Chloral Hydrate	194	0.1	2.0
Butisol®	94	0.0	1.0

[1]In descending order of prevalence.
[2]Respondents were asked about their use of barbiturates and were given the following as examples: Nembutal®, pentobarbital, Seconal®, secobarbital, or butalbital. However, respondents were not given an exhaustive list of examples of barbiturates.

Source: SAMHSA, Office of Applied Studies, National Survey on Drug Use and Health, 2002, 2003, and 2004.

Demographic Differences

Using the average for 2002 through 2004, the prevalence of lifetime nonmedical use of specific sedatives was examined among males and females and among adolescents aged 12 to 17, young adults aged

289

18 to 25, and adults aged 26 or older. Lifetime misuse of any sedative was higher among males (4.9%) than females (3.4%). This pattern predominated across the specific sedatives, although the differences were not always statistically significant. Methaqualone, Sopor®, or Quaalude®, the most frequently reported specific sedative, was misused by 3.8% of males compared with 2.3% of females. In the selected groups of specific sedatives, lifetime barbiturate misuse also was higher for males than females (2.1% versus 1.2%).

The rate of lifetime sedative misuse increased with age and was clearly higher for adults aged 26 or older than for younger adults aged 18 to 25 or youths aged 12 to 17. For example, lifetime misuse of methaqualone, Sopor®, or Quaalude® was reported by 0.2% of youths, 0.9% of young adults, and 3.8% of older adults. Because methaqualone and its brand-name equivalents were withdrawn from the U.S. market several years ago and assigned to Schedule I in the Drug Enforcement Administration's (DEA) list of controlled substances, use by younger people would be expected to be rare. However, the same pattern of differences in prevalence is found for the barbiturates as a group, for which lifetime misuse was highest for adults aged 26 or older (2.0%), followed by young adults aged 18 to 25 (0.6%) and youths aged 12 to 17 (0.3%). This difference across age groups also could be due to changes in drug availability or prescribing practices, as formulations of oral barbiturates are discontinued or replaced by sedatives that have been approved for medical use more recently.

Use of Sedative Drugs among Past Year Initiates of Any Drug in Class

An estimated 214,000 persons initiated nonmedical use of prescription-type sedatives in the 12 months prior to the survey; this is 2.2% of the estimated total of 9.8 million nonmedical users of any prescription-type sedative. The most frequently reported specific sedative among new initiates was Restoril® or temazepam, which was reported by 17.4% of new initiates. Methaqualone, Sopor®, or Quaalude®, then barbiturates, occupied the next two ranks, with 11.0% and 10.8%, respectively. Among all lifetime nonmedical users of sedatives, methaqualone, Sopor®, or Quaalude® ranked first (73.0%). The lower rate among new initiates may reflect the withdrawal of these products from the U.S. market several years ago; the fact that there were an estimated 23,000 persons who initiated misuse of methaqualone or its brand-name equivalents in the year prior to the survey suggests that there is an illicit market in this product, even though it is assigned to the DEA's schedule I category (not approved for medical use). Large discrepancies between rates among all lifetime users and new initiates also were found for Tuinal® (11.9% among all lifetime users, 0.1% among new initiates) and Placidyl® (9.2% among lifetime users versus 0.3% among new initiates). These two drugs also are no longer approved for marketing in the United States.

Chapter 52

Mixing Alcohol and Other Drugs

Chapter Contents

Section 52.1—Risk of Substance Dependence
        following Initial Use of
        Alcohol or Illicit Drugs 294

Section 52.2—Simultaneous Polydrug Use 298

Section 52.3—Alcohol Abuse Makes Prescription
        Drug Abuse More Likely 302

Section 52.1

Risk of Substance Dependence following Initial Use of Alcohol or Illicit Drugs

This section is excerpted from "Substance Use and Dependence Following Initiation of Alcohol or Illicit Drug Use," Substance Abuse and Mental Health Services Administration (SAMHSA), March 27, 2008.

A series of recent research reports has examined the characteristics associated with the development of dependence soon after the initiation of alcohol, marijuana, cocaine, and hallucinogen use.[1-4] These studies suggest that each drug class has a different trajectory from first use to cessation of use, continuation of use without dependence, or dependence upon the drug.

The National Survey on Drug Use and Health (NSDUH) asks persons aged 12 or older to report on their use of alcohol and illicit drugs during their lifetime and in the past year. Illicit drugs refer to marijuana/hashish, cocaine (including crack), inhalants, hallucinogens, heroin, or prescription-type drugs used nonmedically.[5] Respondents who reported use of a given substance were asked when they first used it;[6] responses to these questions were used to determine the number of months since they initiated use of the substance. NSDUH also asks questions to assess symptoms of substance dependence during the past year. NSDUH defines substance dependence using criteria specified by the *Diagnostic and Statistical Manual of Mental Disorders, 4th Edition (DSM-IV)*.[7] It includes such symptoms as withdrawal, tolerance, unsuccessful attempts to cut down on use, and continued use despite health and emotional problems caused by the substance.

This report examines the development of dependence upon a substance in the two years following substance use initiation (1–24 months after initiation). For the purposes of this report, persons who initiated use of a substance 13 to 24 months prior to the interview are referred to as "year-before-last initiates." Year-before-last initiates were assigned to three mutually exclusive categories reflecting their substance use trajectories following initiation: those who had not used the substance in the past 12 months (past year), those who had used the substance during the past year but were not dependent on the substance during the past year, and those who had used the substance and were dependent on the substance during the past year.

Comparisons are made across substance classes in terms of the percentages of these year-before-last initiates classified in each of these three past year categories. All findings presented in this report are annual averages based on combined 2004, 2005, and 2006 NSDUH data.

Among year-before-last initiates of specific substances, over two-thirds of crack cocaine, inhalant, and heroin initiates did not use the drug in the past year. Alcohol and marijuana were the only substances for which the majority of year-before-last initiates used the substance in the past year.

Risk for Developing Alcohol Dependence following Initiation

Among year-before-last initiates of alcohol, one fourth (25.7%) had not used alcohol during the past year, 71.1% had used alcohol in the past year but were not dependent on alcohol, and 3.2% were both using and dependent on alcohol during the past year (Table 52.1).

Risk for Developing Marijuana Dependence following Initiation

Among year-before-last initiates of marijuana, 42.4% had not used marijuana during the past year, 51.8% had used marijuana in the past year but were not dependent on marijuana, and 5.8% were both using and dependent on marijuana in the past year.

Risk for Developing Cocaine Dependence following Initiation

Year-before-last initiates of cocaine were examined in two subgroups: initiates of crack and initiates of cocaine other than crack. Approximately 9.2% of year-before-last crack initiates were dependent on any type of cocaine in the past year, whereas 3.7% of initiates of cocaine other than crack were dependent on any type of cocaine in the past year.

Risk for Developing Other Drug Dependence following Initiation

More than one-tenth (13.4%) of year-before-last initiates of heroin were dependent on heroin in the past year, while less than 1% (0.9%)

of year-before-last inhalant initiates were dependent on inhalants in the past year and less than 2% (1.9%) of year-before-last halluci-nogen initiates were dependent on hallucinogens in the past year. About 5% (4.7%) of year-before-last initiates of nonmedical use of stimulants were dependent on stimulants in the past year, whereas in the past year, 3.1% of year-before-last initiates of nonmedical pain reliever use were dependent on pain relievers, 2.4% of initiates of nonmedical sedative use were dependent on sedatives, and 1.2% of initiates of nonmedical tranquilizer use were dependent on tranquil-izers.

Table 52.1. Percentages of Past Year Use and/or Dependence among Year-Before-Last Initiates Aged 12 or Older, by Substance: 2004–2006

Substance	No Use in Past 12 Months (%)	Use in Past 12 Months but Not Dependent (%)	Use in Past 12 Months and Dependent in Past 12 Months
Alcohol	25.7%	71.1%	3.2%
Marijuana	42.4%	51.8%	5.8%
Cocaine use			
Cocaine (not including crack)*	57.5%	38.8%	3.7%
Crack*	75.6%	15.2%	9.2%
Heroin	69.4%	17.2%	13.4%
Hallucinogens	61.5%	36.6%	1.9%
Inhalants	72.6%	26.5%	0.9%
Nonmedical use of psychotherapeutics			
Pain relievers	56.6%	40.2%	3.1%
Tranquilizers	58.8%	40.0%	1.2%
Stimulants	59.1%	36.2%	4.7%
Sedatives	63.7%	33.9%	2.4%

*Dependence for cocaine not specific to form.

Source: SAMHSA, 2004–2006 NSDUHs.

End Notes

1. Stone, A. L., O'Brien, M. S., De La Torre, A., and Anthony, J. C. (2007). Who is becoming hallucinogen dependent soon after hallucinogen use starts? *Drug and Alcohol Dependence*, 87, 153–163.

2. Wagner, F. A., and Anthony, J. C. (2007). Male-female differences in the risk of progression from first use to dependence upon cannabis, cocaine, and alcohol. *Drug and Alcohol Dependence*, 86, 191–198.

3. O'Brien, M. S., and Anthony, J. C. (2005). Risk of becoming cocaine dependent: Epidemiological estimates for the United States, 2000–2001. *Neuropsychopharmacology*, 30, 1006–1018.

4. Chen, C. Y., O'Brien, M. S., and Anthony, J. C. (2005). Who becomes cannabis dependent soon after onset of use? Epidemiological evidence from the United States: 2000–2001. *Drug and Alcohol Dependence*, 79, 11–22.

5. NSDUH measures the nonmedical use of prescription-type pain relievers, sedatives, stimulants, or tranquilizers. Nonmedical use is defined as the use of prescription-type drugs not prescribed for the respondent by a physician or used only for the experience or feeling they caused. Nonmedical use of any prescription-type pain reliever, sedative, stimulant, or tranquilizer does not include over-the-counter drugs. Nonmedical use of stimulants includes methamphetamine use.

6. Respondents whose age at first use was equal to or one year less than their current age were asked to indicate the month in which they initiated their use of that drug.

7. American Psychiatric Association. (1994). *Diagnostic and statistical manual of mental disorders (4th ed.)*. Washington, DC: Author.

Section 52.2

Simultaneous Polydrug Use

Text in this section is excerpted from "Timing of Alcohol and Other Drug Use," National Institute on Alcohol Abuse and Alcoholism (NIAAA), 2008. The complete text of this document, including references, is available online at http://pubs.niaaa.nih.gov/publications/ahr312/96-99.htm.

Many Americans who drink alcohol are polydrug users—that is, they also use other psychoactive drugs, such as nicotine, pharmaceuticals, cannabis, and other illicit substances. Polydrug use is a general term that describes a wide variety of substance use behaviors. Different types of polydrug use can be described with regard to the timing of the ingestion of multiple substances. Concurrent polydrug use (CPU) is the use of two or more substances within a given time period, such as a month or a year. Simultaneous polydrug use (SPU) is the use of two or more substances in combination (at the same time or in temporal proximity) (Grant and Harford 1990a). Thus, although all simultaneous polydrug users are, by definition, concurrent users, concurrent users may or may not be simultaneous users. This section describes the functions of SPU for substance users, as well as the measurement, prevalence, patterns, and consequences of SPU.

Functions of SPU

SPU varies according to the user's intentions regarding the pharmacological and subjective effects of mixing drugs (Ives and Ghelani 2006; Schensul et al. 2005). Although some SPU may reflect an indiscriminate or haphazard pattern of use, the vast majority of users report a great deal of intentionality regarding their choice of drug combinations (Wibberley and Price 2000). Many experienced substance users demonstrate substantial knowledge of the pharmacology of various drugs and how to combine them to produce certain desired types of intoxication (Merchant and Macdonald 1994; Uys and Niesink 2005).

People often use multiple substances at the same time to produce additive or interactive (synergistic) subjective drug effects (Wibberley and Price 2000). Perceptions of enhanced or potentiated subjective effects among those who engage in SPU have a pharmacologic basis. Pharmacological evidence exists for the synergistic effects of some drug combinations, such as alcohol and certain classes of sedatives. Another example is the production of the psychoactive compound cocaethylene in those who use alcohol in combination with cocaine (Jatlow et al. 1991). In many cases, more research is needed to determine whether different drug combinations have additive or interactive effects on intoxication and impairment.

Some people also use one drug to reduce or offset some or all of the effects of another substance. In such cases, the user often staggers the timing of ingesting different substances. For example, sedatives may be used to reduce anxiety and allow sleep subsequent to a cocaine binge. A time lag is not always necessary, however, to have one substance counteract or offset the effects of another. For example, some people who are not regular smokers nevertheless smoke while drinking alcohol. The nicotine may help them to maintain a level of alertness, which allows them to better enjoy or prolong an episode of alcohol intoxication (Istvan and Matarazzo 1984).

Measuring SPU

Most substance use measures do not assess combined use and, therefore, can only provide information about CPU and not SPU. Simultaneous use is more difficult and time consuming to measure than concurrent use (Schensul et al. 2005) and requires the assessment of the temporal proximity of multiple drug use. The specific time frame that ensures combined pharmacologic effects is difficult to determine and depends on factors such as the quantity consumed and the rate of metabolism for each substance.

Prevalence of SPU

Alcohol with tobacco undoubtedly is the most common drug combination used in the United States, although their simultaneous use has not been directly assessed in large epidemiological studies. Using data from the National Epidemiologic Survey on Alcohol and Related Conditions (NESARC), Falk and colleagues (2006) found that 21.7% of adults (27.5% of men and 16.4% of women) reported the use of alcohol and nicotine in the past year. Although not measured in the NESARC, it is likely that the large majority of these individuals also used these two drugs simultaneously.

Marked increases in the combined use of alcohol and illicit drugs have occurred over the past 40 years, although little research has focused on the prevalence of specific patterns of SPU. A consistent finding is that SPU is more common in males and among teens and young adults. Marijuana is by far the most common illicit drug used in combination with alcohol in the United States. A national survey conducted in the early 1980s of people ages 12 and older showed that 11% of males and 4% of females reported combined (simultaneous) alcohol and marijuana use in the past month. Among 18- to 25-year-olds, the percentages were 24% for men and 12% for women (Norton and Colliver 1988). Using a representative sample of 12th graders studied in the 1990s, Collins and colleagues (1998) reported that 27.6% had engaged in combined alcohol and marijuana use in the past year. National survey data collected in 2000 show that 7% of those ages 18 and older (8.5% of men and 5.5% of women) reported past-year simultaneous use of alcohol and marijuana (Midanik et al. 2007).

The prevalence of other alcohol and drug combinations is lower but substantial. Using a representative 1985 adult sample, Grant and Harford (1990a, b) reported past-year rates of combined use of 1.6% for alcohol with sedatives, 3.3% for alcohol with tranquilizers, and for 4.7% for alcohol with cocaine. National survey data from 2000 showed lower rates, with 1.7% of adults reporting the combined use of alcohol with an illicit drug other than marijuana in the past year (Midanik et al. 2007). Among 12th-graders in the 1990s, Collins and colleagues (1998) found past-year rates of 2.3% for alcohol with sedatives, 6.7% for alcohol with stimulants, 5.3% for cocaine with other drugs, and 9.9% for any substance combination that included an illicit drug other than marijuana. McCabe and colleagues (2006) found that 6.9% of a college student sample reported the use of alcohol in combination with nonprescribed pharmaceutical drugs in the past year.

Patterns of SPU

Those few studies that have assessed the temporal proximity of polydrug use have consistently shown that the majority of concurrent polydrug users also report simultaneous use. This has been found in general population surveys (Grant and Harford 1990; Midanik et al. 2007; Norton and Colliver 1988), among high school and college students (Collins et al. 1998; Martin et al. 1992), among clubgoers (Lankenau and Clatts 2005), and in treatment samples of adults (Martin et al. 1996a; Petry 2001) and adolescents (Martin et al. 1996b).

There are large individual differences, however, in the frequency of simultaneous use. For example, some people report using illicit drugs only rarely while drinking, whereas others use drugs nearly every time they drink (Martin et al., 1996a).

The use of three or more substances concurrently and sometimes simultaneously is common among people in addictions treatment. In a treatment sample of adults, Martin and colleagues (1996a) found that of those who reported SPU in the past 120 days (61% of the sample), about 25% consumed alcohol and two illicit drugs in combination, with an average frequency of about once per week, and about 10% sometimes drank alcohol in combination with three or more illicit drugs. Similarly, about 17% of adolescents in addiction treatment who had an alcohol use disorder reported the use of two or more illicit drugs in combination with alcohol in the past year (Martin et al. 1996b).

SPU patterns show age-related differences (Midanik et al. 2007), regional and ethnic differences (Epstein et al. 1999, 2002), and changing trends over time. Research has highlighted extensive use of alcohol and prescription drugs among college students (McCabe et al. 2006), as well as relatively recent trends of youth and young adults using ecstasy, ketamine, and other club drugs in combination with alcohol and other illicit substances (Lankenau and Clatts 2005; Pedersen and Skrondal 1999). The field needs to continue its surveillance efforts to understand new emerging patterns of SPU, especially among youth.

Consequences of SPU

SPU can have particularly dangerous consequences because alcohol and/or other drugs (AOD) combinations can have additive or interactive effects on acute intoxication and impairment. The majority of deaths attributed to heroin overdose involve significant levels of other drugs such as alcohol or benzodiazepines; opiate levels appear to be similar in both fatal and nonfatal overdoses (Darke and Zador 1996). Similarly, about two-thirds of oxycodone-related deaths were found to involve the use of alcohol and/or other drugs (Cone et al. 2003, 2004). Finally, fatalities and injuries reported to be alcohol-related often involve other drug use (Gossop 2001).

Aside from the acute effects associated with intoxication and impairment, little research has examined SPU in relation to health and psychosocial functioning. Although alcohol and tobacco have additive and occasionally interactive effects on health outcomes, such as cardiovascular disease and cancer (Mukamal 2006; Pelucchi et al. 2006), it is unclear whether such effects are related specifically to simultaneous use. Earleywine and Newcomb (1997) found that in a community study of young adults, those who engaged in certain patterns of SPU had more subsequent physical health problems and psychological distress than those who engaged only in concurrent use. Midanik and colleagues (2007) found that compared with concurrent use only, the simultaneous use of alcohol with marijuana, as well as alcohol with other drugs, was associated with increased social problems. Although more research is needed to understand the consequences of SPU, there is little doubt that such behavior represents a major public health problem

Section 52.3

Alcohol Abuse Makes Prescription Drug Abuse More Likely

This section includes text from "Alcohol Abuse Makes Prescription Drug Abuse More Likely," *Research Findings* Vol. 21, No. 5, National Institute on Drug Abuse (NIDA), March 2008.

Men and women with alcohol use disorders (AUDs) are 18 times more likely to report nonmedical use of prescription drugs than people who don't drink at all, according to researchers at the University of Michigan. Dr. Sean Esteban McCabe and colleagues documented this link in two National Institute on Drug Abuse (NIDA)-funded studies; they also discovered that young adults were most at risk for concurrent or simultaneous abuse of both alcohol and prescription drugs.

"The message of these studies is that clinicians should conduct thorough drug use histories, particularly when working with young adults," says Dr. McCabe. "Clinicians should ask patients with alcohol use disorders about nonmedical use of prescription drugs [NMUPD] and in turn ask nonmedical users of prescription medications about their drinking behaviors." The authors also recommend that college staff educate students about the adverse health outcomes associated with using alcohol and prescription medications at the same time.

Two Studies

The authors' first study looked at the prevalence of AUDs and NMUPD in 43,093 individuals 18 and older who participated in the National Epidemiologic Survey on Alcohol and Related Conditions (NESARC) between 2001 and 2005. Participants lived across the United States in a broad spectrum of household arrangements and represented White, African-American, Asian, Hispanic, and Native American populations. Although people with AUDs constituted only 9% of NESARC's total sample, they accounted for more than a third of those who reported NMUPD.

Since the largest group of alcohol and prescription drug abusers were between the ages of 18 and 24, the team's second study focused entirely on this population and involved 4,580 young adults at a large, public, Midwestern university. The participants completed a self-administered online survey, which revealed that 12% of them had used both alcohol and prescription drugs nonmedically within the last year but at different times (concurrent use), and seven percent had taken them at the same time (simultaneous use).

When alcohol and prescription drugs are used simultaneously, severe medical problems can result, including alcohol poisoning, unconsciousness, respiratory depression, and sometimes death. In addition, college students who drank and took prescription drugs simultaneously were more likely than those who did not to blackout, vomit, and engage in other risky behaviors such as drunk driving and unplanned sex.

Who, What, and When

The prescription drugs that were combined with alcohol in order of prevalence included prescription opiates (Vicodin®, OxyContin®, Tylenol 3 with codeine®, Percocet®), stimulant medication (Ritalin®, Adderall®, Concerta®), sedative/anxiety medication (Ativan®, Xanax®, Valium®), and sleeping medication (Ambien®, Halcion®, Restoril®). The college study asked about the respondent's use of medications prescribed for other people while the NESARC explored both use of someone else's prescription medications as well as the use of one's own prescription medications in a manner not intended by the prescribing clinician (to get high).

The researchers found that the more alcohol a person drank and the younger he or she started drinking, the more likely he or she was to report NMUPD. Compared with people who did not drink at all, drinkers who did not binge were almost twice as likely to engage in NMUPD; binge drinkers with no AUD were three times as likely; people who abused alcohol but were not dependent on alcohol were nearly seven times as likely; and people who were dependent on alcohol were 18 times as likely to report NMUPD.

While the majority of the respondents in both studies were White (71% in NESARC and 65% in the college group), an even higher percentage of the simultaneous polydrug users in the college study were White males who had started drinking in their early teens. The NESARC study also found that Whites in general were two to five times more likely than African-Americans to report NMUPD during the past year. Native Americans were at increased risk for NMUPD, and the authors indicated that this subpopulation should receive greater research attention in the future.

Dr. McCabe emphasizes that many people who simultaneously drink alcohol and use prescription medications have no idea how dangerous the interactions between these substances can be. "Passing out is a protective mechanism that stops people from drinking when they are approaching potentially dangerous blood alcohol concentrations," he explains. "But if you take stimulants when you drink, you can potentially override this mechanism and this could lead to life-threatening consequences."

Dr. James Colliver, formerly of NIDA's Division of Epidemiology, Services and Prevention Research, offers perspective on these studies. "Prescription sedatives, tranquilizers, painkillers, and stimulants are generally safe and effective medications for patients who take them as prescribed by a clinician," Dr. Colliver states. "They are used to treat acute and chronic pain, attention deficit hyperactivity disorder, anxiety disorders, and sleep disorders. The problem is that many people think that, because prescription drugs have been tested and approved by the Food and Drug Administration, they are always safe to use; but they are safe only when used under the direction of a physician for the purpose for which they are prescribed."

Chapter 53

Am I an Addict?

Only you can answer this question.

This may not be an easy thing to do. All through our using, we told ourselves, "I can handle it." Even if this was true in the beginning, it is not so now. The drugs handled us. We lived to use and used to live. Very simply, an addict is a person whose life is controlled by drugs.

Perhaps you admit you have a problem with drugs, but you don't consider yourself an addict. All of us have preconceived ideas about what an addict is. There is nothing shameful about being an addict once you begin to take positive action. If you can identify with our problems, you may be able to identify with our solution. The following questions were written by recovering addicts in Narcotics Anonymous. If you have doubts about whether or not you're an addict, take a few moments to read the questions below and answer them as honestly as you can.

1. Do you ever use alone?   __Yes __No

2. Have you ever substituted one drug for
   another, thinking that one particular drug
   was the problem?   __Yes __No

3. Have you ever manipulated or lied to a
   doctor to obtain prescription drugs?   __Yes __No

4. Have you ever stolen drugs or stolen to
   obtain drugs? __Yes __No

5. Do you regularly use a drug when you
   wake up or when you go to bed? __Yes __No

6. Have you ever taken one drug to overcome
   the effects of another? __Yes __No

7. Do you avoid people or places that do not
   approve of you using drugs? __Yes __No

8. Have you ever used a drug without knowing
   what it was or what it would do to you? __Yes __No

9. Has your job or school performance ever
   suffered from the effects of your drug use? __Yes __No

10. Have you ever been arrested as a result of
    using drugs? __Yes __No

11. Have you ever lied about what or how
    much you use? __Yes __No

12. Do you put the purchase of drugs ahead of
    your financial responsibilities? __Yes __No

13. Have you ever tried to stop or control
    your using? __Yes __No

14. Have you ever been in a jail, hospital, or drug
    rehabilitation center because of your using? __Yes __No

15. Does using interfere with your sleeping or
    eating? __Yes __No

16. Does the thought of running out of drugs
    terrify you? __Yes __No

17. Do you feel it is impossible for you to live
    without drugs? __Yes __No

18. Do you ever question your own sanity? __Yes __No

19. Is your drug use making life at home
    unhappy? __Yes __No

20. Have you ever thought you couldn't fit in or
    have a good time without drugs? __Yes __No

21. Have you ever felt defensive, guilty, or
    ashamed about your using? __Yes __No

22. Do you think a lot about drugs?   __Yes __No

23. Have you had irrational or indefinable fears?   __Yes __No

24. Has using affected your sexual relationship?   __Yes __No

25. Have you ever taken drugs you didn't prefer?   __Yes __No

26. Have you ever used drugs because of
    emotional pain or stress?   __Yes __No

27. Have you ever overdosed on any drugs?   __Yes __No

28. Do you continue to use despite negative
    consequences?   __Yes __No

29. Do you think that you have a drug problem?   __Yes __No

"Am I an addict?" This is a question only you can answer. We found that we all answered different numbers of these questions "yes." The actual number of yes responses wasn't as important as how we felt inside and how addiction had affected our lives.

Some of these questions don't even mention drugs. This is because addiction is an insidious disease that affects all areas of our lives—even those areas which seem at first to have little to do with drugs. The different drugs we used were not as important as why we used them and what they did to us.

When we first read these questions, it was frightening for us to think we might be addicts. Some of us tried to dismiss these thoughts by saying:

- "Oh, those questions don't make sense;" or

- "I'm different. I know I take drugs, but I'm not an addict. I have real emotional/family/job problems;" or

- "I'm just having a tough time getting it together right now;" or

- "I'll be able to stop when I find the right person/get the right job, and so forth."

If you are an addict you must first admit that you have a problem with drugs before any progress can be made toward recovery. These questions, when honestly approached, may help to show you how using drugs has made your life unmanageable. Addiction is a disease which, without recovery, ends in jails, institutions and death. Many of us came to Narcotics Anonymous (NA) because drugs had stopped doing what we needed them to do. Addiction takes our pride, self-esteem, family, loved ones, and even our desire to live. If you have not reached this point in your addiction, you don't have to. We have found that our own private hell was within us. If you want help, you can find it in the Fellowship of Narcotics Anonymous.

"We were searching for an answer when we reached out and found Narcotics Anonymous. We came to our first NA meeting in defeat and didn't know what to expect. After sitting in a meeting, or several meetings, we began to feel that people cared and were willing to help. Although our minds told us we would never make it, the people in the fellowship gave us hope by insisting that we could recover. Surrounded by fellow addicts, we realized that we were not alone anymore. Recovery is what happens in our meetings. Our lives are at stake. We found that by putting recovery first, the program works. We faced three disturbing realizations:

1. We are powerless over addiction and our lives are unmanageable.

2. Although we are not responsible for our disease, we are responsible for our recovery.

3. We can no longer blame people, places and things for our addiction. We must face our problems and our feelings.

The ultimate weapon for recovery is the recovering addict."[1]

[1]*Narcotics Anonymous, 5th edition* (Van Nuys, CA: Narcotics Anonymous World Services, Inc., 1988), p. 15.

Chapter 54

Medical Consequences of Drug Addiction

Individuals who suffer from addiction often have one or more accompanying medical issues, including lung and cardiovascular disease, stroke, cancer, and mental disorders. Imaging scans, chest x-rays, and blood tests show the damaging effects of drug abuse throughout the body. For example, tests show that tobacco smoke causes cancer of the mouth, throat, larynx, blood, lungs, stomach, pancreas, kidney, bladder, and cervix. In addition, some drugs of abuse, such as inhalants, are toxic to nerve cells and may damage or destroy them either in the brain or the peripheral nervous system.

Does drug abuse cause mental disorders, or vice versa?

Drug abuse and mental disorders often coexist. In some cases, mental diseases may precede addiction; in other cases, drug abuse may trigger or exacerbate mental disorders, particularly in individuals with specific vulnerabilities.

What harmful consequences to others result from drug addiction?

Beyond the harmful consequences for the addicted individual, drug abuse can cause serious health problems for others. Three of the more devastating and troubling consequences of addiction include the following:

This chapter includes text from "Drugs, Brains, and Behavior: The Science of Addiction (Part IV)," National Institute on Drug Abuse (NIDA), April 2007.

Negative effects of prenatal drug exposure on infants and children: It is likely that some drug-exposed children will need educational support in the classroom to help them overcome what may be subtle deficits in developmental areas such as behavior, attention, and cognition. Ongoing work is investigating whether the effects of prenatal exposure on brain and behavior extend into adolescence to cause developmental problems during that time period.

Negative effects of second-hand smoke: Second-hand tobacco smoke, also referred to as environmental tobacco smoke (ETS), is a significant source of exposure to a large number of substances known to be hazardous to human health, particularly to children. According to the Surgeon General's 2006 Report, *The Health Consequences of Involuntary Exposure to Tobacco Smoke*, involuntary smoking increases the risk of heart disease and lung cancer in never-smokers by 25–30% and 20–30%, respectively.

Increased spread of infectious diseases: Injection of drugs such as heroin, cocaine, and methamphetamine accounts for more than a third of new acquired immunodeficiency syndrome (AIDS) cases. Injection drug use is also a major factor in the spread of hepatitis C, a serious, potentially fatal liver disease and a rapidly growing public health problem. Injection drug use is not the only way that drug abuse contributes to the spread of infectious diseases. All drugs of abuse cause some form of intoxication, which interferes with judgment and increases the likelihood of risky sexual behaviors. This, in turn, contributes to the spread of human immunodeficiency virus (HIV)/AIDS, hepatitis B and C, and other sexually transmitted diseases. Four out of ten U.S. AIDS deaths are related to drug abuse.

What are some effects of specific abused substances?

Nicotine is an addictive stimulant found in cigarettes and other forms of tobacco. Tobacco smoke increases a user's risk of cancer, emphysema, bronchial disorders, and cardiovascular disease. The mortality rate associated with tobacco addiction is staggering. Tobacco use killed approximately 100 million people during the 20th century and, if current smoking trends continue, the cumulative death toll for this century has been projected to reach one billion.

Alcohol consumption can damage the brain and most body organs. Areas of the brain that are especially vulnerable to alcohol-related damage are the cerebral cortex (largely responsible for our higher brain functions, including problem solving and decision making), the hippocampus (important for memory and learning), and the cerebellum (important for movement coordination).

Marijuana is the most commonly abused illicit substance. This drug impairs short-term memory and learning, the ability to focus attention, and coordination. It also increases heart rate, can harm the lungs, and can cause psychosis in those at risk.

Inhalants are volatile substances found in many household products, such as oven cleaners, gasoline, spray paints, and other aerosols, that induce mind-altering effects. Inhalants are extremely toxic and can damage the heart, kidneys, lungs, and brain. Even a healthy person can suffer heart failure and death within minutes of a single session of prolonged sniffing of an inhalant.

Cocaine is a short-acting stimulant, which can lead abusers to binge (to take the drug many times in a single session). Cocaine abuse can lead to severe medical consequences related to the heart, and the respiratory, nervous, and digestive systems.

Amphetamines, including methamphetamine, are powerful stimulants that can produce feelings of euphoria and alertness. Methamphetamine effects are particularly long lasting and harmful to the brain. Amphetamines can cause high body temperature and can lead to serious heart problems and seizures.

Ecstasy (MDMA) produces both stimulant and mind-altering effects. It can increase body temperature, heart rate, blood pressure, and heart wall stress. Ecstasy may also be toxic to nerve cells.

Lysergic acid diethylamide (LSD) is one of the most potent hallucinogenic, or perception altering, drugs. Its effects are unpredictable, and abusers may see vivid colors and images, hear sounds, and feel sensations that seem real but do not exist. Abusers also may have traumatic experiences and emotions that can last for many hours. Some short-term effects can include increased body temperature, heart rate, and blood pressure; sweating; loss of appetite; sleeplessness; dry mouth; and tremors.

Heroin is a powerful opiate drug that produces euphoria and feelings of relaxation. It slows respiration and can increase risk of serious infectious diseases, especially when taken intravenously. Other opioid drugs include morphine, OxyContin®, Vicodin®, and Percodan®, which have legitimate medical uses; however, their nonmedical use or abuse can result in the same harmful consequences as abusing heroin.

Prescription medications are increasingly being abused or used for nonmedical purposes. This practice cannot only be addictive, but in some cases also lethal. Commonly abused classes of prescription drugs include painkillers, sedatives, and stimulants. Among the most disturbing aspects of this emerging trend is its prevalence among teenagers and young adults, and the common misperception that because these medications are prescribed by physicians, they are safe even when used illicitly.

Steroids, which can also be prescribed for certain medical conditions, are abused to increase muscle mass and to improve athletic performance or physical appearance. Serious consequences of abuse can include severe acne, heart disease, liver problems, stroke, infectious diseases, depression, and suicide.

Drug combinations: A particularly dangerous and not uncommon practice is the combining of two or more drugs. The practice ranges from the co-administration of legal drugs, like alcohol and nicotine, to the dangerous random mixing of prescription drugs, to the deadly combination of heroin or cocaine with fentanyl (an opioid pain medication). Whatever the context, it is critical to realize that because of drug–drug interactions, such practices often pose significantly higher risks than the already harmful individual drugs.

Chapter 55

Club Drugs' Health Effects

Club drugs are a pharmacologically heterogeneous group of psychoactive compounds that tend to be abused by teens and young adults at a nightclub, bar, rave, or trance scene. Gamma hydroxybutyrate (GHB), Rohypnol, and ketamine are some of the drugs in this group.

GHB (Xyrem) is a central nervous system (CNS) depressant that was approved by the Food and Drug Administration (FDA) in 2002 for use in the treatment of narcolepsy (a sleep disorder). This approval came with severe restrictions, including its use only for the treatment of narcolepsy, and the requirement for a patient registry monitored by the FDA. GHB is also a metabolite of the inhibitory neurotransmitter gamma-aminobutyric acid (GABA); thus, it is found naturally in the brain, but at concentrations much lower than doses that are abused.

Rohypnol (flunitrazepam) started appearing in the United States in the early 1990s. It is a benzodiazepine (chemically similar to Valium® or Xanax®), but it is not approved for medical use in this country, and its importation is banned.

Ketamine is a dissociative anesthetic, mostly used in veterinary practice.

This chapter is excerpted from "NIDA InfoFacts: Club Drugs (GHB, Ketamine, and Rohypnol)," National Institute on Drug Abuse (NIDA), August 2008.

How are club drugs abused?

Raves and trance events are generally night-long dances, often held in warehouses. Many who attend raves and trances do not use club drugs, but those who do may be attracted to their generally low cost and the intoxicating highs that are said to deepen the rave or trance experience.

- Rohypnol is usually taken orally, although there are reports that it can be ground up and snorted.

- GHB and Rohypnol have both been used to facilitate date rape (also known as drug rape, acquaintance rape, or drug-assisted assault). They can be colorless, tasteless, and odorless, and can be added to beverages and ingested unbeknownst to the victim. When mixed with alcohol, Rohypnol can incapacitate victims and prevent them from resisting sexual assault.

- GHB also has anabolic effects (it stimulates protein synthesis) and has been sought by bodybuilders to aid in fat reduction and muscle building.

- Ketamine is usually snorted or injected intramuscularly.

How do club drugs affect the brain?

GHB acts on at least two sites in the brain: the GABAB receptor and a specific GHB binding site. At high doses, GHB's sedative effects may result in sleep, coma, or death. Rohypnol, like other benzodiazepines, acts at the GABAA receptor. It can produce anterograde amnesia, in which individuals may not remember events they experienced while under the influence of the drug.

Ketamine is a dissociative anesthetic, so called because it distorts perceptions of sight and sound and produces feelings of detachment from the environment and self. Ketamine acts on a type of glutamate receptor (NMDA receptor) to produce its effects, similar to those of the drug PCP.[1] Low-dose intoxication results in impaired attention, learning ability, and memory. At higher doses, ketamine can cause dreamlike states and hallucinations; and at higher doses still, ketamine can cause delirium and amnesia.

Addictive Potential

Repeated use of GHB may lead to withdrawal effects, including insomnia, anxiety, tremors, and sweating. Severe withdrawal reactions have been reported among patients presenting from an overdose of

GHB or related compounds, especially if other drugs or alcohol are involved.[2] Like other benzodiazepines, chronic use of Rohypnol can produce tolerance and dependence. There have been reports of people binging on ketamine, a behavior that is similar to that seen in some cocaine- or amphetamine-dependent individuals. Ketamine users can develop signs of tolerance and cravings for the drug.[3]

What other adverse effects do club drugs have on health?

Uncertainties about the sources, chemicals, and possible contaminants used to manufacture many club drugs make it extremely difficult to determine toxicity and associated medical consequences.

- Coma and seizures can occur following use of GHB. Combined use with other drugs such as alcohol can result in nausea and breathing difficulties. GHB and two of its precursors, gamma butyrolactone (GBL) and 1,4 butanediol (BD), have been involved in poisonings, overdoses, date rapes, and deaths.

- Rohypnol may be lethal when mixed with alcohol and/or other CNS depressants.

- Ketamine, in high doses, can cause impaired motor function, high blood pressure, and potentially fatal respiratory problems.

What treatment options exist?

There is very little information in scientific literature about treatment for persons who abuse or are dependent upon club drugs.

- There are no GHB detection tests for use in emergency rooms, and as many clinicians are unfamiliar with the drug, many GHB incidents likely go undetected. According to case reports, however, patients who abuse GHB appear to present both a mixed picture of severe problems upon admission and good response to treatment, which often involves residential services.[2]

- Treatment for Rohypnol follows accepted protocols for any benzodiazepine, which may consist of a three- to five-day inpatient detoxification program with 24-hour intensive medical monitoring and management of withdrawal symptoms, since withdrawal from benzodiazepines can be life-threatening.[2]

- Patients with a ketamine overdose are managed through supportive care for acute symptoms, with special attention to cardiac and respiratory functions.[4]

How widespread is club drug abuse?

According to results of the 2007 Monitoring the Future (MTF) survey, 0.7% of students in the 8th grade reported past-year use of GHB, as did 0.6% and 0.9% of students in grades 10 and 12, respectively. This is consistent with use reported in 2006.

Past-year use of ketamine did not change significantly from 2006 to 2007—use was reported by 1.0% of 8th-graders, 0.8% of 10th-graders, and 1.3% of 12th-graders in 2007.

There was no significant change in the illicit use of Rohypnol from 2006 to 2007, according to 2007 MTF results, which report consistently low levels of Rohypnol use since the drug was added to the survey in 1996. Annual prevalence of use stands now at around 0.5% in all three grades surveyed.

End Notes

1. Maeng S, Zarate CA Jr. The role of glutamate in mood disorders: Results from the ketamine in major depression study and the presumed cellular mechanism underlying its antidepressant effects. *Curr Psychiatry Rep* 9(6):467–474, 2007.

2. Maxwell JC, Spence RT. Profiles of club drug users in treatment. *Subst Use Misuse* 40(9–10):1409–1426, 2005.

3. Jansen KL, Darracot-Cankovic R. The nonmedical use of ketamine, part two: A review of problem use and dependence. *J Psychoactive Drugs* 33(2):151–158, 2001.

4. Smith KM, Larive LL, Romanelli F. Club Drugs: Methylenedioxymethamphetamine, flunitrazepam, ketamine hydrochloride, and y–hydroxybutyrate. *Am J Health-Syst Pharm* 59(11):1067–1076, 2002.

Chapter 56

Health Effects of Hallucinogens: Ecstasy, LSD, Peyote, Psilocybin, and PCP

Use of Specific Hallucinogens: 2006

- In 2006, young adults aged 18 to 25 were more likely than youths aged 12 to 17 and adults aged 26 or older to be past year users of lysergic acid diethylamide (LSD), ecstasy, and *Salvia divinorum*.

- Among youths, females were more likely than males to be past year users of ecstasy, but males were more likely than females to be past year users of *Salvia divinorum*.

- Young adult males were more likely than young adult females to be past year users of LSD, ecstasy, and *Salvia divinorum*.

Hallucinogens are drugs that distort a person's perception of reality. Hallucinogens such as lysergic acid diethylamide (LSD), phencyclidine (PCP), ketamine, and methylenedioxymethamphetamine (MDMA or ecstasy) are man-made chemicals, while others, such as psilocybin mushrooms and the herb *Salvia divinorum*, occur in nature. These drugs can produce visual and auditory hallucinations, feelings of detachment from one's environment and oneself, and distortions in time and perception. Other effects can include mood swings, elevated

---

This chapter begins with an excerpt from "Use of Specific Hallucinogens: 2006," Substance Abuse and Mental Health Services Administration (SAMHSA), February 14, 2008; and continues with text from "Hallucinogens: LSD, Peyote, Psilocybin, and PCP," National Institute on Drug Abuse (NIDA), June 2009.

body temperature and blood pressure, psychotic-like effects, seizures, and intense feelings of sensory detachment. Although some indicators of hallucinogen use have shown decreases in the past several years, the number of persons who first used ecstasy in the past 12 months increased from 2005 to 2006, and the past year prevalence of this drug is showing signs of increase among young people. In addition, there is evidence suggesting the emergence of new hallucinogens, such as *Salvia divinorum*, which has been marketed as an herbal high.

Table 56.1. Estimated Numbers (in Thousands) of Persons Aged 12 or Older Who Used LSD, PCP, or Ecstasy in Their Lifetime and in the Past Year: 2006

Hallucinogen	Lifetime	Past Year
LSD	23,346	666
PCP	6,618	187
Ecstasy	12,262	2,130

Source: SAMHSA, 2006 NSDUH.

Hallucinogens: LSD, Peyote, Psilocybin, and PCP

Almost all hallucinogens contain nitrogen and are classified as alkaloids. Many hallucinogens have chemical structures similar to those of natural neurotransmitters (for example, acetylcholine-, serotonin-, or catecholamine-like). While the exact mechanisms by which hallucinogens exert their effects remain unclear, research suggests that these drugs work, at least partially, by temporarily interfering with neurotransmitter action or by binding to their receptor sites. Four common types of hallucinogens include the following:

LSD (d-lysergic acid diethylamide) is one of the most potent mood-changing chemicals. It was discovered in 1938 and is manufactured from lysergic acid, which is found in ergot, a fungus that grows on rye and other grains.

Peyote is a small, spineless cactus in which the principal active ingredient is mescaline. This plant has been used by natives in northern Mexico and the southwestern United States as a part of religious ceremonies. Mescaline can also be produced through chemical synthesis.

Psilocybin (4-phosphoryloxy-N,N-dimethyltryptamine) is obtained from certain types of mushrooms that are indigenous to tropical and subtropical regions of South America, Mexico, and the United States. These mushrooms typically contain less than 0.5 percent psilocybin plus trace amounts of psilocin, another hallucinogenic substance.

PCP (phencyclidine) was developed in the 1950s as an intravenous anesthetic. Its use has since been discontinued due to serious adverse effects.

How do hallucinogens affect the brain?

LSD, peyote, psilocybin, PCP, and ecstasy are drugs that cause hallucinations, which are profound distortions in a person's perception of reality. Under the influence of hallucinogens, people see images, hear sounds, and feel sensations that seem real but are not. Some hallucinogens also produce rapid, intense emotional swings. LSD, peyote, and psilocybin cause their effects by initially disrupting the interaction of nerve cells and the neurotransmitter serotonin. Distributed throughout the brain and spinal cord, the serotonin system is involved in the control of behavioral, perceptual, and regulatory systems, including mood, hunger, body temperature, sexual behavior, muscle control, and sensory perception. On the other hand, PCP acts mainly through a type of glutamate receptor in the brain that is important for the perception of pain, responses to the environment, and learning and memory.

There have been no properly controlled research studies on the specific effects of these drugs on the human brain, but smaller studies and several case reports have been published documenting some of the effects associated with the use of hallucinogens.

LSD: Sensations and feelings change much more dramatically than the physical signs in people under the influence of LSD. The user may feel several different emotions at once or swing rapidly from one emotion to another. If taken in large enough doses, the drug produces delusions and visual hallucinations. The user's sense of time and self is altered. Experiences may seem to cross over different senses, giving the user the feeling of hearing colors and seeing sounds. These changes can be frightening and can cause panic. Some LSD users experience severe, terrifying thoughts and feelings of despair, fear of losing control, or fear of insanity and death while using LSD.

LSD users can also experience flashbacks, or recurrences of certain aspects of the drug experience. Flashbacks occur suddenly, often without warning, and may do so within a few days or more than a year after LSD use. In some individuals, the flashbacks can persist and cause significant distress or impairment in social or occupational functioning, a condition known as hallucinogen-induced persisting perceptual disorder (HPPD).

Most users of LSD voluntarily decrease or stop its use over time. LSD is not considered an addictive drug since it does not produce compulsive drug-seeking behavior. However, LSD does produce tolerance, so some users who take the drug repeatedly must take progressively higher doses to achieve the state of intoxication that they had previously achieved. This is an extremely dangerous practice, given the unpredictability of the drug. In addition, cross-tolerance between LSD and other hallucinogens has been reported.

Peyote: The long-term residual psychological and cognitive effects of mescaline, peyote's principal active ingredient, remain poorly understood. A recent study found no evidence of psychological or cognitive deficits among Native Americans that use peyote regularly in a religious setting. It should be mentioned, however, that these findings may not generalize to those who repeatedly abuse the drug for recreational purposes. Peyote abusers may also experience flashbacks.

Psilocybin: The active compounds in psilocybin-containing "magic" mushrooms have LSD-like properties and produce alterations of autonomic function, motor reflexes, behavior, and perception. The psychological consequences of psilocybin use include hallucinations, an altered perception of time, and an inability to discern fantasy from reality. Panic reactions and psychosis also may occur, particularly if a user ingests a large dose. Long-term effects such as flashbacks, risk of psychiatric illness, impaired memory, and tolerance have been described in case reports.

PCP: The use of PCP as an approved anesthetic in humans was discontinued in 1965 because patients often became agitated, delusional, and irrational while recovering from its anesthetic effects. PCP is a dissociative drug, meaning that it distorts perceptions of sight and sound and produces feelings of detachment (dissociation) from the environment and self. First introduced as a street drug in the 1960s, PCP quickly gained a reputation as a drug that could cause bad reactions and was not worth the risk. However, some abusers continue to use PCP due to the feelings of strength, power, and invulnerability as well as a numbing effect on the mind that PCP can induce. Among the adverse psychological effects reported are the following:

- Symptoms that mimic schizophrenia, such as delusions, hallucinations, paranoia, disordered thinking, and a sensation of distance from one's environment.

- Mood disturbances: Approximately 50 percent of individuals brought to emergency rooms because of PCP-induced problems—related to use within the past 48 hours—report significant elevations in anxiety symptoms.

- People who have abused PCP for long periods of time have reported memory loss, difficulties with speech and thinking, depression, and weight loss. These symptoms can persist up to one year after stopping PCP abuse.

- Addiction: PCP is addictive—its repeated abuse can lead to craving and compulsive PCP-seeking behavior, despite severe adverse consequences.

What other adverse effects do hallucinogens have on health?

Unpleasant adverse effects as a result of the use of hallucinogens are not uncommon. These may be due to the large number of psychoactive ingredients in any single source of hallucinogen.

LSD: The effects of LSD depend largely on the amount taken. LSD causes dilated pupils; can raise body temperature and increase heart rate and blood pressure; and can cause profuse sweating, loss of appetite, sleeplessness, dry mouth, and tremors.

Peyote: Its effects can be similar to those of LSD, including increased body temperature and heart rate, uncoordinated movements (ataxia), profound sweating, and flushing. The active ingredient mescaline has also been associated, in at least one report, to fetal abnormalities.

Psilocybin: It can produce muscle relaxation or weakness, ataxia, excessive pupil dilation, nausea, vomiting, and drowsiness. Individuals who abuse psilocybin mushrooms also risk poisoning if one of many existing varieties of poisonous mushrooms is incorrectly identified as a psilocybin mushroom.

PCP: At low-to-moderate doses, physiological effects of PCP include a slight increase in breathing rate and a pronounced rise in blood pressure and pulse rate. Breathing becomes shallow; flushing and profuse sweating, generalized numbness of the extremities, and loss of muscular coordination may occur.

At high doses, blood pressure, pulse rate, and respiration drop. This may be accompanied by nausea, vomiting, blurred vision, flicking up and down of the eyes, drooling, loss of balance, and dizziness. PCP abusers are often brought to emergency rooms because of overdose or because of the drug's severe untoward psychological effects. While intoxicated, PCP abusers may become violent or suicidal and are therefore dangerous to themselves and others. High doses of PCP can also cause seizures, coma, and death (though death more often results from accidental injury or suicide during PCP intoxication). Because PCP can also have sedative effects, interactions with other central nervous system depressants, such as alcohol and benzodiazepines, can also lead to coma.

How widespread is the abuse of hallucinogens?

According to the National Survey on Drug Use and Health (NSDUH), there were approximately 1.1 million persons aged 12 or older in 2007 who reported using hallucinogens for the first time within the past 12 months.

Chapter 57

Impact of Inhalants
on the Brain and Health

Facts about Inhalants

Inhalants are a diverse group of volatile substances whose chemical vapors can be inhaled to produce psychoactive (mind-altering) effects. While other abused substances can be inhaled, the term inhalant is used to describe substances that are rarely, if ever, taken by any other route of administration. A variety of products common in the home and workplace contain substances that can be inhaled to get high; however, people do not typically think of these products (for example, spray paints, glues, and cleaning fluids) as drugs because they were never intended to induce intoxicating effects. Yet young children and adolescents can easily obtain these extremely toxic substances and are among those most likely to abuse them. In fact, more 8th-graders have tried inhalants than any other illicit drug.

What types of products are abused as inhalants?

Inhalants generally fall into the following categories:

This chapter includes text from "NIDA InfoFacts: Inhalants," National Institute on Drug Abuse (NIDA), June 2009; an excerpt from "Inhalant Use and Major Depressive Episode among Youths Aged 12 to 17: 2004 to 2006," Substance Abuse and Mental Health Services Administration (SAMHSA), August 21, 2008; and text from "Adolescent Admissions Reporting Inhalants: 2006," SAMHSA, March 13, 2008.

- **Volatile solvents:** Liquids that vaporize at room temperature.

- **Aerosols:** Sprays that contain propellants and solvents.

- **Gases:** Found in household or commercial products and used as medical anesthetics.

- **Nitrites:** A special class of inhalants that are used primarily as sexual enhancers.

These various products contain a wide range of chemicals such as:

- toluene (spray paints, rubber cement, gasoline),

- chlorinated hydrocarbons (dry-cleaning chemicals, correction fluids),

- hexane (glues, gasoline),

- benzene (gasoline),

- methylene chloride (varnish removers, paint thinners),

- butane (cigarette lighter refills, air fresheners), and

- nitrous oxide (whipped cream dispensers, gas cylinders).

Adolescents tend to abuse different products at different ages. Among new users ages 12–15, the most commonly abused inhalants are glue, shoe polish, spray paints, gasoline, and lighter fluid. Among new users age 16 or 17, the most commonly abused products are nitrous oxide or whippets. Nitrites are the class of inhalants most commonly abused by adults.

How do inhalants affect the brain?

The effects of inhalants are similar to those of alcohol, including slurred speech, lack of coordination, euphoria, and dizziness. Inhalant abusers may also experience lightheadedness, hallucinations, and delusions. With repeated inhalations, many users feel less inhibited and less in control. Some may feel drowsy for several hours and experience a lingering headache. Chemicals found in different types of inhaled products may produce a variety of additional effects, such as confusion, nausea, or vomiting.

By displacing air in the lungs, inhalants deprive the body of oxygen, a condition known as hypoxia. Hypoxia can damage cells throughout the body, but the cells of the brain are especially sensitive to it. The symptoms of brain hypoxia vary according to which regions of the brain are affected: for example, the hippocampus helps control memory, so someone who repeatedly uses inhalants may lose the ability to learn new things or may have a hard time carrying on simple conversations.

Long-term inhalant abuse can also breakdown myelin, a fatty tissue that surrounds and protects some nerve fibers. Myelin helps nerve fibers carry their messages quickly and efficiently, and when damaged, can lead to muscle spasms and tremors or even permanent difficulty with basic actions such as walking, bending, and talking.

Although not very common, addiction to inhalants can occur with repeated abuse. According to the 2006 Treatment Episode Data Set, inhalants were reported as the primary substance abused by less than 0.1% of all individuals admitted to substance abuse treatment. However, of those individuals who reported inhalants as their primary, secondary, or tertiary drug of abuse, nearly half were adolescents aged 12 to 17. This age group represents only 8% of total admissions to treatment.

What other adverse effects do inhalants have on health?

Lethal effects: Sniffing highly concentrated amounts of the chemicals in solvents or aerosol sprays can directly induce heart failure and death within minutes of a session of repeated inhalation. This syndrome, known as sudden sniffing death, can result from a single session of inhalant use by an otherwise healthy young person. Sudden sniffing death is particularly associated with the abuse of butane, propane, and chemicals in aerosols.

High concentrations of inhalants may also cause death from suffocation by displacing oxygen in the lungs, causing the user to lose consciousness and stop breathing. Deliberately inhaling from a paper or plastic bag or in a closed area greatly increases the chances of suffocation. Even when using aerosols or volatile products for their legitimate purposes (for example: painting, cleaning), it is wise to do so in a well-ventilated room or outdoors.

Harmful irreversible effects include:

- hearing loss from spray paints, glues, dewaxers, dry-cleaning chemicals, or correction fluids;

- peripheral neuropathies or limb spasms from glues, gasoline, whipped cream dispensers, or gas cylinders;

- central nervous system or brain damage from spray paints, glues, or dewaxers; and

- bone marrow damage from gasoline.

Serious but potentially reversible effects include:

- liver and kidney damage from correction fluids and dry-cleaning fluids, and

- blood oxygen depletion from varnish removers and paint thinners.

Human immunodeficiency virus/acquired immunodeficiency syndrome (HIV/AIDS), hepatitis, and other infectious diseases: Because nitrites are abused to enhance sexual pleasure and performance, they can be associated with unsafe sexual practices that greatly increase the risk of contracting and spreading infectious diseases such as HIV/AIDS and hepatitis.

Inhalant Use and Major Depressive Episode among Youths Aged 12 to 17: 2004 to 2006

- In 2004 to 2006, 1.1 million youths aged 12 to 17 (4.5%) used inhalants in the past year, and 2.1 million (8.5%) had experienced major depressive episode (MDE) in the past year.

- The rate of past year inhalant use was higher among youths aged 12 to 17 who had MDE in the past year than among those who did not (10.2% versus 4.0%); an estimated 218,000 youths had used inhalants and experienced MDE in the past year.

- Among the youths aged 12 to 17 who had used inhalants and experienced MDE in their lifetime, 43.1% had their first episode of MDE before initiating inhalant use, 28.3% used inhalants before they had their first episode of MDE, and 28.5% started using inhalants and had their first episode of MDE at about the same time.

Were youths with MDE more likely to use inhalants?

Of the youths aged 12 to 17 who had experienced past year MDE, 10.2% used inhalants in the past year compared with 4.0% of the youths aged 12 to 17 who had not had past year MDE. Males with past year MDE were about twice as likely as those without past year MDE to have used inhalants (9.6% versus 4.0%). Females with past year MDE were about three times as likely as those without past year MDE to have used inhalants (10.5% versus 3.9%). In each age group, youths with past year MDE were more likely than youths without past year MDE to have used inhalants in the past year.

Which comes first, inhalant use or MDE?

An estimated 218,000 (0.9%) youths aged 12 to 17 used inhalants and experienced MDE in the past year. Among those who had used inhalants and had also experienced MDE in the past year, 43.1% experienced their first episode of MDE before initiating inhalant use, 28.3% used inhalants before they experienced their first episode of MDE, and 28.5% started using inhalants and experienced their first episode of MDE at about the same time.

Do youths with MDE use inhalants more frequently than youths without MDE?

Regardless of whether youths aged 12 to 17 experienced MDE in the past year, the majority of youths who used inhalants did so on one to eleven days in that time frame. However, among youths who used inhalants in the past year, those with past year MDE were more likely than those without past year MDE to have used inhalants on 100 days or more per year (12.3% versus 7.9%).

Conclusion

Inhalant use continues to be a serious public health problem that can have potentially dire consequences for young people, including damage to major organ systems and cognitive processes. When combined with a major episode of depression, inhalant use can have devastating consequences for adolescents and their families. These findings suggest that clinicians and parents monitoring adolescents for depression should be alert to the potential for the initiation of substance abuse, including the use of inhalants. Similarly, the data suggest that adolescents using or abusing inhalants might benefit from screening to determine the presence of co-occurring mental health issues such as depression.

Chapter 58

Adverse Health Effects of Marijuana Use

Marijuana is the most commonly abused illicit drug in the United States. It is a dry, shredded green and brown mix of flowers, stems, seeds, and leaves derived from the hemp plant Cannabis sativa. The main active chemical in marijuana is delta-9-tetrahydrocannabinol (THC).

How does marijuana affect the brain?

Scientists have learned a great deal about how THC acts in the brain to produce its many effects. When someone smokes marijuana, THC rapidly passes from the lungs into the bloodstream, which carries the chemical to the brain and other organs throughout the body.

THC acts upon specific sites in the brain, called cannabinoid receptors, kicking off a series of cellular reactions that ultimately lead to the high that users experience when they smoke marijuana. Some brain areas have many cannabinoid receptors; others have few or none. The highest density of cannabinoid receptors are found in parts of the brain that influence pleasure, memory, thoughts, concentration, sensory and time perception, and coordinated movement.[1]

Not surprisingly, marijuana intoxication can cause distorted perceptions, impaired coordination, difficulty in thinking and problem solving, and problems with learning and memory. Research has shown that marijuana's adverse impact on learning and memory can last for days or weeks after the acute effects of the drug wear off.[2] As a result,

This chapter includes text from "NIDA InfoFacts: Marijuana," National Institute on Drug Abuse (NIDA), July 2009.

someone who smokes marijuana every day may be functioning at a suboptimal intellectual level all of the time.

Research on the long-term effects of marijuana abuse indicates some changes in the brain similar to those seen after long-term abuse of other major drugs. For example, cannabinoid withdrawal in chronically exposed animals leads to an increase in the activation of the stress-response system[3] and changes in the activity of nerve cells containing dopamine.[4] Dopamine neurons are involved in the regulation of motivation and reward, and are directly or indirectly affected by all drugs of abuse.

Addictive Potential

Long-term marijuana abuse can lead to addiction; that is, compulsive drug seeking and abuse despite its known harmful effects upon social functioning in the context of family, school, work, and recreational activities. Long-term marijuana abusers trying to quit report irritability, sleeplessness, decreased appetite, anxiety, and drug craving, all of which make it difficult to quit. These withdrawal symptoms begin within about one day following abstinence, peak at 2–3 days, and subside within 1–2 weeks following drug cessation.[5]

Marijuana and Mental Health

A number of studies have shown an association between chronic marijuana use and increased rates of anxiety, depression, suicidal ideation, and schizophrenia. Some of these studies have shown age at first use to be a factor, where early use is a marker of vulnerability to later problems. However, at this time, it not clear whether marijuana use causes mental problems, exacerbates them, or is used in attempt to self-medicate symptoms already in existence. Chronic marijuana use, especially in a very young person, may also be a marker of risk for mental illnesses, including addiction, stemming from genetic or environmental vulnerabilities, such as early exposure to stress or violence. At the present time, the strongest evidence links marijuana use and schizophrenia and/or related disorders.[6] High doses of marijuana can produce an acute psychotic reaction; in addition, use of the drug may trigger the onset or relapse of schizophrenia in vulnerable individuals.

What other adverse effect does marijuana have on health?

Effects on the heart: Marijuana increases heart rate by 20–100% shortly after smoking; this effect can last up to three hours. In one study, it was estimated that marijuana users have a 4.8-fold increase in the risk of heart attack in the first hour after smoking the drug.[7] This may be due to the increased heart rate as well as effects of marijuana on heart rhythms, causing palpitations and arrhythmias. This risk may be greater in aging populations or those with cardiac vulnerabilities.

Effects on the lungs: Numerous studies have shown marijuana smoke to contain carcinogens and to be an irritant to the lungs. In fact, marijuana smoke contains 50–70% more carcinogenic hydrocarbons than does tobacco smoke. Marijuana users usually inhale more deeply and hold their breath longer than tobacco smokers do, which further increase the lungs' exposure to carcinogenic smoke. Marijuana smokers show dysregulated growth of epithelial cells in their lung tissue, which could lead to cancer;[8] however, a recent case-controlled study found no positive associations between marijuana use and lung, upper respiratory, or upper digestive tract cancers.[9] Thus, the link between marijuana smoking and these cancers remains unsubstantiated at this time.

Nonetheless, marijuana smokers can have many of the same respiratory problems as tobacco smokers, such as daily cough and phlegm production, more frequent acute chest illness, and a heightened risk of lung infections. A study of 450 individuals found that people who smoke marijuana frequently but do not smoke tobacco have more health problems and miss more days of work than nonsmokers.[10] Many of the extra sick days among the marijuana smokers in the study were for respiratory illnesses.

Effects on daily life: Research clearly demonstrates that marijuana has the potential to cause problems in daily life or make a person's existing problems worse. In one study, heavy marijuana abusers reported that the drug impaired several important measures of life achievement including physical and mental health, cognitive abilities, social life, and career status.[11] Several studies associate workers' marijuana smoking with increased absences, tardiness, accidents, workers' compensation claims, and job turnover.

End Notes

1. Herkenham M, Lynn A, Little MD, et al. Cannabinoid receptor localization in the brain. *Proc Natl Acad Sci, USA* 87(5):1932–1936, 1990.

2. Pope HG, Gruber AJ, Hudson JI, Huestis MA, Yurgelun-Todd D. Neuropsychological performance in long-term cannabis users. *Arch Gen Psychiatry* 58(10):909–915, 2001.

3. Rodríguez de Fonseca F, Carrera MRA, Navarro M, Koob GF, Weiss F. Activation of corticotropin-releasing factor in the limbic system during cannabinoid withdrawal. *Science* 276(5321):2050–2054, 1997.

4. Diana M, Melis M, Muntoni AL, Gessa GL. Mesolimbic dopaminergic decline after cannabinoid withdrawal. *Proc Natl Acad Sci, USA* 95(17):10269–10273, 1998.

5. Budney AJ, Vandrey RG, Hughes JR, Thostenson JD, Bursac Z. Comparison of cannabis and tobacco withdrawal: Severity and contribution to relapse. *J Subst Abuse Treat*, e-publication ahead of print, March 12, 2008.

6. Moore TH, Zammit S, Lingford-Hughes A, et al. Cannabis use and risk of psychotic or affective mental health outcomes: A systematic review. *Lancet* 370 (9584):319–328, 2007.

7. Mittleman MA, Lewis RA, Maclure M, Sherwood JB, Muller JE. Triggering myocardial infarction by marijuana. *Circulation* 103(23):2805–2809, 2001.

8. Tashkin DP. Smoked marijuana as a cause of lung injury. *Monaldi Arch Chest Dis* 63(2):92–100, 2005.

9. Hashibe M, Morgenstern H, Cui Y, et al. Marijuana use and the risk of lung and upper aerodigestive tract cancers: Results of a population-based case-control study. *Cancer Epidemiol Biomarkers Prev* 15(10):1829–1834, 2006.

10. Polen MR, Sidney S, Tekawa IS, Sadler M, Friedman GD. Health care use by frequent marijuana smokers who do not smoke tobacco. *West J Med* 158(6):596–601, 1993.

11. Gruber AJ, Pope HG, Hudson JI, Yurgelun-Todd D. Attributes of long-term heavy cannabis users: A case control study. *Psychological Med* 33(8):1415–1422, 2003.

Chapter 59

Drug Abuse and Infectious Disease

Chapter Contents

Section 59.1—Link to Human Immunodeficiency
Virus (HIV)/Acquired Immunodeficiency Syndrome (AIDS)
and Other Infectious Diseases 334

Section 59.2—Syringe Exchange Programs 337

Section 59.1

Link to Human Immunodeficiency Virus (HIV)/Acquired Immunodeficiency Syndrome (AIDS) and Other Infectious Diseases

This section includes text from "NIDA InfoFacts: Drug Abuse and the link to HIV/AIDS and Other Infectious Diseases," National Institute on Drug Abuse (NIDA), August 2008.

The human immunodeficiency virus (HIV), which causes acquired immunodeficiency syndrome (AIDS), is a virus that lives and multiplies primarily in white blood cells (CD4+ lymphocytes), which are part of the immune system. HIV ultimately causes severe depletion of these cells. An HIV-infected person may look and feel fine for many years and may therefore be unaware of the infection. However, as the immune system weakens, the individual becomes more vulnerable to illnesses and common infections. Over time, a person with untreated HIV is likely to develop AIDS and succumb to multiple, concurrent illnesses. Because HIV/AIDS is a condition characterized by a defect in the body's natural immunity to diseases, infected individuals are at risk for severe illnesses that are not usually a threat to anyone whose immune system is working properly. Behaviors associated with drug abuse, such as sharing drug injection equipment and/or engaging in risky sexual behavior while intoxicated (from drugs or alcohol), have been central to the spread of HIV/AIDS since the pandemic began more than 25 years ago. As yet, there is no cure for AIDS, and there is no vaccine to prevent a person from acquiring HIV, although there are effective medications to treat HIV infection and help prevent the progression to AIDS.

HIV can be transmitted by contact with the blood or other body fluids of an infected person. In addition, infected pregnant women can pass HIV to their infants during pregnancy, delivery, and breastfeeding. Among drug users, HIV transmission can occur through sharing needles and other injection paraphernalia such as cotton swabs, rinse water, and cookers. However, another way people are at risk for HIV is simply by using drugs, regardless of whether a needle and syringe is involved. Drugs and alcohol can interfere with judgment and can lead to risky sexual behaviors that put people in danger of contracting or transmitting HIV.

Is HIV/AIDS preventable?

Early detection can help prevent HIV transmission. Research indicates that routine HIV screening in health care settings among populations with a prevalence rate as low as one percent is as cost effective as screening for other conditions such as breast cancer and high blood pressure. These findings suggest that HIV screening can lower health care costs by preventing high-risk practices and decreasing virus transmission.

For drug abusing populations, cumulative research has shown that comprehensive HIV prevention—drug abuse treatment, community-based outreach, testing and counseling for HIV and other infections, and HIV treatment—is the most effective way to reduce the risk of blood-borne infections.

Combined pharmacological and behavioral treatments for drug abuse have a demonstrated impact on HIV risk behaviors and acquisition of HIV infection. For example, recent research showed that when behavioral therapies were combined with methadone treatment, about half of the study participants who reported injection drug use at intake reported no such use at study exit, and over 90% of all participants reported no needle sharing at study exit. Although these findings show great promise for achieving reductions in HIV risk behaviors, studies are now underway to improve the long-term effectiveness of such interventions.

Is HIV/AIDS treatable?

Since the mid-1990s, the lives of people with HIV/AIDS have been prolonged and symptoms decreased through the use of highly active antiretroviral therapy (HAART). HAART is a customized combination of different classes of medications prescribed for individual patients based on such factors as their viral load, CD4+ lymphocyte count, and clinical symptoms.

Behavioral treatments for drug abuse have shown promise for enhancing patient adherence to HAART. Interventions aimed at increasing HIV treatment adherence are crucial to treatment success, but they usually require dramatic lifestyle changes to counter the often irregular lifestyle created by drug abuse and addiction. Adequate medical care for HIV/AIDS and related illnesses is also critical to reducing and preventing the spread of new infections.

What other infectious diseases are associated with HIV/AIDS?

Besides increasing their risk of HIV infection, individuals who take drugs or engage in high-risk behaviors associated with drug use also put themselves and others at risk for contracting or transmitting hepatitis C (HCV), hepatitis B (HBV), tuberculosis (TB), as well as a number of sexually transmitted diseases, including syphilis, chlamydia, trichomoniasis, gonorrhea, and genital herpes. Injecting drug users (IDUs) are also commonly susceptible to skin infections at the site of injection and to bacterial and viral infections, such as bacterial pneumonia and endocarditis, which, if left untreated, can lead to serious health problems.

HCV, HBV, and HIV/AIDS: HCV, the leading cause of liver disease, is highly prevalent among IDUs and often co-occurs with HIV; HBV is also common among drug abusers. These are two of several viruses that cause inflammation of the liver. Chronic infection with HCV or HBV can result in cirrhosis (liver scarring) or primary liver cancer. A vaccine does not yet exist for HCV; however, HBV infection can be prevented by an effective vaccine.

HCV is highly transmissible through blood-borne exposure. NIDA-funded studies have found that, within three years of beginning injection drug use, most IDUs contract HCV—and up to 90% of HIV-infected IDUs may also be infected with HCV. The effects of HCV infection on HIV disease are not well understood; however, the course of HCV infection is accelerated in dually infected individuals, with higher rates of progressive liver disease and death in those with both HIV and HCV than in those with HCV alone.

While treatment can be effective, management of co-occurring HIV and HCV presents certain challenges. HIV therapy can slow progression of liver disease in co-infected persons, but treatment response rates to HCV therapy in these individuals are reduced. Assessment of stage of disease is important to the timing of therapy initiation for both infections, as is long-term medical followup in order to improve quality of life.

Tuberculosis (TB) and HIV/AIDS: TB is a chronic and infectious lung disease. Through major public health detection and treatment initiatives, its prevalence declined in the United States for several years—in 2005, 14,000 cases were reported, the lowest number since surveillance began in 1953. However, the decline of TB prevalence has slowed by half in recent years, and TB infection remains intertwined with HIV/AIDS and drug abuse.

People with latent TB infection do not have symptoms, may not develop active disease, and cannot spread TB. However, if such individuals do not receive preventive therapy, they may develop active TB, which is contagious. NIDA research has shown that IDUs have high rates of latent TB infection. Because HIV infection severely weakens the immune system, people infected with both HIV and latent TB are at increased risk of developing active TB and becoming highly infectious. Effective treatment for HIV and TB can reduce TB/HIV-associated disease and the risk of transmission to others.

Section 59.2

Syringe Exchange Programs

"Syringe Exchange Programs—United States, 2005," *MMWR Weekly*,
November 9, 2007, Centers for Disease Control and Prevention (CDC).

Syringe exchange programs (SEPs) provide free sterile syringes in exchange for used syringes to reduce transmission of bloodborne pathogens among injection-drug users (IDUs). SEPs in the United States began as a way to prevent the spread of human immunodeficiency virus (HIV) and other bloodborne infections such as hepatitis B and hepatitis C. The National Institute on Drug Abuse (NIDA) recommends that persons who continue to inject drugs use a new, sterile syringe for each injection. Monitoring syringe exchange activity is an important part of assessing HIV prevention measures in the United States. As of November 2007, a total of 185 SEPs were operating in 36 states, the District of Columbia (DC), and Puerto Rico (North American Syringe Exchange Network [NASEN], unpublished data, 2007). The report summarizes a survey of SEP activities in the United States during 2005 and compares the findings with previous SEP surveys. The findings indicated an increase in overall funding for SEPs, including an increase in public funding, and a stabilization in both the number of SEPs operating and the number of syringes exchanged since 2004. The report also documents an expansion of services offered by SEPs, a trend that resulted from an increase in state and local funding. These expanded services are helping protect IDUs and their communities from the spread of bloodborne pathogens and are providing access to health services for a population at high risk.

SEP size was determined by the number of syringes exchanged during 2005; 117 SEPs reported exchanging a total of 22,472,168 syringes (one SEP did not track the number of syringes exchanged in 2005). The 12 largest programs exchanged 11,863,932 (53% of all the syringes exchanged).

In addition to exchanging syringes, SEPs provided various supplies, services, and referrals in 2005. Nearly all SEPs provided alcohol pads (117 [99%]), male condoms (115 [97%]), and referrals to substance-abuse treatment (102 [86%]). Certain medical services also were offered by SEPs, including counseling and testing for HIV (96 [81%]) and hepatitis C (66 [56%]). Vaccinations for hepatitis B were provided by 46 (39%) SEPs, and hepatitis A vaccinations were provided by 43 (37%). Thirty-four (29%) SEPs offered other on-site medical care.

In 2005, many SEPs operated multiple sites, including fixed sites and mobile van routes. The total number of hours that clients were served by SEPs was summed for all sites operated by each program. This total number of hours per program ranged from 1–168 hours per week (mean: 26 hours per week; median: 20 hours per week). Delivery of syringes and other risk-reduction supplies to residences or meeting spots was reported by 56 (47%) SEPs. A total of 110 (93%) SEPs allowed persons to exchange syringes on behalf of other persons (secondary exchange).

From the period 1994–1995, when the first national survey of SEPs was conducted, to 2002, the number of SEPs and the number of syringes exchanged by these programs increased consistently. However, in 2005, a reduction was observed in the number of SEPs and syringes exchanged. In 2005, eight fewer SEPs were operating than previously indicated by results from the 2004 survey, and two fewer states had SEPs operating. However, four additional cities had SEPs operating in 2005, compared with 2004. The number of syringes exchanged decreased from approximately 24.0 million in 2004 to 22.5 million in 2005.

Compared with data from previous national SEP surveys, the findings in this report indicate an overall stabilization in the number of SEPs operating in the United States. Total funding of SEPs increased in 2005 despite a reduction in the number of SEPs. Increases in funding, particularly public funding, provided opportunities for SEPs to expand the types of services they provide. As a result of these increases, many SEPs have evolved into larger, community-based organizations that provide numerous social and medical services to IDUs and their communities (for example, testing for HIV and hepatitis A, hepatitis B, and hepatitis C; vaccinations for hepatitis A and hepatitis B; and general medical care). These more costly services have been added to many SEPs during the past several years, and continued increases in funding might make these services more available. By expanding such services, SEPs are becoming part of a comprehensive approach to the prevention of bloodborne infections among IDUs and their communities.

The findings in this report are subject to at least three limitations. First, the extent of SEP activity in the United States is likely underestimated because 48 (29%) of the SEPs known to NASEN did not complete the survey. Other SEPs might exist but are not known to NASEN. Second, certain SEPs operating within larger organizations were not able to report exact budget information because of difficulties in allocating shared costs across administrative units. Finally, data collected were based on self-reports by program directors and were not verified independently.

Although the number of SEPs in the United States has stabilized, many SEPs are providing a wider range of services than initially offered. On-site medical services are being provided by an increasing number of SEPs. IDUs often encounter problems in accessing health care, and offering these services in SEP locations increases the likelihood that IDUs will receive these services.

Chapter 60

Comorbidity (Dual Diagnosis): Addiction and Other Mental Illnesses

When two disorders or illnesses occur in the same person, simultaneously or sequentially, they are called comorbid. Comorbidity also implies interactions between the illnesses that affect the course and prognosis of both.

Is drug addiction a mental illness?

Yes, because addiction changes the brain in fundamental ways, disturbing a person's normal hierarchy of needs and desires and substituting new priorities connected with procuring and using the drug. The resulting compulsive behaviors that override the ability to control impulses despite the consequences are similar to hallmarks of other mental illnesses.

In fact, the *Diagnostic and Statistical Manual of Mental Disorder, 4th Ed.* (DSM-IV), the definitive resource of diagnostic criteria for all mental disorders, includes criteria for drug use disorders, distinguishing between two types: drug abuse and drug dependence. Drug dependence is synonymous with addiction. By comparison, the criteria for drug abuse hinge on the harmful consequences of repeated use but do not include the compulsive use, tolerance (needing higher doses to achieve the same effect), or withdrawal (symptoms that occur when use is stopped) that can be signs of addiction.

This chapter includes text from "Comorbidity: Addiction and Other Mental Illnesses," National Institute on Drug Abuse (NIDA), December 2008.

How common are comorbid drug use and other mental disorders?

Many people who regularly abuse drugs are also diagnosed with mental disorders and vice versa. The high prevalence of this comorbidity has been documented in multiple national population surveys since the 1980s. Data show that persons diagnosed with mood or anxiety disorders were about twice as likely to suffer also from a drug use disorder (abuse or dependence) compared with respondents in general. The same was true for those diagnosed with an antisocial syndrome, such as antisocial personality or conduct disorder. Similarly, persons diagnosed with drug disorders were roughly twice as likely to suffer also from mood and anxiety disorders.

Gender is also a factor in the specific patterns of observed comorbidities. For example, the overall rates of abuse and dependence for most drugs tend to be higher among males than females, and males are more likely to suffer also from antisocial personality disorder. In contrast, women have higher rates of amphetamine dependence and higher rates of mood and anxiety disorders.

Why do drug use disorders often co-occur with other mental illnesses?

The high prevalence of comorbidity between drug use disorders and other mental illnesses does not mean that one caused the other, even if it appeared first. In fact, establishing causality or directionality is difficult for several reasons. Some symptoms of a mental disorder may not be recognized until the illness has substantially progressed, and imperfect recollections of when drug use/abuse started can also present timing issues. Still, three scenarios deserve consideration:

1. Drugs of abuse can cause abusers to experience one or more symptoms of another mental illness. The increased risk of psychosis in some marijuana abusers has been offered as evidence for this possibility.

2. Mental illnesses can lead to drug abuse. Individuals with overt, mild, or even subclinical mental disorders may abuse drugs as a form of self-medication. For example, the use of tobacco products by patients with schizophrenia is believed to lessen the symptoms of the disease and improve cognition.

3. Both drug use disorders and other mental illnesses are caused by overlapping factors such as underlying brain deficits, genetic vulnerabilities, and/or early exposure to stress or trauma.

All three scenarios probably contribute, in varying degrees, to how and whether specific comorbidities manifest themselves.

Common Factors

Overlapping genetic vulnerabilities: A particularly active area of comorbidity research involves the search for genes that might predispose individuals to develop both addiction and other mental illnesses, or to have a greater risk of a second disorder occurring after the first appears. It is estimated that 40–60% of an individual's vulnerability to addiction is attributable to genetics; most of this vulnerability arises from complex interactions among multiple genes and from genetic interactions with environmental influences. In some instances, a gene product may act directly, as when a protein influences how a person responds to a drug (whether the drug experience is pleasurable or not) or how long a drug remains in the body. But genes can also act indirectly by altering how an individual responds to stress or by increasing the likelihood of risk-taking and novelty-seeking behaviors, which could influence the development of both drug use disorders and other mental illnesses. Several regions of the human genome have been linked to increased risk of both, including associations with greater vulnerability to adolescent drug dependence and conduct disorders.

Involvement of similar brain regions: Some areas of the brain are affected by both drug use disorders and other mental illnesses. For example, the circuits in the brain that use the neurotransmitter dopamine—a chemical that carries messages from one neuron to another—are typically affected by addictive substances and may also be involved in depression, schizophrenia, and other psychiatric disorders.

Indeed, some antidepressants and essentially all antipsychotic medications target the regulation of dopamine in this system directly, whereas others may have indirect effects. Importantly, dopamine pathways have also been implicated in the way in which stress can increase vulnerability to drug addiction. Stress is also a known risk factor for a range of mental disorders and therefore provides one likely common neurobiological link between the disease processes of addiction and those of other mental disorders.

The overlap of brain areas involved in both drug use disorders and other mental illnesses suggests that brain changes stemming from one may affect the other. For example, drug abuse that precedes the first symptoms of a mental illness may produce changes in brain structure and function that kindle an underlying propensity to develop that mental illness. If the mental disorder develops first, associated changes in brain activity may increase the vulnerability to abusing substances by enhancing their positive effects, reducing awareness of their negative effects, or alleviating the unpleasant effects associated with the mental disorder or the medication used to treat it.

The Influence of Developmental Stage

Adolescence—a vulnerable time: Although drug abuse and addiction can happen at any time during a person's life, drug use typically starts in adolescence, a period when the first signs of mental illness commonly appear. It is therefore not surprising that comorbid disorders can already be seen among youth. Significant changes in the brain occur during adolescence, which may enhance vulnerability to drug use and the development of addiction and other mental disorders. Drugs of abuse affect brain circuits involved in reward, decision making, learning and memory, and behavioral control, all of which are still maturing into early adulthood. Thus, understanding the long-term impact of early drug exposure is a critical area of comorbidity research.

Early occurrence increases later risk: Strong evidence has emerged showing early drug use to be a risk factor for later substance abuse problems; additional findings suggest that it may also be a risk factor for the later occurrence of other mental illnesses. However, this link is not necessarily a simple one and may hinge upon genetic vulnerability, psychosocial experiences, and/or general environmental influences. A recent study highlights this complexity, with the finding that frequent marijuana use during adolescence can increase the risk of psychosis in adulthood, but only in individuals who carry a particular gene variant.

It is also true that having a mental disorder in childhood or adolescence can increase the risk of later drug abuse problems, as frequently occurs with conduct disorder and untreated attention-deficit hyperactivity disorder (ADHD). This presents a challenge when treating children with ADHD, since effective treatment often involves prescribing stimulant medications with abuse potential. This issue has generated strong interest from the research community, and although the results are not yet conclusive, most studies suggest that ADHD medications do not increase the risk of drug abuse among children with ADHD.

Regardless of how comorbidity develops, it is common in youth as well as adults. Given the high prevalence of comorbid mental disorders and their likely adverse impact on substance abuse treatment outcomes, drug abuse programs for adolescents should include screening and, if needed, treatment for comorbid mental disorders.

How can comorbidity be diagnosed?

The high rate of comorbidity between drug use disorders and other mental illnesses argues for a comprehensive approach to intervention that identifies, evaluates, and treats each disorder concurrently. The needed approach calls for broad assessment tools that are less likely to result in a missed diagnosis. Accordingly, patients entering treatment for psychiatric illnesses should also be screened for substance use disorders and vice versa. Accurate diagnosis is complicated, however, by the similarities between drug-related symptoms such as withdrawal and those of potentially comorbid mental disorders. Thus, when people who abuse drugs enter treatment, it may be necessary to observe them after a period of abstinence in order to distinguish the effects of substance intoxication or withdrawal from the symptoms of comorbid mental disorders—this would allow for a more accurate diagnosis.

How should comorbid conditions be treated?

A fundamental principle emerging from scientific research is the need to treat comorbid conditions concurrently—which can be a difficult proposition. Patients who have both a drug use disorder and another mental illness often exhibit symptoms that are more persistent, severe, and resistant to treatment compared with patients who have either disorder alone. Nevertheless, steady progress is being made through research on new and existing treatment options for comorbidity and through health services research on implementation of appropriate screening and treatment within a variety of settings.

Note: See Chapter 72 for examples of treatment therapies for comorbid conditions.

Chapter 61

Serious Psychological Distress (SPD) and Substance Use Disorder

Chapter Contents

Section 61.1—SPD and Substance Use
            among Veterans 348

Section 61.2—Higher Rates of Substance
            Use among Young Adult
            Men with SPD 351

Section 61.1

SPD and Substance Use among Veterans

Excerpted from "Serious Psychological Distress and Substance Use Disorder among Veterans," Substance Abuse and Mental Health Services Administration (SAMHSA), December 30, 2008.

Every year, thousands of troops depart from military service and rejoin their families and civilian communities. Given the demanding environments of the military and traumatizing experiences of combat, many veterans experience psychological distress that can be further complicated by substance use and related disorders. Research indicates that male veterans in the general U.S. population are at an elevated risk of suicide. In addition, among veterans of the wars in Iraq and Afghanistan who received care from the Department of Veterans Affairs between 2001 and 2005, nearly one-third were diagnosed with mental health and/or psychosocial problems and one-fifth were diagnosed with a substance use disorder (SUD).

The National Survey on Drug Use and Health (NSDUH) includes questions to assess serious psychological distress (SPD) and substance use disorders. SPD is an overall indicator of nonspecific psychological distress. NSDUH measures past year SPD using the K6 distress questions. The K6 questions measure symptoms of psychological distress during the one month in the past 12 months when respondents were at their worst emotionally. NSDUH also asks respondents to report on their use of illicit drugs and alcohol, as well as symptoms of substance dependence or abuse during the past year. NSDUH defines dependence on or abuse of alcohol or illicit drugs using criteria specified in the American Psychiatric Association's *Diagnostic and Statistical Manual of Mental Disorders, 4th Ed. (DSM-IV)*. Substance dependence or abuse includes such symptoms as withdrawal, tolerance, use in dangerous situations, trouble with the law, and interference in major obligations at work, school, or home during the past year. Individuals who meet the criteria for either dependence or abuse are said to have an SUD. NSDUH respondents also are asked about their military veteran status. A veteran is defined as an individual who has served in any of the U.S. Armed Forces but who is not currently serving in the military.

This report examines past year SPD, SUD, and co-occurring SPD and SUD among veterans aged 18 or older by demographic characteristics. For the purpose of this report, individuals with both SPD and SUD in the past year are said to have co-occurring SPD and SUD. All findings presented in this report are based on combined 2004, 2005, and 2006 NSDUH data. According to NSDUH estimates, 25.9 million military veterans were living in the United States during this 3-year period.

Serious Psychological Distress

Combined data from 2004 to 2006 indicate that an annual average of 7.0% of veterans aged 18 or older (an estimated 1.8 million persons annually) experienced SPD in the past year. Veterans aged 18 to 25 were more likely to have had SPD (20.9%) than veterans aged 26 to 54 (11.2%) or those aged 55 or older (4.3%). Female veterans were twice as likely as male veterans to have had SPD in the past year (14.5% versus 6.5%). Veterans with family incomes of less than $20,000 per year were more likely to have had SPD in the past year than veterans with higher family incomes.

Table 61.1. Prevalence of Serious Psychological Distress (SPD), Substance Use Disorder (SUD), and Co-Occurring SPD and SUD in the Past Year among Veterans, by Age: 2004 to 2006

Disorder	Aged 18 to 25	Aged 26 to 54	Aged 55 or Older
SPD	20.9%	11.2%	4.3%
SUD	25.0%	11.3%	4.4%
Co-occurring SPD and SUD	8.4%	2.7%	0.7%

Source: SAMHSA, 2004, 2005, and 2006 NSDUHs.

Substance Use Disorder

Combined data from 2004 to 2006 indicate that an annual average of 7.1% of veterans aged 18 or older (an estimated 1.8 million persons) met the criteria for SUD in the past year. One quarter of veterans aged 18 to 25 met the criteria for SUD in the past year compared with 11.3% of veterans aged 26 to 54 and 4.4% of veterans aged 55 or older. There was no difference in SUD between male and female veterans (7.2% versus 5.8%). Veterans with a family income of less than $20,000 per year (10.8%) were more likely to have met the criteria for SUD in the past year than veterans with a family income of $20,000–$49,999 (6.6%), $50,000–$74,999 (6.3%), or $75,000 or more (6.7%).

Table 61.2. Prevalence of Serious Psychological Distress (SPD), Substance Use Disorder (SUD), and Co-Occurring SPD and SUD in the Past Year among Veterans, by Family Income: 2004 to 2006

Disorder	Less than $20,000	$20,000 –$49,999	$50,000– $74,999	$75,000 or More
SPD	15.1%	6.9%	5.9%	4.2%
SUD	10.8%	6.6%	6.3%	6.7%
Co-occurring SPD and SUD	4.1%	1.4%	1.2%	0.7%

Source: SAMHSA, 2004, 2005, and 2006 NSDUHs.

Co-Occurring SPD and SUD

From 2004 to 2006, approximately 1.5% of veterans aged 18 or older (an estimated 395,000 persons) had co-occurring SPD and SUD. Increasing age was associated with lower rates of past year co-occurring SPD and SUD, with veterans aged 18 to 25 having the highest rate (8.4%) and veterans aged 55 or older having the lowest rate (0.7%). There was no significant difference in co-occurring disorders among males and females (1.5% versus 2.0%, respectively). Veterans with family incomes of less than $20,000 per year were more likely to have had co-occurring SPD and SUD in the past year than veterans with higher family incomes.

Section 61.2

Higher Rates of Substance Use among Young Adult Men with SPD

Excerpted from "Serious Psychological Distress and Substance Use among Young Adult Males," Substance Abuse and Mental Health Services Administration (SAMHSA), May 16, 2008.

The transition from adolescence to adulthood is a time when individuals assume new social roles and form new identities that provide the foundations for later life. It is also a time of great risk for substance use and mental health problems. Research has shown that substance use and mental health problems tend to be highest among persons in their late adolescent and young adult years, with substance use generally being higher among males and mental health problems generally being higher among females.

The National Survey on Drug Use and Health (NSDUH) includes questions to assess serious psychological distress (SPD) and substance use. SPD is an overall indicator of nonspecific psychological distress. NSDUH measures past year SPD using the K6 distress questions. The K6 questions measure symptoms of psychological distress during the one month in the past 12 months when respondents were at their worst emotionally.

NSDUH asks persons aged 12 or older about their use of illicit drugs and alcohol, including binge and heavy alcohol use, in the past month. Binge alcohol use is defined as drinking five or more drinks on the same occasion (at the same time or within a couple of hours of each other) on at least one day in the past 30 days. Heavy alcohol use is defined as drinking five or more drinks on the same occasion on each of five or more days in the past 30 days; all heavy alcohol users are also binge alcohol users. NSDUH defines any illicit drug as marijuana/hashish, cocaine (including crack), inhalants, hallucinogens, heroin, or prescription-type drugs used nonmedically.

This report examines SPD and substance use among young adult males aged 18 to 25, a relatively understudied group with respect to mental health issues. All findings are annual averages based on combined 2002, 2003, and 2004 NSDUH data.

351

Serious Psychological Distress

An estimated 10.3% of males aged 18 to 25 (1.6 million persons) experienced SPD during the past year. Males aged 18 to 22 were more likely to have had past year SPD than males aged 23 to 25 (10.8% versus 9.3%). Males aged 18 to 25 who were divorced or separated were more likely to have experienced SPD than their counterparts who were married or never married There were no statistically significant differences in the rate of past year SPD across racial/ethnic groups.

For males aged 18 to 22, the prevalence of SPD among those who were full-time college students was 9.4%; the prevalence was 14.3% among those who were part-time students, and 11.6% among those not enrolled in college.

In the month prior to the interview, an estimated 21.4% of males aged 18 to 25 met the criteria for heavy alcohol use, 50.6% engaged in binge alcohol use, and 23.5% had used an illicit drug. Males aged 23 to 25 were more likely to have engaged in binge drinking in the past month than males aged 18 to 22 (53.6% versus 49.0%), while males aged 18 to 22 were more likely to have used an illicit drug than those aged 23 to 25 (25.1% versus 20.5%). American Indians/Alaska Natives had the highest rate of past month illicit drug use, whereas Whites had the highest rates of heavy alcohol use and binge alcohol use. Males aged 18 to 25 who were married had lower rates of past month heavy alcohol use, binge alcohol use, and illicit drug use (12.4%, 42.2%, and 12.4%, respectively) than their peers who were divorced or separated (17.4%, 53.0%, and 20.6%) and those who had never married (22.6%, 51.5%, and 24.9%).

Among males aged 18 to 22, full-time college students were less likely to have used an illicit drug in the past month than those who were not attending college (23.6% versus 26.7%); however, full-time college students were more likely to have engaged in heavy alcohol use in the past month than those attending college part-time or those who were not attending college (25.9% versus 17.3% and 20.9%, respectively).

Co-Occurrence of SPD and Substance Use

Males aged 18 to 25 with past year SPD had higher rates of heavy alcohol use, binge alcohol use, and illicit drug use in the past month than those without past year SPD.

The National Survey on Drug Use and Health (NSDUH) is an annual survey sponsored by the Substance Abuse and Mental Health

Services Administration (SAMHSA). Prior to 2002, this survey was called the National Household Survey on Drug Abuse (NHSDA). For this report, the 2002, 2003, and 2004 data are based on information obtained from 26,921 males aged 18 to 25. The survey collects data by administering questionnaires to a representative sample of the population through face-to-face interviews at their place of residence.

Chapter 62

Suicide, Severe Depression, and Substance Use

Suicide is a major public health problem in the United States. In 2003, suicide was the 11th leading cause of death among adults and accounted for 30,559 deaths among people aged 18 or older. Suicide rates vary across demographic groups, with some of the highest rates occurring among males, whites, and the older population. Suicide also is strongly associated with mental illness and substance use disorders.

Individuals who die from suicide, however, represent a fraction of those who consider or attempt suicide. In 2003, there were 348,830 nonfatal emergency department (ED) visits by adults aged 18 or older who had harmed themselves. Research suggests that there may be between eight and 25 attempted suicides for every suicide death. As with suicide completions, risk factors for attempted suicide in adults include depression and substance use.

The mission of the Office of Applied Studies (OAS) in the Substance Abuse and Mental Health Services Administration (SAMHSA) is to collect, analyze, and disseminate critical public health data. OAS manages two national surveys that offer insight into suicidal ideation and attempts and, in particular, drug-related suicide attempts: the

This chapter includes excerpts from "Suicidal Thoughts, Suicide Attempts, Major Depressive Episode, and Substance Use among Adults," Substance Abuse and Mental Health Services Administration (SAMHSA), December 30, 2008.

National Survey on Drug Use and Health (NSDUH) and the Drug Abuse Warning Network (DAWN).

NSDUH is the nation's primary source of information on the prevalence of illicit drug use among the civilian, noninstitutionalized population aged 12 or older and also provides estimates of alcohol and tobacco use and mental health problems in that population. NSDUH data provide information about the relationships between suicidal thoughts, suicide attempts, and substance use among adults aged 18 or older who have had at least one major depressive episode (MDE) during the past year.

DAWN is a public health surveillance system that measures some of the health consequences of drug use by monitoring drug-related visits to hospital emergency departments (EDs) in the United States. Data from DAWN provide information about the patients, types of drugs, and other characteristics of suicide-related DAWN ED visits.

NSDUH Methods and Findings

NSDUH asks adults aged 18 or older questions to assess lifetime and past year major depressive episodes (MDEs). MDE is defined using diagnostic criteria from the 4th edition of the *Diagnostic and Statistical Manual of Mental Disorders (DSM-IV)*, which specifies a period of two weeks or longer during which there is either depressed mood or loss of interest or pleasure and at least four other symptoms that reflect a change in functioning, such as problems with sleep, eating, energy, concentration, and self-image. Suicide-related questions are administered to respondents who report having had a period of two weeks or longer during which they experienced either depressed mood or loss of interest or pleasure. These questions ask if (during their worst or most recent episode of depression) respondents thought it would be better if they were dead, thought about committing suicide, and, if they had thought about committing suicide, whether they made a suicide plan and whether they made a suicide attempt.

NSDUH also asks all respondents about their use of alcohol and illicit drugs during the 12 months prior to the interview. Binge alcohol use is defined as drinking five or more drinks on the same occasion (at the same time or within a couple of hours of each other) on at least one day in the past 30 days. Any illicit drug refers to marijuana/hashish, cocaine (including crack), inhalants, hallucinogens, heroin, or prescription-type drugs used nonmedically.

This chapter examines the prevalence of suicidal thoughts among adults who experienced at least one MDE during the past year. Because mental illness and substance use commonly co-occur, the prevalence of past year MDE, suicidal thoughts, and suicide attempts is also examined by substance use status.

Prevalence of MDE: In 2004–2005, 14.5% of persons aged 18 or older (31.2 million adults) experienced at least one MDE in their lifetime, and 7.6% (16.4 million adults) experienced an MDE in the past year. Females were almost twice as likely as males to have experienced a past year MDE (9.8% versus 5.4%). Rates of past year MDE varied by age group, with adults aged 55 or older being less likely to have had a past year MDE than adults in all other age groups.

Table 62.1. Percentages of Adults Aged 18 or Older Reporting a Past Year Major Depressive Episode, by Age Group: 2004 and 2005 NSDUHs

Age	Percentage
18 to 20	10.2
21 to 24	9.9
25 to 34	8.7
35 to 54	9.1
55 or older	4.0

Source: SAMHSA, 2004 and 2005 NSDUHs.

Suicidal thoughts among adults with MDE: Among adults aged 18 or older who experienced a past year MDE, 56.3% thought, during their worst or most recent MDE, that it would be better if they were dead, and 40.3% thought about committing suicide. There were some differences in suicidal thoughts by gender and age. Although males and females with past year MDE did not differ significantly in the percentage who thought that it would be better if they were dead, males were more likely than females to have thought about committing suicide (45.5% versus 37.6%). Among adults with a past year MDE, those aged 55 or older were less likely than individuals in all other age groups to have thought that it would be better if they were dead and to have thought about committing suicide. There were no significant differences in the prevalence of suicidal thoughts by region or urban city.

Table 62.2. Percentages Reporting Suicidal Thoughts among Adults Aged 18 or Older with a Past Year Major Depressive Episode, by Age Group: 2004 and 2005 NSDUHs

Age

	18 to 20	21 to 24	25 to 34	35 to 54	55 or Older
Thought better if dead	64.3	62.8	57.5	56.5	46.2
Thought about committing suicide	52.6	46.8	41.9	40.6	27.1

Source: SAMHSA, 2004 and 2005 NSDUHs.

Suicide plans and attempts among adults with MDE: Among persons aged 18 or older with a past year MDE, 14.5% made a suicide plan during their worst or most recent MDE. Also, 10.4% (1.7 million adults) made a suicide attempt during such an episode. There were no significant differences between males and females in attempting suicide, but males were more likely than females to have made a suicide plan (17.9% versus 12.7%). There were also a few differences by age. Adults aged 55 or older with past year MDE were less likely than their counterparts in other age groups to have made a suicide plan. Adults aged 18 to 20 were more likely than adults in all other age groups to have attempted suicide. Among adults aged 18 or older with past year MDE, there were no significant differences in suicide planning or attempts by region or urban city.

Table 63.3. Percentages Reporting Suicide Plans and Attempts among Adults Aged 18 or Older with a Past Year Major Depressive

Age

	18 to 20	21 to 24	25 to 34	35 to 54	55 or Older
Made suicide plan	22.3	18.0	17.4	13.5	7.3
Attempted suicide	19.5	14.7	10.9	9.8	3.9

Source: SAMHSA, 2004 and 2005 NSDUHs.

Past month substance use, MDE, and suicidal thoughts and behaviors: Adults aged 18 or older who reported binge alcohol use were more likely to report past year MDE than their counterparts who had not engaged in binge drinking (8.7% versus 7.3%). In addition, adults with past year MDE and past month binge alcohol use were more likely to report past year suicidal thoughts and past year suicide attempts than those with MDE who did not binge drink.

Similarly, adults aged 18 or older who reported having used illicit drugs during the past month were more likely to report past year MDE than adults who had not used illicit drugs during the past month (14.2% versus 7.1%). Rates of past year suicidal thoughts and suicide attempts were also higher among adults with past year MDE who had used illicit drugs during the past month than adults with past year MDE who had not used illicit drugs.

Table 62.4. Percentages Reporting Suicidal Thoughts and Suicide Attempts among Adults Aged 18 or Older with a Past Year Major Depressive Episode, by Past Month Illicit Drug Use: 2004 and 2005 NSDUHs

	Past Month Illicit Drug Use	No Past Month Illicit Drug Use
Past year suicidal thoughts	67.0	56.9
Past year suicide attempt	19.0	8.9

Source: SAMHSA, 2004 and 2005 NSDUHs.

DAWN Methods and Findings

DAWN is a public health surveillance system that monitors drug-related ED visits in the United States. Data are collected from a nationally representative sample of short-stay, general, non-federal hospitals that operate 24-hour EDs. In DAWN, a drug-related ED visit is defined as any ED visit related to drug use. The drug must be implicated in the ED visit, either as the direct cause or as a contributing factor. For each drug-related ED visit, information is gathered from medical records about the number and types of drugs involved. These include illegal or illicit drugs, such as cocaine, heroin, and marijuana; prescription drugs; over-the-counter medications; dietary supplements;

inhalants; and alcohol. DAWN differs from NSDUH in that it captures medical as well as nonmedical use of pharmaceuticals and includes pharmaceuticals sold over the counter as well as by prescription. DAWN also collects demographic information about the patients, their diagnoses, and their disposition (outcome) at the time of their discharge from the ED.

In this report, ED visits associated with drug-related suicide attempts among persons aged 18 or older are examined. Although DAWN includes only those suicide attempts that involve drugs, these attempts are not limited to overdoses. Also included are suicide attempts made by other means (for example, by firearm) when drugs are involved. National estimates of the number of ED visits involving drug-related suicide attempts in 2004 are presented, along with percentages of visits and visit rates per 100,000 population.

Characteristics of patients involved in ED visits for drug-related suicide attempts: In 2004, an estimated 106,079 ED visits were the result of drug-related suicide attempts by persons aged 18 or older. Females had a higher rate of these drug-related suicide attempts (57 visits per 100,000 population) than males (39 visits per 100,000 population). Comparing age groups, adults aged 18 to 34 had the highest rates of drug-related suicide attempts treated in the ED (from 75 to 90 visits per 100,000 population), while adults aged 55 or older had the lowest rate (10 visits per 100,000 population). A psychiatric condition was diagnosed in 41% (43,176) of the drug-related suicide attempts treated in the ED. The most frequent psychiatric diagnosis was depression, which was documented in 36% of the total visits (37,886 visits).

Substances involved in drug-related suicide attempts treated in EDs: In 2004, an average of 2.3 drugs were implicated in suicide attempts by adults aged 18 or older that were treated in the ED. Over 33% (35,560 visits) involved only one drug, 51.3% involved two or three drugs, and 15.2% involved four or more drugs.

About one-third of the drug-related suicide attempts treated in the ED involved alcohol. Alcohol is always reported to DAWN if the patient was younger than age 21. If the patient was aged 21 or older, alcohol is reported only if it was used with another drug. Although it is an illegal substance for persons under age 21, alcohol was involved in approximately 25% (2,504 visits) of the suicide-related DAWN ED visits by patients aged 18 to 20 and frequently was combined with another drug (2,504 visits). The suicide-related

DAWN ED visits involving patients aged 55 or older had the lowest rate of alcohol involvement, although it should be noted that DAWN only captured these visits for adults if alcohol was used with another drug.

Illicit drugs were involved in an estimated 28.4% (30,109 visits) of the drug-related suicide attempts treated in the ED. The most frequently reported illicit drug was cocaine (13,620 visits), followed by marijuana (8,490 visits).

Almost 59% (62,502) of the drug-related suicide attempts treated in the ED involved a psychotherapeutic drug. Among these, drugs used to treat anxiety and sleeplessness (anxiolytics, sedatives, and hypnotics) were involved in 38.8% (41,188) of the drug-related suicide attempts; most of the drugs reported in these visits were benzodiazepines. Antidepressants were involved in 22.0% (23,359) of the visits. It should be noted that it is not possible in the DAWN system

Table 62.5. Selected Drugs Involved in Emergency Department (ED) Visits for Drug-Related Suicide Attempts among Persons Aged 18 or Older: National Estimates, 2004 DAWN

Selected Drug Category/Drug	Estimated ED Visits	Percentage of ED Visits
Alcohol	35,242	33.2
Illicit drugs	30,109	28.4
Cocaine	13,620	12.8
Marijuana	8,490	8.0
Psychotherapeutic medications	62,502	58.9
Antidepressants	23,359	22.0
Anxiolytics/sedatives/hypnotics	41,188	38.8
Antipsychotics	11,968	11.3
Pain medications	38,238	36.0
Opioids	15,706	14.8
Nonsteroidal anti-inflammatory agents (NSAIDs)	8,167	7.7
Acetaminophen/combinations	14,410	13.6
Anticonvulsants	7,961	7.5
Cardiovascular medications	5,859	5.5

Source: SAMHSA, 2004 DAWN (September 2005 update).

to distinguish the patients who had been prescribed antidepressants to treat preexisting depression and other mental health problems from those who obtained antidepressants by other means.

Pain medications (analgesics) were involved in 36.0% (38,238) of the drug-related suicide attempts treated in the ED. Analgesics containing opiates were involved in an estimated 15,706 suicide attempts. They were followed in frequency by drugs containing acetaminophen (14,410 visits) and nonsteroidal anti-inflammatory agents (NSAIDs) (8,167 visits).

Part Four

Drug Abuse Treatment and Recovery

Chapter 63

Recognizing Drug Use

Chapter Contents

Section 63.1—Signs and Symptoms of Drug Use 366

Section 63.2—Drug Paraphernalia 372

Section 63.1

Signs and Symptoms of Drug Use

This section includes text from "Signs and Symptoms of Teen Drinking and Drug Use," and "Detailed Signs and Symptoms," National Youth Anti-Drug Media Campaign; and "Behavior," Drug Enforcement Administration (DEA), 2009.

Signs and Symptoms of Teen Drinking and Drug Use

How can you tell if your child is using drugs or alcohol? It is difficult because changes in mood or attitudes, unusual temper outbursts, changes in sleeping habits and changes in hobbies or other interests are common in teens. What should you look for? You can also look for signs of depression, withdrawal, carelessness with grooming, or hostility. Also ask yourself, is your child doing well in school, getting along with friends, taking part in sports or other activities?

Watch List for Parents

- Changes in friends

- Negative changes in schoolwork, missing school, or declining grades

- Increased secrecy about possessions or activities

- Use of incense, room deodorant, or perfume to hide smoke or chemical odors

- Subtle changes in conversations with friends, (being more secretive, using coded language)

- Change in clothing choices: new fascination with clothes that highlight drug use

- Increase in borrowing money

- Evidence of drug paraphernalia such as pipes, rolling papers, and so forth

- Evidence of use of inhalant products (such as hairspray, nail polish, correction fluid, common household products)—rags and paper bags are sometimes used as accessories

- Bottles of eye drops, which may be used to mask bloodshot eyes or dilated pupils

- New use of mouthwash or breath mints to cover up the smell of alcohol

- Missing prescription drugs—especially narcotics and mood stabilizers

These changes often signal that something harmful is going on—and often involves alcohol or drugs. You may want to take your child to the doctor and ask him or her about screening your child for drugs and alcohol. This may involve the health professional asking your child a simple question, or it may involve a urine or blood drug screen. However, some of these signs also indicate there may be a deeper problem with depression, gang involvement, or suicide. Be on the watch for these signs so that you can spot trouble before it goes too far.

Detailed Signs and Symptoms

Alcohol use signs and symptoms include: Odor on the breath; intoxication/drunkenness; difficulty focusing—glazed appearance of the eyes; uncharacteristically passive behavior or combative and argumentative behavior; gradual decline in personal appearance and hygiene; gradual development of difficulties, especially in school work or job performance; absenteeism (particularly on Monday); unexplained bruises and accidents; irritability; flushed skin; loss of memory (blackouts); availability and consumption of alcohol becomes the focus of social activities; changes in peer-group associations and friendships; and impaired interpersonal relationships (unexplainable termination of relationships, and separation from close family members).

Cocaine/crack/methamphetamines/stimulants use signs and symptoms include: Extremely dilated pupils; dry mouth and nose, bad breath, frequent lip licking; excessive activity; difficulty sitting still, lack of interest in food or sleep; irritable, argumentative, nervous; talkative, but conversation often lacks continuity; changes subjects rapidly; runny nose, cold or chronic sinus/nasal problems, nose bleeds; use or possession of paraphernalia including small spoons, razor blades, mirror, little bottles of white powder and plastic, glass or metal straws.

Depressants use symptoms include: Symptoms of alcohol intoxication with no alcohol odor on breath (remember that depressants are frequently used with alcohol); lack of facial expression or animation; flat affect; limp appearance; slurred speech. (Note: There are few readily apparent symptoms. Abuse may be indicated by activities such as frequent visits to different physicians for prescriptions to treat nervousness, anxiety, stress, and so forth.)

Ecstasy use signs and symptoms include: Confusion, blurred vision, rapid eye movement, chills or sweating, high body temperature, sweating profusely, dehydrated, confusion, faintness, paranoia or severe anxiety, panic attacks, trance-like state, transfixed on sites and sounds, unconscious clenching of the jaw, grinding teeth, muscle tension, very affectionate. Depression, headaches, dizziness (from hangover/after effects), possession of pacifiers (used to stop jaw clenching), lollipops, candy necklaces, mentholated vapor rub, vomiting, or nausea (from hangover/after effects).

Hallucinogens/LSD/acid use symptoms include: Extremely dilated pupils; warm skin, excessive perspiration, and body odor; distorted sense of sight, hearing, touch; distorted image of self and time perception; mood and behavior changes, the extent depending on emotional state of the user and environmental conditions; unpredictable flashback episodes even long after withdrawal (although these are rare). With the exception of PCP, all hallucinogens seem to share common effects of use. Any portion of sensory perceptions may be altered to varying degrees. Synesthesia, or the seeing of sounds, and the hearing of colors, is a common side effect of hallucinogen use. Depersonalization, acute anxiety, and acute depression resulting in suicide have also been noted as a result of hallucinogen use.

Inhalants use signs and symptoms include: Substance odor on breath and clothes; runny nose; watering eyes; drowsiness or unconsciousness; poor muscle control; prefers group activity to being alone; presence of bags or rags containing dry plastic cement or other solvent at home, in locker at school or at work; discarded whipped cream, spray paint or similar chargers (users of nitrous oxide); small bottles labeled incense (users of butyl nitrite).

Marijuana/pot use signs and symptoms include: Rapid, loud talking and bursts of laughter in early stages of intoxication; sleepy or daze in the later stages; forgetfulness in conversation; inflammation in whites of eyes; pupils unlikely to be dilated; odor similar to burnt rope on clothing or breath; brown residue on fingers; tendency to drive slowly—below speed limit; distorted sense of time passage—tendency to overestimate time intervals; use or possession of paraphernalia including roach clip, packs of rolling papers, pipes, or bongs. Marijuana users are difficult to recognize unless they are under the influence of the drug at the time of observation. Casual users may show none of the general symptoms. Marijuana does have a distinct odor and may be the same color or a bit greener than tobacco.

Narcotics/prescription drugs/ heroin/ opium/ codeine/Oxy-Contin® use signs and symptoms include: Lethargy or drowsiness; constricted pupils fail to respond to light; redness and raw nostrils from inhaling heroin in power form; scars (tracks) on inner arms or other parts of body, from needle injections; use or possession of paraphernalia, including syringes, bent spoons, bottle caps, eye droppers, rubber tubing, cotton, and needles; slurred speech. While there may be no readily apparent symptoms of analgesic abuse, it may be indicated by frequent visits to different physicians or dentists for prescriptions to treat pain of non-specific origin. In cases where patient has chronic pain and abuse of medication is suspected, it may be indicated by amounts and frequency taken.

PCP signs and symptoms include: Unpredictable behavior; mood may swing from passiveness to violence for no apparent reason; symptoms of intoxication; disorientation; agitation and violence if exposed to excessive sensory stimulation; fear or terror; rigid muscles; strange gait; deadened sensory perception (may experience severe injuries while appearing not to notice); pupils may appear dilated; mask-like facial appearance; floating pupils, appear to follow a moving object; comatose (unresponsive) if large amount consumed; eyes may be open or closed.

Solvents, Aerosols, Glue, Petrol signs and symptoms include: Slurred speech, impaired coordination, nausea, vomiting, slowed breathing; brain damage; pains in the chest, muscles, joints, heart trouble, severe depression, fatigue, loss of appetite, bronchial spasm, sores on nose or mouth, nosebleeds, diarrhea, bizarre or reckless behavior, sudden death, suffocation.

Be Involved

If you have increased your monitoring of your child and you suspect that he or she may be using drugs or alcohol, it's time to have a conversation about substance abuse. In a caring, gentle way, let your child know that in your family you have a policy of no drug use. And know that you should have this conversation not just once in your child's life, but often. If you continue to spot the signs and symptoms of drug use, you may want to take your child to the doctor and ask him or her to screen for the use of illicit substances. This may involve a urine or blood drug screen. There are also over-the-counter drug tests available in some pharmacies. However, the analysis will have to done by a professional.

Behavior

Is it just a bad day at school or a fight with a friend, or is there something else going on? Is your child using his computer to complete his homework and a drug transaction? How can you tell?

When you notice behavioral changes in your child, you want to be able to identify if these changes are due to adolescent stress and typical growing up—or due to something darker, like drug abuse. Learn what types of behaviors can be monitored in the quest to keep the family drug free:

Use Your Senses

When you are trying to figure out what your teen has been up to, it makes sense to make use of all of your senses.

Sight: Take a look at your teen—do you notice that his eyes and cheeks are red and that he's having trouble focusing on you? He may have been drinking alcohol. Are his eyes red and his pupils constricted? That can be a sign of marijuana use. Does he have a strange burn on his mouth or fingers? That can signify smoking something through a metal or glass pipe. Is he wearing long sleeves in the middle of the summer? He may be trying to hide puncture marks that would indicate intravenous drug use. Has he begun developing nosebleeds? That can be one of the first signs of cocaine abuse.

Smell: Marijuana, cigarettes, and alcohol or beer all have very telltale smells. And whether you notice them on your teen's breath or on her clothing, they are reason for alarm—simply being around other teens who may be drinking or smoking makes it more likely that your teen will, too. Follow your nose—and don't forget that excessive good smells, like breath fresheners, heavy perfumes and freshly laundered clothing (for a teen who's never run the washing machine in her life) can be as telling as the smells they're trying to mask. And make sure too that you take a whiff of your teen's car—the smell of stale beer or marijuana smoke may linger in the car's upholstery.

Sound: Listen for the clues that your teen is giving you by the things that he's saying, the things that he's laughing at, or the fact that he isn't saying anything at all. Silence can speak volumes about the fact that something's going on in your teen's life. By continuing to listen over time, you'll be able to identify which behaviors are the result of a short-term mood swing and which are indicative of a more serious underlying issue.

Considerations: Is there a potentially rational explanation for many of these scenarios? Certainly—your teen may be suffering from a cold, trying to mask eczema on his arms, or may just be tired. He may be feeling stressed by a difficult class in school, or may be having issues in his love life. By observing your teen using all of your senses combined with your gut instinct, you'll better be able to determine if a certain behavior is typical or indicative of drug use. Other signs to look for that may indicate drug use include the following:

Stories don't add up, and social circles change: When your teen says she's going to the football game but can't tell you which team won, or when she's staying at Jenny's house and Jenny just called your house asking for her, it's time to be concerned. No matter how much she denies there's anything going on, it's up to you to confront her and get to the heart of the issue.

The same thing holds true if you see a sudden change in your child's social circle. If they are no longer associating with childhood friends, seem to be only interested in hanging out with kids who are older, or are simply spending time with new friends that give you a bad feeling, you should follow your instincts. And don't accept sullen silence as an answer—make sure the conversation occurs.

School goes downhill: Declining grades can be a stark indicator that drug abuse is occurring—especially if your teen typically performs well. If he seems to have lost his motivation, is missing homework, skipping school, or foregoing the extracurricular activities that he used to be passionate about, that's a sign that there may be a drug issue.

Lying and stealing: Your six-pack of beer has suddenly turned into a five-pack. Your after-dinner aperitif tastes suspiciously watered-down.

You're missing cash from your wallet, or a gold ring from your jewelry box. When a teen wants to get drunk or high, one of the first places they're going to go looking for resources is right within your house. If you begin to notice missing items, you must immediately confront your teen with your suspicions and let them know that stealing—whether it be $5 from your purse or a $500 necklace—will not be tolerated.

Remember: When it comes to identifying the signs of drug abuse, the best rule to follow is this: No one knows their kids better than you. If you think something's going on, take the steps necessary to find out for certain.

Section 63.2

Drug Paraphernalia

"What Kinds of Things Are Paraphernalia?" Drug Enforcement Administration (DEA), 2009.

Drug paraphernalia typically used to smoke marijuana, crack, cocaine, and methamphetamine, like pipes and bongs are easily identifiable drug paraphernalia. Syringes are also widely known to be used to inject a wide variety of drugs such as heroin, methamphetamine, ketamine, and steroids. These forms of drug paraphernalia are often marketed specifically to youth—with colorful logos, celebrity pictures and designs like smiley faces on the products, the items are meant to look harmless and minimize the dangers of taking controlled substances.

Drug paraphernalia, like magic markers, can conceal pipes, and small, hand-painted blown glass items look more like pretty trinkets than pipes or stash containers. Parents need to be aware that these kinds of products often conceal drug use. Identifying drug paraphernalia can be extremely challenging because they are ordinary items, or things that are disguised to resemble ordinary items. For example, a soda can, lipstick dispenser, felt tip marker, or a pager—all normal things that you may find in your child's room—could be used as paraphernalia to hide or use drugs. The soda can could have a false bottom to hide drugs; the lipstick dispenser could hide a drug pipe; the felt tip marker might be an internal drug pipe; and the pager could be hollowed out to conceal drugs. Other items that can be used to conceal drugs include the following:

- Plastic bag
- Small paper bags
- Make-up kits
- Change bottles
- Plastic film canisters
- Cigarette packs
- Small glass vials
- Pill bottles
- Breath mint containers
- Inside candy or gum wrappers

Examples of Paraphernalia Associated with Using Specific Drugs

Ecstasy Paraphernalia

- Pacifiers and lollipops are often used to help ecstasy users guard against the teeth grinding that comes from involuntary jaw clenching.
- Candy necklaces are sometimes used to hide ecstasy pills (bags of small candies also are good for this purpose).
- Glow sticks, mentholated rub, and surgical masks are often used by kids on ecstasy to overstimulate their senses.
- Water bottles are used to bring alcohol to parties or to transport liquid drugs, such as GHB.

Cocaine Paraphernalia

- Pipes to smoke crack
- Small mirrors and short plastic straws or rolled-up paper tubes
- Razor blades
- Small spoons (coke spoons)
- Lighters

Marijuana Paraphernalia

- Rolling papers
- Cigars to make a blunt
- Small plastic bag and stash cans
- Deodorizers, incense, room deodorizers used to disguise the smell of marijuana
- Pipes (metal, wooden, acrylic, glass, stone, plastic, or ceramic)
- Bongs
- Roach clips

Inhalant Paraphernalia

- Rags used for sniffing
- Empty spray cans
- Tubes of glue
- Plastic bags
- Balloons
- Nozzles
- Bottles or cans with hardened glue, sprays, paint, or chemical odors inside of them

Be on the lookout for common products that are out of place in your home, including items used to cover up drug use:

- Mouth washes, breathe sprays, and mints are used to cover alcohol or drug odors.

- Eye drops are used to conceal bloodshot eyes, and can occasionally be used to deliver acid or other drugs.

- Sunglasses worn at seemingly inappropriate times may cover up red eyes from smoking drugs, or changes in pupil size or eye movements related to drug use.

- Paraphernalia, clothing, jewelry, temporary or permanent tattoos, teen jargon, publications and other displays may reflect messages associated with the drug culture and be designed to openly flaunt drug culture involvement or identify drug culture involvement to insiders.

Chapter 64

Drug Abuse First Aid

Definition: Drug abuse is the misuse or overuse of any medication or drug, including alcohol. This chapter discusses first aid for drug overdose and withdrawal.

Considerations: Many street drugs have no therapeutic benefits. Any use of these drugs is a form of drug abuse. Legitimate medications can be abused by people who take more than the recommended dose or who intentionally take them with alcohol or other drugs. Drug interactions may also produce adverse effects. Therefore, it is important to let your doctor know about all the drugs you are taking.

Many drugs are addictive. Sometimes the addiction is gradual. However, some drugs (such as cocaine) can cause addiction after only a few doses. Someone who has become addicted to a drug usually will have withdrawal symptoms when the drug is suddenly stopped. Withdrawal is greatly assisted by professional help.

A drug dose that is large enough to be toxic is called an overdose. Prompt medical attention may save the life of someone who accidentally or deliberately takes an overdose.

Causes: An overdose of narcotics can cause sleepiness and even unconsciousness. Uppers (stimulants) produce excitement, increased rate of heartbeat, and rapid breathing. Downers (depressants) do just the opposite. Mind-altering drugs are called hallucinogens.

They include lysergic acid diethylamide (LSD), PCP (angel dust), and other street drugs. Using such drugs may cause paranoia, hallucinations, aggressive behavior, or extreme social withdrawal. Cannabis-containing drugs such as marijuana may cause relaxation, impaired motor skills, and increased appetite. Legal prescription drugs are sometimes taken in higher-than-recommended amounts to achieve a feeling other than the therapeutic effects for which they were intended. This may lead to serious side effects. The use of any of the mentioned drugs may result in impaired judgment and decision-making skills.

Symptoms: Drug overdose symptoms vary widely depending on the specific drug(s) used, but may include the following:

- Abnormal pupil size
- Agitation
- Convulsions
- Death
- Delusional or paranoid behavior
- Difficulty breathing
- Drowsiness
- Hallucinations
- Nausea and vomiting
- Nonreactive pupils (pupils that do not change size when exposed to light)
- Staggering or unsteady gait (ataxia)
- Sweating or extremely dry, hot skin
- Tremors
- Unconsciousness (coma)
- Violent or aggressive behavior

Drug withdrawal symptoms also vary widely depending on the specific drug(s) used, but may include these:

- Abdominal cramping
- Agitation
- Cold sweat

- Convulsions
- Delusions
- Depression
- Diarrhea
- Hallucinations
- Nausea and vomiting
- Restlessness
- Shaking
- Death

First Aid

1. Check the patient's airway, breathing, and pulse. If necessary, begin cardiopulmonary resuscitation (CPR). If the patient is unconscious but breathing, carefully place him or her in the recovery position. If the patient is conscious, loosen the clothing, keep the person warm, and provide reassurance. Try to keep the patient calm. If an overdose is suspected, try to prevent the patient from taking more drugs. Call for immediate medical assistance.

2. Treat the patient for signs of shock, if necessary. Signs include: weakness, bluish lips and fingernails, clammy skin, paleness, and decreasing alertness.

3. If the patient is having seizures, give convulsion first aid.

4. Keep monitoring the patient's vital signs (pulse, rate of breathing, blood pressure) until emergency medical help arrives.

5. If possible, try to determine which drug(s) were taken and when. Save any available pill bottles or other drug containers. Provide this information to emergency medical personnel.

Do Not

- Do not jeopardize your own safety. Some drugs can cause violent and unpredictable behavior. Call for professional assistance.

- Do not try to reason with someone who is on drugs. Do not expect them to behave reasonably.

- Do not offer your opinions when giving help. You don't need to know why drugs were taken in order to give effective first aid.

When to Contact a Medical Professional

Drug emergencies are not always easy to identify. If you suspect someone has overdosed, or if you suspect someone is experiencing withdrawal, give first aid and seek medical assistance. Try to find out what drug the person has taken. If possible, collect all drug containers and any remaining drug samples or the person's vomit and take them to the hospital.

The National Poison Control Center (800-222-1222) can be called from anywhere in the United States. They will give you further instructions. This is a free and confidential service. All local poison control centers in the United States use this national number. You should call if you have any questions about poisoning or poison prevention. It does not need to be an emergency. You can call for any reason, 24 hours a day, seven days a week.

References

Hantsch CE. Opioids. In: Marx J, ed. *Rosen's Emergency Medicine: Concepts and Clinical Practice. 6th ed.* St. Louis, Mo.: Mosby; 2006: chap 160.

Chapter 65

How People View
Addictions and Recovery

The Summary Report of the *CARAVAN® Survey for SAMHSA on Addictions and Recovery* presents the findings of eleven global questions related to addiction, prevention, recovery, and stigma related to addictions. These questions were part of a nationally representative CARAVAN® telephone survey conducted from August 29 to September 1, 2008. The target audience was a national probability sample of 1,010 adults, 18 years of age and older living in private households in the continental United States. All results in this report are weighted by four variables (age, sex, geographic region, and race) to ensure reliable and accurate representation of the total population, 18 years of age and older.

Findings

Half of all adults 18 and older know someone in recovery from addiction to alcohol, illicit drugs, or prescription drugs.

Age: Respondents age 65 and older are least likely to state they know someone in recovery from addiction. In general, the older a person is, the more likely he or she is to think less of someone who is in recovery from drugs or alcohol, and the less likely he or she is to feel comfortable with someone in recovery from alcohol or drug abuse.

Text in this chapter is from "Summary Report CARAVAN® Survey for SAMHSA on Addictions and Recovery," Substance Abuse and Mental Health Services Administration (SAMHSA), September 2008. The complete report is available at http://www.samhsa.gov/attitudes/CARAVAN_LongReport.pdf.

Respondents age 65 and older are least likely to believe that substance addictions can be prevented. However, more than half do believe they can be prevented. Respondents in the 25- to 34-year age bracket are the most positive that a person in recovery from addiction could go on to live a productive life. Those age 65 and older were the least so.

Stigma: Less than one-fifth of the respondents agree that they would think less of a friend or relative if they discovered that person is in recovery from addiction. Almost one-third would think less of a person with a current addiction.

Almost three-quarters of young adults agree with the statement that people who are addicted to alcohol could stop if they had enough willpower. Twice as many young adults age 18 to 24 believe that willpower could play a decisive role in recovery from addiction than does the general population.

Prevention: Almost two-thirds of respondents agree that addiction to illicit drugs such as cocaine and heroin can be prevented. Respondents age 25 to 34 are the most positive that substance addictions can be prevented. Respondents from households with children are more likely than those in households without children to agree that substance addictions can be prevented.

Drugs versus alcohol: People tend to view addiction to drugs differently than alcohol. In general, respondents are more comfortable with someone in recovery from alcohol abuse than drug addiction. Overall, respondents feel that persons who are addicted to illicit drugs such as cocaine and heroin are much more of a danger to society than those addicted to alcohol, prescription drugs, or marijuana.

Gender: Females are much more likely than males to agree that individuals who are addicted to any of the substances mentioned in the survey are dangers to society. This is particularly true in relation to alcohol addictions. Women are more likely than men to agree that a person in recovery from an addiction to prescription drugs or illicit drugs can live a productive life.

Marijuana: Marijuana appears to be less of an immediate issue with respondents than the other substances mentioned. Less than one-fifth (18%) of respondents mentioned knowing anyone in recovery from marijuana, compared to twice that (41%) for alcohol. In the list of substances that pose a danger to society, marijuana ranked last among all demographic groups (age, race, gender, ethnicity, and income).

Recovery Perceptions

Approximately three-quarters of the population believe that recovery is possible from marijuana, alcohol, and prescription drugs. However, only 58% believe that a person can fully recover from addiction to other illicit drugs such as cocaine, heroin, or methamphetamines.

In general, as Americans grow older, they are less likely to agree that recovery from substance addiction is possible. Women are more likely (62%) than men (54%) to agree that a person can fully recover from addiction to illicit drugs such as cocaine, heroin, or methamphetamines.

The majority of respondents agree with the statement that people in recovery from addictions can live a productive life. Respondents felt most positive about people in recovery from addictions to marijuana, alcohol, and prescription drugs (82%, 78%, and 76%, respectively) than those in recovery from addiction to other illicit drugs such as cocaine, heroin, or methamphetamines (61%).

The percentage of Americans who agree that treatment programs can help people with substance addictions is slightly higher than the percentage of those who agree that people in recovery can live a productive life. Respondents see programs to help people with addictions to alcohol, marijuana, and prescription drugs more favorably than treatment programs designed to help people with addictions to illicit drugs such as heroin, cocaine, or methamphetamines.

Chapter 66

Brief Guide to Intervention

Middle School Interventions Reduce Nonmedical Use of Prescription Drugs

The rates of nonmedical use of prescription drugs among adolescents and young adults in the United States are alarmingly high. Researchers examined whether several universal drug abuse preventive interventions for middle school-age youth could reduce their future nonmedical use of prescription drugs. The interventions, which were administered to both middle school-aged children and their families, were tested in two randomized, controlled studies conducted in the rural Midwest. The first study tested two different family-based interventions, the Preparing for the Drug Free Years (PDFY) program and the Iowa Strengthening Families Program (ISFP), which focus on teaching families about risk and protective factors for substance use. The second study compared the school-based Life Skills Training (LST) intervention program with the Strengthening Family Program for Parents and Youth 10–14 (SFP), a revised version of the family-based ISFP, plus the school-based LST programs. Both studies

---

This chapter begins with an excerpt from "NIDA NewsScan: Middle School Interventions Reduce Nonmedical Use of Prescription Drugs," National Institute on Drug Abuse (NIDA), June 2, 2009; and continues with "If Your Child Is Using: How to Step In and Help," © 2009 Partnership for Drug-Free America (www.drugfree .org). Used with permission. The chapter concludes with text from "NIDA Launches Drug Use Screening Tools for Physicians," NIDA, April 20, 2009.

followed participants until the age of 21 and also included control groups of students that did not receive any of the interventions being tested. Beginning in the 9th or 10th grade, students were asked about prescription drug abuse. Results from both studies showed that teens and young adults who had received the interventions in middle school reported less prescription drug abuse compared with participants who had not received the interventions. The magnitude of the difference depended on the specific intervention received, with the ISFP (in study 1) and SFP programs (in study 2) producing significant decreases in rates of prescription drug abuse. Whether these results can be generalized to other populations (such as non-rural or international populations) and whether the effects of the interventions persist into emerging adulthood years will need to be examined in further studies.

Source: Spoth R, Trudeau L, Shin C, Redmond C. Long-term effects of universal preventive interventions on prescription drug misuse. *Addiction*. 2008;103(7):1160–1168.

If Your Child Is Using: How to Step In and Help

Intervention is not always a formal process involving drug counselors and group confrontation. Substance abuse treatment can actually start right at the kitchen table with a conversation. Here are ten steps you can take right now if your child is using drugs:

1. Discuss—and agree to—a plan of action for your child's substance abuse treatment with your spouse or his other parent or guardian. Ask questions to find out the extent of the problem.

2. Pick a time to talk to your child when he or she is not high or drunk, or extremely upset or angry.

3. Make it clear that you love your child, and that by bringing up substance abuse treatment you are showing your concern for his safety and wellbeing.

4. Point out to your child that, as parents, it is your job to make sure he or she reaches adulthood as safely as possible.

5. Spell out the warning signs of alcohol and drug use that you've observed in your child's behavior. Explain that the problem warrants serious attention and family support, as

well as professional help because without substance abuse treatment it can get out of control and can even be fatal. You may want to detail the negative effects of the person's substance use on you and your family but it's important to remain neutral and non-judgmental in tone. To sum up the warning signs at this step, you should state that the pursuit of substance use despite adverse effects on yourself or others is actually the definition of drug addiction. Don't press the child to agree on this assessment of the problem.

6. Actively listen to anything and everything your child has to say in response. The listening step is crucial, to establish empathy and to convey that you really see and hear your child. If he or she brings up related problems, they should be listened to with a promise of being addressed separately. Reiterate that what you are addressing at the moment is substance abuse which is serious and can be at the core of other problems.

7. Then, to empower your child and get him to think about his substance use in a new way, ask him questions about what he wants out of his life and how things are going with school, his friends, his parents, siblings, job, activities, and so forth.

8. Prompt your child to consider the link between substance use and where her life is not matching up to her dreams and wishes.

9. Ask the child—in light of what he or she is concluding in this conversation about the substance abuse effect on his or her life—to reassess the problem. Set a goal for getting well. Together, plan out some concrete steps to find information about addiction, recovery, and resources, and identify any necessary professional substance abuse treatment.

10. Understand that the conversation you just had is actually a successful intervention, a first concrete step toward interrupting the progression of the problem and getting well. It is a good idea to reiterate again your love and caring concern for your child. Acknowledge yourselves, knowing that you need and deserve strong encouragement and support, and have the power to solve this problem together.

NIDAMED Helps Doctors Provide the Best in Medical Care

The National Institute on Drug Abuse (NIDA), part of the National Institutes of Health, has unveiled its first comprehensive Physicians' Outreach Initiative, NIDAMED, which gives medical professionals tools and resources to screen their patients for tobacco, alcohol, illicit, and nonmedical prescription drug use. The NIDAMED resources include an online screening tool, a companion quick reference guide, and a comprehensive resource guide for clinicians. The initiative stresses the importance of the patient-doctor relationship in identifying unhealthy behaviors before they evolve into life-threatening conditions.

The NIDAMED tools—targeting primary care clinicians—were launched April 20, 2009. "Many patients do not discuss their drug use with their physicians, and do not receive treatment even when their drug abuse escalates," said NIDA Director Dr. Nora D. Volkow. "NIDAMED enables physicians to be the first line of defense against substance abuse and addiction and to increase awareness of the impact of substance use on a patient's overall health."

In 2007, an estimated 19.9 million Americans aged 12 or older (around 8% of the population) were current (past month) users of illegal drugs—nearly one in five of those being 18 to 25 years old—and many more are current tobacco or binge alcohol users. The consequences of this drug use can be far-reaching, playing a role in the cause and progression of many medical disorders, including addiction. Yet only a fraction of people who need addiction treatment receive it.

The NIDAMED tools were developed because doctors are in a unique position to discuss drug-taking behaviors with their patients before they lead to serious medical problems. Research shows that screening, brief intervention, and referral to treatment by clinicians in general medical settings, can promote significant reductions in alcohol and tobacco use.

A growing body of literature also suggests potential reductions in illegal and nonmedical prescription drug use. Yet many primary care physicians express concern that they do not have the experience or diagnostic tools to identify drug use in their patients. "Not only will these tools potentially help clinicians identify the use of drugs such as cocaine and heroin, they can also identify patients who are misusing prescription medications," said Dr. Steven K. Galson, a rear admiral in the U.S. Public Health Service. "In 2007, 16.3 million Americans age 12 and older had taken a prescription pain reliever, tranquilizer, stimulant, or sedative for nonmedical purposes at least once in the past year—behaviors that can lead to serious health problems, including addiction."

NIDAMED's screening tool was adapted from the Alcohol, Smoking and Substance Involvement Screening Test (ASSIST), developed, validated, and published by the World Health Organization (WHO) as an effective screening tool for identifying substance use. NIDA-modified ASSIST tools are specifically designed to fit into today's busy clinical practices. Doctors can access the new tools at www.drugabuse.gov by clicking on the NIDAMED icon.

The online screening tool is an interactive website that guides clinicians through a short series of questions and, based on the patient's responses, generates a substance involvement score that suggests the level of intervention needed. A physician can use this interactive tool during routine office visits. NIDAMED also includes an online resource guide with detailed instructions on how to implement the screening tool, discuss screening results, offer a brief intervention, and make necessary referrals. In addition, a quick reference guide has been developed to serve as a prompt to medical professionals to initiate screening. This abbreviated guide provides a snapshot of the NIDA-modified ASSIST, briefly summarizing the questions, scoring, and next steps.

For More Information

NIDAMED
Website: http://www.drugabuse.gov/nidamed

Chapter 67

Treatment Approaches for Drug Addiction

Drug addiction is a complex illness characterized by intense and, at times, uncontrollable drug craving, along with compulsive drug seeking and use that persist even in the face of devastating consequences. While the path to drug addiction begins with the voluntary act of taking drugs, over time a person's ability to choose not to do so becomes compromised, and seeking and consuming the drug becomes compulsive. This behavior results largely from the effects of prolonged drug exposure on brain functioning. Addiction is a brain disease that affects multiple brain circuits, including those involved in reward and motivation, learning and memory, and inhibitory control over behavior.

Because drug abuse and addiction have so many dimensions and disrupt so many aspects of an individual's life, treatment is not simple. Effective treatment programs typically incorporate many components, each directed to a particular aspect of the illness and its consequences. Addiction treatment must help the individual stop using drugs, maintain a drug-free lifestyle, and achieve productive functioning in the family, at work, and in society. Because addiction is typically a chronic disease, people cannot simply stop using drugs for a few days and be cured. Most patients require long-term or repeated episodes of care to achieve the ultimate goal of sustained abstinence and recovery of their lives.

Text in this chapter is from "Treatment Approaches for Drug Addiction," National Institute on Drug Abuse (NIDA), September 2009.

Too often, addiction goes untreated: According to SAMHSA's National Survey on Drug Use and Health (NSDUH), 23.2 million persons (9.4% of the U.S. population) aged 12 or older needed treatment for an illicit drug or alcohol use problem in 2007. Of these individuals, 2.4 million (10.4% of those who needed treatment) received treatment at a specialty facility (hospital, drug or alcohol rehabilitation, or mental health center). Thus, 20.8 million persons (8.4% of the population aged 12 or older) needed treatment for an illicit drug or alcohol use problem but did not receive it. These estimates are similar to those in previous years.[1]

Principles of Effective Treatment

Scientific research since the mid-1970s shows that treatment can help patients addicted to drugs stop using, avoid relapse, and successfully recover their lives. Based on this research, key principles have emerged that should form the basis of any effective treatment programs:

- Addiction is a complex but treatable disease that affects brain function and behavior.

- No single treatment is appropriate for everyone.

- Treatment needs to be readily available.

- Effective treatment attends to multiple needs of the individual, not just his or her drug abuse.

- Remaining in treatment for an adequate period of time is critical.

- Counseling—individual and/or group—and other behavioral therapies are the most commonly used forms of drug abuse treatment.

- Medications are an important element of treatment for many patients, especially when combined with counseling and other behavioral therapies.

- An individual's treatment and services plan must be assessed continually and modified as necessary to ensure that it meets his or her changing needs.

- Many drug-addicted individuals also have other mental disorders.

- Medically assisted detoxification is only the first stage of addiction treatment and by itself does little to change long-term drug abuse.

- Treatment does not need to be voluntary to be effective.

- Drug use during treatment must be monitored continuously, as lapses during treatment do occur.

- Treatment programs should assess patients for the presence of human immunodeficiency virus (HIV)/acquired immune deficiency syndrome (AIDS), hepatitis B and C, tuberculosis, and other infectious diseases as well as provide targeted risk-reduction counseling to help patients modify or change behaviors that place them at risk of contracting or spreading infectious diseases.

Effective Treatment Approaches

Medication and behavioral therapy, especially when combined, are important elements of an overall therapeutic process that often begins with detoxification, followed by treatment and relapse prevention. Easing withdrawal symptoms can be important in the initiation of treatment; preventing relapse is necessary for maintaining its effects. And sometimes, as with other chronic conditions, episodes of relapse may require a return to prior treatment components. A continuum of care that includes a customized treatment regimen—addressing all aspects of an individual's life, including medical and mental health services—and follow-up options (for example, community- or family-based recovery support systems) can be crucial to a person's success in achieving and maintaining a drug-free lifestyle.

Medications

Medications can be used to help with different aspects of the treatment process.

Withdrawal: Medications offer help in suppressing withdrawal symptoms during detoxification. However, medically assisted detoxification is not in itself treatment—it is only the first step in the treatment process. Patients who go through medically assisted withdrawal but do not receive any further treatment show drug abuse patterns similar to those who were never treated.

Treatment: Medications can be used to help reestablish normal brain function and to prevent relapse and diminish cravings. Currently, we have medications for opioids (heroin, morphine), tobacco (nicotine), and alcohol addiction and are developing others for treating stimulant (cocaine, methamphetamine) and cannabis (marijuana) addiction. Most people with severe addiction problems, however, are polydrug users (users of more than one drug) and will require treatment for all of the substances that they abuse.

- **Opioids:** Methadone, buprenorphine, and for some individuals naltrexone are effective medications for the treatment of opiate addiction. Acting on the same targets in the brain as heroin and morphine, methadone and buprenorphine suppress withdrawal symptoms and relieve cravings. Naltrexone works by blocking the effects of heroin or other opioids at their receptor sites and should only be used in patients who have already been detoxified. Because of compliance issues, naltrexone is not as widely used as the other medications. All medications help patients disengage from drug seeking and related criminal behavior and become more receptive to behavioral treatments.

- **Tobacco:** A variety of formulations of nicotine replacement therapies now exist—including the patch, spray, gum, and lozenges—that are available over the counter. In addition, two prescription medications have been Food and Drug Administration (FDA)-approved for tobacco addiction: bupropion and varenicline. They have different mechanisms of action in the brain, but both help prevent relapse in people trying to quit. Each of the above medications is recommended for use in combination with behavioral treatments, including group and individual therapies, as well as telephone quit lines.

- **Alcohol:** Three medications have been FDA-approved for treating alcohol dependence: naltrexone, acamprosate, and disulfiram. A fourth, topiramate, is showing encouraging results in clinical trials. Naltrexone blocks opioid receptors that are involved in the rewarding effects of drinking and in the craving for alcohol. It reduces relapse to heavy drinking and is highly effective in some but not all patients—this is likely related to genetic differences. Acamprosate is thought to reduce symptoms of protracted withdrawal, such as insomnia, anxiety, restlessness, and dysphoria (an unpleasant or uncomfortable emotional state, such as depression, anxiety, or irritability). It may be more effective in patients with severe dependence. Disulfiram interferes with the degradation of alcohol, resulting in the accumulation of acetaldehyde, which, in turn, produces a very unpleasant reaction that includes flushing, nausea, and palpitations if the patient drinks alcohol. Compliance can be a problem, but among patients who are highly motivated, disulfiram can be very effective.

Behavioral Treatments

Behavioral treatments help patients engage in the treatment process, modify their attitudes and behaviors related to drug abuse, and increase healthy life skills. These treatments can also enhance the effectiveness of medications and help people stay in treatment longer. Treatment for drug abuse and addiction can be delivered in many different settings using a variety of behavioral approaches.

Outpatient behavioral treatment encompasses a wide variety of programs for patients who visit a clinic at regular intervals. Most of the programs involve individual or group drug counseling. Some programs also offer other forms of behavioral treatment such as:

- Cognitive-behavioral therapy which seeks to help patients recognize, avoid, and cope with the situations in which they are most likely to abuse drugs.

- Multidimensional family therapy which was developed for adolescents with drug abuse problems—as well as their families— addresses a range of influences on their drug abuse patterns and is designed to improve overall family functioning.

- Motivational interviewing which capitalizes on the readiness of individuals to change their behavior and enter treatment.

- Motivational incentives (contingency management) which uses positive reinforcement to encourage abstinence from drugs.

Residential treatment programs can also be very effective, especially for those with more severe problems. For example, therapeutic communities (TCs) are highly structured programs in which patients remain at a residence, typically for 6–12 months. TCs differ from other treatment approaches principally in their use of the community—treatment staff and those in recovery—as a key agent of change to influence patient attitudes, perceptions, and behaviors associated with drug use. Patients in TCs may include those with relatively long histories of drug addiction, involvement in serious criminal activities, and seriously impaired social functioning. TCs are now also being designed to accommodate the needs of women who are pregnant or have children. The focus of the TC is on the resocialization of the patient to a drug-free, crime-free lifestyle.

Treatment within the Criminal Justice System

Treatment in a criminal justice setting can succeed in preventing an offender's return to criminal behavior, particularly when treatment continues as the person transitions back into the community. Studies show that treatment does not need to be voluntary to be effective.

[1]Data is from the National Survey on Drug Use and Health (formerly known as the National Household Survey on Drug Abuse), which is an annual survey of Americans age 12 and older conducted by the Substance Abuse and Mental Health Services Administration. This survey is available online at www.samhsa.gov and from NIDA at 877-643-2644.

Chapter 68

Detoxification: One Part of Substance Abuse Treatment

Detoxification is a set of interventions aimed at managing acute intoxication and withdrawal. It denotes a clearing of toxins from the body of the patient who is acutely intoxicated and/or dependent on substances of abuse. Detoxification seeks to minimize the physical harm caused by the abuse of substances. The acute medical management of life-threatening intoxication and related medical problems generally is not included within the term detoxification.

Supervised detoxification may prevent potentially life-threatening complications that might appear if the patient were left untreated. At the same time, detoxification is a form of palliative care (reducing the intensity of a disorder) for those who want to become abstinent or who must observe mandatory abstinence as a result of hospitalization or legal involvement. Finally, for some patients it represents a point of first contact with the treatment system and the first step to recovery. Treatment/rehabilitation, on the other hand, involves a constellation of ongoing therapeutic services ultimately intended to promote recovery for substance abuse patients.

This chapter includes text excerpted from "Detoxification and Substance Abuse Treatment: A Treatment Improvement Protocol TIP 45," Substance Abuse and Mental Health Services Administration (SAMHSA), DHHS Publication No. (SMA) 06–4131, 2006. The complete text, including references, is available online at http://download.ncadi.samhsa.gov/prevline/pdfs/DTXTIP 45(3-30-06).PDF.

Guiding Principles Recognized by the Treatment Improvement Protocol (TIP) 45 Consensus Panel

1. Detoxification does not constitute substance abuse treatment but is one part of a continuum of care for substance-related disorders.

2. The detoxification process consists of evaluation, stabilization, and fostering patient readiness for and entry into treatment— three sequential and essential components: A detoxification process that does not incorporate all three critical components is considered incomplete and inadequate by the consensus panel.

3. Detoxification can take place in a wide variety of settings and at a number of levels of intensity within these settings. Placement should be appropriate to the patient's needs.

4. Persons seeking detoxification should have access to the components of the detoxification process described, no matter what the setting or the level of treatment intensity.

5. All persons requiring treatment for substance use disorders should receive treatment of the same quality and appropriate thoroughness and should be put into contact with a substance abuse treatment program after detoxification, if they are not going to be engaged in a treatment service provided by the same program that provided them with detoxification services. There can be no wrong door to treatment for substance use disorders.

6. Ultimately, insurance coverage for the full range of detoxification services is cost-effective. If reimbursement systems do not provide payment for the complete detoxification process, patients may be released prematurely, leading to medically or socially unattended withdrawal. Ensuing medical complications ultimately drive up the overall cost of health care.

7. Patients seeking detoxification services have diverse cultural and ethnic backgrounds as well as unique health needs and life situations. Organizations that provide detoxification services need to ensure that they have standard practices in place to address cultural diversity. It also is essential that care providers possess the special clinical skills necessary to provide culturally competent comprehensive assessments. Detoxification

program administrators have a duty to ensure that appropriate training is available to staff.

8. A successful detoxification process can be measured, in part, by whether an individual who is substance dependent enters, remains in, and is compliant with the treatment protocol of a substance abuse treatment/rehabilitation program after detoxification.

Assessment for Placement Decisions

The *Patient Placement Criteria, Second Edition, Revised* (PPC-2R) identifies six "assessment dimensions to be evaluated in making placement decisions" (American Society of Addiction Medicine [ASAM] 2001, p. 4). They are as follows:

- Acute intoxication and/or withdrawal potential
- Biomedical conditions and complications
- Emotional, behavioral, or cognitive conditions and complications
- Readiness to change
- Relapse, continued use, or continued problem potential
- Recovery/living environment

The ASAM PPC-2R describes both the settings in which services may take place and the intensity of services (for example, level of care) that patients may receive in particular settings. It is important to reiterate, however, that the ASAM PPC-2R criteria do not characterize all the details that may be essential to the success of treatment (Gastfriend et al. 2000). Moreover, traditional assumptions that certain treatment can be delivered only in a particular setting may not be applicable or valuable to patients.

Clinical judgment and consideration of the patient's particular situation are required for appropriate detoxification and treatment. In addition to the general placement criteria for treatment for substance-related disorders, ASAM also has developed a second set of placement criteria—the five adult detoxification placement levels of care within Dimension 1 (ASAM 2001).

Adult Detoxification Placement Levels

1. **Level I-D:** Ambulatory detoxification without extended onsite monitoring (physician's office, home health care agency). This

level of care is an organized outpatient service monitored at predetermined intervals.

2. **Level II-D:** Ambulatory detoxification with extended onsite monitoring (day hospital service). This level of care is monitored by appropriately licensed nurses with credentials.

3. **Level III.2-D:** Clinically managed residential detoxification (nonmedical or social detoxification setting). This level emphasizes peer and social support and is intended for patients whose intoxication and/or withdrawal is sufficient to warrant 24-hour support.

4. **Level III.7-D:** Medically monitored inpatient detoxification (freestanding detoxification center). Unlike Level III.2.D, this level provides 24-hour medically supervised detoxification services.

5. **Level IV-D:** Medically managed intensive inpatient detoxification (psychiatric hospital inpatient center). This level provides 24-hour care in an acute care inpatient settings.

Least Restrictive Care

Least restrictive refers to patients' civil rights and their right to choice of care. There are four specific themes of historical and clinical importance:

1. Patients should be treated in those settings that least interfere with their civil rights and freedom to participate in society.

2. Patients should be able to disagree with clinician recommendations for care. While this includes the right to refuse any care at all, it also includes the right to obtain care in a setting of their choice (as long as considerations of dangerousness and mental competency are satisfied). It implies a patient's right to seek a higher or different level of care than that which the clinician has planned.

3. Patients should be informed participants in defining their care plan. Such planning should be done in collaboration with their healthcare providers.

4. Careful consideration of state laws and agency policies is required for patients who are unable to act in their own self-interests. Because the legal complexities of this issue will vary

from state to state definitive guidance cannot be provided here, but providers need to consider whether or not the person is gravely incapacitated, suicidal, or homicidal; likely to commit grave bodily injury; or, in some states, likely to cause injury to property. In such cases, state law and/or case law may hold providers responsible if they do not commit the patient to care, but in other cases programs may be open to lawsuits for forcibly holding a patient.

Overarching Principles for Care during Detoxification Services

- Detoxification services do not offer a cure for substance use disorders. They often are a first step toward recovery and the first door through which patients pass to treatment.

- Substance use disorders are treatable, and there is hope for recovery.

- Substance use disorders are brain disorders and not evidence of moral weaknesses.

- Patients are treated with respect and dignity at all times.

- Patients are treated in a nonjudgmental and supportive manner.

- Services planning is completed in partnership with the patient and his or her social support network, including such persons as family, significant others, or employers.

- All health professionals involved in the care of the patient will maximize opportunities to promote rehabilitation and maintenance activities and to link her or him to appropriate substance abuse treatment immediately after the detoxification phase.

- Active involvement of the family and other support systems while respecting the patient's rights to privacy and confidentiality is encouraged.

- Patients are treated with due consideration for individual background, culture, preferences, sexual orientation, disability status, vulnerabilities, and strengths.

Chapter 69

Withdrawal from Drugs

Withdrawal

Withdrawal occurs because your brain works like a spring when it comes to addiction. Drugs and alcohol are brain depressants that push down the spring. They suppress your brain's production of neurotransmitters like noradrenaline. When you stop using drugs or alcohol it is like taking the weight off the spring, and your brain rebounds by producing a surge of adrenaline that causes withdrawal symptoms.

Every drug is different: Some drugs produce significant physical withdrawal (alcohol, opiates, and tranquilizers). Some drugs produce little physical withdrawal, but more emotional withdrawal (cocaine, marijuana, and ecstasy). Every person's physical withdrawal pattern is also different. You may experience little physical withdrawal. That does not mean that you are not addicted. You may experience more emotional withdrawal.

Following are two lists of withdrawal symptoms. The first list is the emotional withdrawal symptoms produced by all drugs. You can experience them whether you have physical withdrawal symptoms or not. The second list is the physical withdrawal symptoms that usually occur with alcohol, opiates, and tranquilizers.

Information in this chapter is reprinted with permission from "Withdrawal" and "Post-Acute Withdrawal," by Dr. Steven M. Melemis, © 2009. For additional information, visit www.AddictionsAndRecovery.org.

Emotional Withdrawal Symptoms

- Anxiety
- Restlessness
- Irritability
- Insomnia
- Headaches
- Poor concentration
- Depression
- Social isolation

Physical Withdrawal Symptoms

- Sweating
- Racing heart
- Palpitations
- Muscle tension
- Tightness in the chest
- Difficulty breathing
- Tremor
- Nausea, vomiting, or diarrhea

Dangerous Withdrawal Symptoms

Alcohol and tranquilizers produce the most dangerous physical withdrawal: Suddenly stopping alcohol or tranquilizers can lead to seizures, strokes, or heart attacks in high risk patients. A medically supervised detox can minimize your withdrawal symptoms and reduce the risk of dangerous complications. Some of the dangerous symptoms of alcohol and tranquilizer withdrawal are:

- grand mal seizures,
- heart attacks,
- strokes,
- hallucinations, and
- delirium tremens (DTs).

Withdrawal from opiates like heroin and OxyContin® is extremely uncomfortable, but not dangerous unless they are mixed with other drugs. Heroin withdrawal on its own does not produce seizures, heart attacks, strokes, or delirium tremens. (Reference: www.AddictionsAnd Recovery.org)

Post-Acute Withdrawal (PAWS)

There are two stages of withdrawal. The first stage is the acute stage, which usually lasts at most a few weeks. During this stage, you may experience physical withdrawal symptoms. But every drug is different, and every person is different.

The second stage of withdrawal is called the post acute withdrawal syndrome (PAWS). During this stage you will have fewer physical symptoms, but more emotional and psychological withdrawal symptoms.

Post-acute withdrawal occurs because your brain chemistry is gradually returning to normal. As your brain improves the levels of your brain chemicals fluctuate as they approach the new equilibrium causing post-acute withdrawal symptoms.

Most people experience some post-acute withdrawal symptoms: Whereas in the acute stage of withdrawal every person is different, in post-acute withdrawal most people have the same symptoms.

The Symptoms of Post-Acute Withdrawal

The most common post-acute withdrawal symptoms are:

- mood swings,
- anxiety,
- irritability,
- tiredness,
- variable energy,
- low enthusiasm,
- variable concentration, and
- disturbed sleep.

Post-acute withdrawal feels like a roller coaster of symptoms: In the beginning, your symptoms will change minute to minute and hour to hour. Later as you recover further they will disappear for a few weeks or months only to return again. As you continue to recover the good stretches will get longer and longer. But the bad periods of post-acute withdrawal can be just as intense and last just as long.

Each post-acute withdrawal episode usually lasts for a few days: Once you have been in recovery for a while, you will find that each post-acute withdrawal episode usually lasts for a few days. There is no obvious trigger for most episodes. You will wake up one day feeling irritable and have low energy. If you hang on for just a few days, it will lift just as quickly as it started. After a while you will develop confidence that you can get through post-acute withdrawal, because you will know that each episode is time limited.

Post-acute withdrawal usually lasts for two years: This is one of the most important things you need to remember. If you are up for the challenge, you can get though this. But if you think that post-acute withdrawal will only last for a few months, then you will get caught off guard, and when you are disappointed you are more likely to relapse. (Reference: www.AddictionsAndRecovery.org)

How to Survive Post-Acute Withdrawal

Be patient: Two years can feel like a long time if you are in a rush to get through it. You cannot hurry recovery. But you can get through it one day at a time.

If you try to rush your recovery, or resent post-acute withdrawal, or try to bulldoze your way through, you will become exhausted. And when you are exhausted you will think of using to escape.

Post-acute withdrawal symptoms are a sign that your brain is recovering. They are the result of your brain chemistry gradually going back to normal. Therefore don't resent them. But remember, even after one year, you are still only half way there.

Go with the flow: Withdrawal symptoms are uncomfortable. But the more you resent them the worse they will seem. You will have lots of good days over the next two years. Enjoy them. You will also have lots of bad days. On those days, don't try to do too much. Take care of yourself, focus on your recovery, and you will get through this.

Practice self-care: Give yourself lots of little breaks over the next two years. Tell yourself "what I am doing is enough." Be good to yourself. That is what most addicts cannot do, and that is what you must learn in recovery. Recovery is the opposite of addiction.

Sometimes you will have little energy or enthusiasm for anything. Understand this and don't overbook your life. Give yourself permission to focus on your recovery.

Post-acute withdrawal can be a trigger for relapse: You will go for weeks without any withdrawal symptoms, and then one day you will wake up and your withdrawal will hit you like a ton of bricks. You will have slept badly. You will be in a bad mood. Your energy will be low. And if you are not prepared for it, if you think that post-acute withdrawal only lasts for a few months, or if you think that you will be different and it will not be as bad for you, then you will get caught off guard. But if you know what to expect you can do this.

Being able to relax will help you through post-acute withdrawal: When you are tense you tend to dwell on your symptoms and make them worse. When you are relaxed it is easier to not get caught up in them. You are not as triggered by your symptoms which means you are less likely to relapse.

Remember: Every relapse, no matter how small undoes the gains your brain has made during recovery. Without abstinence everything will fall apart. With abstinence everything is possible. (Reference: www.AddictionsAndRecovery.org)

Chapter 70

Mutual Support Groups for Alcohol and Drug Abuse

Mutual Support Groups Aid Recovery from Substance Use Disorders

Mutual support (also called self-help) groups are an important part of recovery from substance use disorders (SUDs). Mutual support groups exist both for persons with an SUD and for their families or significant others and are one of the choices an individual has during the recovery process.

Mutual support groups are nonprofessional groups comprising members who share the same problem and voluntarily support one another in the recovery from that problem. Although mutual support groups do not provide formal treatment, they are one part of a recovery-oriented systems-of-care approach to substance abuse recovery. By providing social, emotional, and informational support for persons throughout the recovery process, mutual support groups help individuals take responsibility for their alcohol and drug problems and for their sustained health, wellness, and recovery. The most widely available mutual support groups are twelve-step groups, such as Alcoholics Anonymous (AA), but other mutual support groups such as

This chapter includes text from "Substance Abuse in Brief Fact Sheet, Vol. 5, Issue 1: An Introduction to Mutual Support Groups for Alcohol and Drug Abuse," Substance Abuse and Mental Health Services Administration (SAMHSA), Spring 2008; and, "Participation in Self-Help Groups for Alcohol and Illicit Drug Use: 2006 and 2007," SAMHSA, November 13, 2008.

Women for Sobriety (WFS), SMART Recovery®, and Secular Organizations for Sobriety/Save Our Selves (SOS) are also available.

Twelve-Step Groups

Twelve-Step groups emphasize abstinence and have 12 core developmental steps to recovering from dependence. Other elements of twelve-step groups include taking responsibility for recovery, sharing personal narratives, helping others, and recognizing and incorporating into daily life the existence of a higher power. Participants often maintain a close relationship with a sponsor, an experienced member with long-term abstinence and lifetime participation is expected.

AA is the oldest and best known twelve-step mutual support group. There are more than 100,000 AA groups worldwide and nearly two million members. The AA model has been adapted for people with dependence on drugs and for their family members. Some groups, such as Narcotics Anonymous (NA) and Chemically Dependent Anonymous, focus on any type of drug use. Other groups, such as Cocaine Anonymous and Crystal Meth Anonymous, focus on abuse of specific drugs. Groups for persons with co-occurring substance use and mental disorders also exist (Double Trouble in Recovery; Dual Recovery Anonymous). Other twelve-step groups—Families Anonymous, Al-Anon/Alateen, Nar-Anon, and Co-Anon—provide support to significant others, families, and friends of persons with SUDs.

Twelve-step meetings are held in locations such as churches and public buildings. Metropolitan areas usually have specialized groups, based on such member characteristics as gender, length of time in recovery, age, sexual orientation, profession, ethnicity, and language spoken. Attendance and membership are free, although people usually give a small donation when they attend a meeting.

Meetings can be open or closed, that is, anyone can attend an open meeting, but attendance at closed meetings is limited to people who want to stop drinking or using drugs. Although meeting formats vary somewhat, most twelve-step meetings have an opening and a closing that are the same at every meeting, such as a twelve-step reading or prayer. The main part of the meeting usually consists of members sharing their stories of dependence, its effect on their lives, and what they are doing to stay abstinent; the study of a particular step or other doctrine of the group; or a guest speaker.

Twelve-step groups are not necessarily for everyone. Some people are uncomfortable with the spiritual emphasis and prefer a more secular approach. Others may not agree with the twelve-step philosophy that addiction is a chronic disease, thinking that this belief can be a self-fulfilling prophesy that weakens the ability to remain abstinent. Still others may prefer gender specific groups.

Mutual support groups that are not based on the twelve-step model typically do not advocate sponsors or lifetime membership. These support groups offer an alternative to traditional twelve-step groups, but the availability of in-person meetings is more limited than that of twelve-step programs. However, many offer literature, discussion boards, and online meetings.

Women for Sobriety (WFS)

WFS is the first national self-help group solely for women wishing to stop using alcohol and drugs. The program is based on *Thirteen Statements* that encourage emotional and spiritual growth, with abstinence as the only acceptable goal. Although daily meditation is encouraged, WFS does not otherwise emphasize God or a higher power. The nearly 300 meetings held weekly are led by experienced, abstinent WFS members and follow a structured format which includes reading the *Thirteen Statements*, an introduction of members, and a moderated discussion.

SMART Recovery

SMART Recovery helps individuals become free from dependence on any substance. Dependence is viewed as a learned behavior that can be modified using cognitive-behavioral approaches. Its four principles are to (1) enhance and maintain motivation to abstain; (2) cope with urges; (3) manage thoughts, feelings, and behaviors; and (4) balance momentary and enduring satisfactions. At the approximately 300 weekly group meetings held worldwide, attendees discuss personal experiences and real-world applications of these SMART Recovery principles. SMART Recovery has online meetings and a message board discussion group on its website.

Secular Organization for Sobriety/Save Our Selves (SOS)

SOS considers recovery from alcohol and drugs an individual responsibility separate from spirituality and emphasizes a cognitive approach to maintaining lifelong abstinence. Meetings typically begin with a reading of the SOS *Guidelines for Sobriety* and introductions, followed by an open discussion of a topic deemed appropriate by the members. However, because each of the approximately 500 SOS groups is autonomous, the meeting format may differ from group to group. SOS also has online support groups, such as the SOS International E-Support Group

LifeRing Secular Recovery

Originally part of SOS, LifeRing is now a separate organization for people who want to stop using alcohol and drugs. The principles of LifeRing are sobriety, secularity, and self-help. LifeRing encourages participants to develop a unique path to abstinence according to their needs and to use the group meetings to facilitate their personal recovery plan. LifeRing meetings are relatively unstructured; attendees discuss what has happened to them in the past week, but some meetings focus on helping members create a personal recovery plan. Although there are fewer than 100 meetings worldwide, LifeRing has a chat room, e-mail lists, and an online forum that provide additional support to its members.

The Effectiveness of Mutual Support Groups

Research on mutual support groups indicates that active participation in any type of mutual support group significantly increases the likelihood of maintaining abstinence. Previous research has shown that participating in twelve-step or other mutual support groups is related to abstinence from alcohol and drug use. An important finding is that these abstinence rates increase with greater group participation. Persons who attend mutual support groups have also been found to have lower levels of alcohol- and drug-related problems.

Another benefit of mutual support group participation is that "helping helps the helper." Helping others by sharing experiences and providing support increases involvement in twelve-step groups, which in turn increases abstinence and lowers binge drinking rates among those who have not achieved abstinence.

Facilitating Mutual Support Group Participation

If a healthcare or social service provider suspects that a patient or client has an SUD, the provider should ensure that the client receives formal treatment. Once the client receives formal treatment—or if he or she refuses or cannot afford treatment—the provider's next step is to facilitate involvement in a mutual support group. Matching clients to treatment based solely on gender, motivation, cognitive impairment, or other such characteristics has not been proven to be effective. Clients who are philosophically well-matched to a mutual support group are more likely to actively participate in that group. Thus, the best way to help a client benefit from mutual support groups is to encourage increased participation in his or her chosen group.

Understanding the needs and beliefs of clients with SUDs helps providers make informed referrals. Providers should find out clients' experiences with mutual support groups, their concerns and misconceptions about mutual support groups, and their personal beliefs. Persons who agree with the group's belief system are more likely to participate and, thus, more likely to have better outcomes.

Participation in Self-Help Groups for Alcohol and Illicit Drug Use: 2006 and 2007

Participation in self-help groups, such as Alcoholics Anonymous and Narcotics Anonymous, is an important adjunct to formal treatment for substance use problems, and it provides valuable peer support throughout the recovery process. The National Survey on Drug Use and Health (NSDUH) includes a question for persons aged 12 or older about their participation in the past 12 months in a self-help group for substance use (alcohol use, illicit drug use, or both). NSDUH also asks questions about past year receipt of treatment for substance use problems in a specialty treatment facility.

Who attended self-help groups for substance use?

An annual average of 5.0 million persons aged 12 or older (2.0% of the population in that age group) attended a self-help group in the past year because of their use of alcohol or illicit drugs. The majority of people who attended a self-help group for their substance use in the past year were male (66.1%). Most attendees (80.2%) were over the age of 25, two-thirds (67.7%) were White, a majority (55.6%) lived in a large metropolitan area, and over two-thirds (68.1%) had a total family income of under $50,000 per year.

Among persons aged 12 or older who attended a self-help group in the past year, 45.3% attended a group because of their alcohol use only, and 21.8% attended a group because of their illicit drug use only. One-third (33.0%) attended a group because of their use of both alcohol and illicit drugs.

411

Table 70.1. Percent distribution of persons aged 12 or older who attended a self-help group in the past year because of their alcohol or illicit drug use* and of total population aged 12 or older, by sociodemographic characteristics: 2006 and 2007

Sociodemographic Characteristic	Percent of Self-Help Group Participants	Percent** of Total Population
Total	100.0%	100.0%
Gender		
Male	66.1%	48.5%
Female	33.9%	51.5%
Age Group in Years		
12 to 17	4.6%	10.3%
18 to 25	15.3%	13.3%
26 to 49	57.4%	40.6%
50 or Older	22.8%	35.9%
Race/Ethnicity		
White	67.7%	68.3%
Black or African American	15.8%	11.8%
Hispanic or Latino	12.9%	13.7%
American Indian or Alaska Native	1.2%	0.5%
Native Hawaiian or Other Pacific Islander	0.3%	0.3%
Asian	0.7%	4.2%
Two or more races	1.4%	1.1%
County Type		
Large metropolitan	55.6%	53.7%
Small metropolitan	28.9%	29.4%
Non-metropolitan	15.4%	16.8%
Family Income		
Less than $20,000	30.5%	18.6%
$20,000 to $49,999	37.6%	33.7%
$50,000 to $74,999	13.4%	17.9%
$75,000 or more	18.5%	29.8%

*These data include respondents who reported attendance at a self-help group, but did not report for which substance(s) (alcohol, illicit drugs, or both) they attended.
**Due to rounding, percentages do not total 100 percent.

Source: SAMHSA, 2006 and 2007 NSDUHs.

How many attendees had stopped using substances, and how many continued to use?

Among past year self-help group participants aged 12 or older, 45.1% abstained from substance use in the past month, and the remaining 54.9% continued to use substances. Rates of abstinence differed depending on the substance(s) for which individuals were attending self-help groups. For example, past month abstinence from alcohol and illicit drug use was reported by 33.3% of those who attended a self-help group for their illicit drug use only. This compares with 47.3% of those who attended a self-help group for their alcohol use only and 52.5% of those who attended a self-help group for their use of both alcohol and illicit drugs.

Specialty Treatment for Alcohol or Illicit Drugs and Self-Help Group Attendance

Almost one-third (32.7%) of individuals aged 12 or older who attended a self-help group for their substance use in the past year also received specialty treatment for substance use in the past year. About one-quarter (26.1%) of persons who attended a self-help group for their alcohol use only also received specialty treatment for any substance use, compared with 43.4% of those who attended a self-help group because of their illicit drug use only and 32.2% of those who attended a self-help group for their use of both alcohol and illicit drugs.

Two-thirds (66.0%) of persons aged 12 or older who received any alcohol or illicit drug use specialty treatment in the past year also attended a self-help group in the same time frame. Three-fourths (75.6%) of the persons who received specialty treatment for both alcohol and illicit drug use also attended a self-help group compared with 65.8% of those who received specialty treatment for illicit drug use only and 63.6% of those who received specialty treatment for alcohol use only.

Recovery from problem substance use and abuse is an ongoing life event that requires long-term support and treatment. A substantial body of research has found that attendance at self-help groups improves substance use outcomes, mainly in the form of reductions in the amount used and increases in rates of abstinence. Self-help groups often are used in conjunction with specialty treatment and also continue beyond treatment as people go through the recovery process.

Chapter 71

Treatment for Methamphetamine Abusers

Methamphetamine abusers can achieve long-term abstinence with the help of standard community-based drug abuse treatment. Nine months after beginning therapy, 87% of patients treated for heavy or long-term methamphetamine abuse in California outpatient and residential programs were abstinent from all drugs, according to a NIDA-supported analysis. "In the public dialogue, and even among professionals in the field, one sometimes hears that meth abuse is not treatable. But that view is not borne out by recent clinical trials or our study, which shows that community-based treatment reduces drug abuse and other problems," says lead investigator Dr. Yih-Ing Hser.

"Because methamphetamine abusers respond to treatment, getting them into therapy is a top priority. For women, there is added urgency to help them avoid exposing the children they may bear to the consequences of prenatal drug exposure." Dr. Hser and colleagues at the University of California, Los Angeles analyzed data from the California Treatment Outcome Project (CalTOP), an ongoing study that has followed the progress of adult substance abusers treated at 43 outpatient and residential programs throughout the state since April 2000. The researchers focused on 1,073 patients who reported that

This chapter includes text from "Community-Based Treatment Benefits Methamphetamine Abusers," *NIDA Notes* Vol. 20, No. 5, National Institute on Drug Abuse (NIDA), April 2006; and excerpts from "Primary Methamphetamine/Amphetamine Admissions to Substance Abuse Treatment: 2005," Substance Abuse and Mental Health Services Administration (SAMHSA), February 7, 2008.

methamphetamine abuse was their primary drug problem (572) or that they had abused the stimulant regularly for at least one year before beginning treatment (501). Most were in their 30s or younger, White or Latino, unemployed, and on public assistance; most had an arrest history. They had abused methamphetamine for about nine years, on average, and nearly one-quarter (22%) reported injecting drugs at least once. Although 64% had children aged 18 or younger, one-third of parents did not live with their children in the month before beginning treatment. One parent in five reported that a child protection court had ordered that his or her children live with someone else, and 6.3% had their parental rights terminated by the state.

The patients received the addiction treatment services routinely provided by each program. These usually included group therapy, with an average of 69 drug-related and 51 alcohol-related sessions during the first three months of treatment. On average, the patients also received 22 sessions on dealing with mental health symptoms and 13 addressing psychosocial problems, including family, parenting, and employment.

More than 60% of the patients completed three months of treatment. Among all the patients in the study—those who finished three months and those who did not—the average reported frequency of methamphetamine abuse fell from 2.7 to 0.5 days per month from the start of treatment to nine months later. The portion who were abstinent from all drugs rose from 55% to 87% in the same interval, and 68% were abstinent and also not incarcerated. Patients improved in all areas—drug and alcohol abuse; mental health symptoms; and employment, family, and legal problems—except one: men's medical problems.

Dr. Thomas Hilton of NIDA's Division of Epidemiology, Services and Prevention Research says these findings should reassure professionals working in the addiction, social services, and criminal justice fields that current therapies work for these troubled patients. "Dr. Hser's findings suggest that treatments available in the community help meth abusers reduce drug abuse and start to get their lives back on track, echoing prior research," he says.

Primary Methamphetamine/Amphetamine Admissions to Substance Abuse Treatment: 2005

Methamphetamine and amphetamines are highly addictive central nervous system stimulants. Methamphetamine and amphetamine abuse can lead to serious health consequences, such as rapid or irregular heartbeats, dental problems, mood disturbances, impaired memory, and chronic psychiatric problems. From 1995 to 2005, the percentage of substance abuse treatment admissions for primary abuse of methamphetamine/amphetamine more than doubled from 4%–9%.

Primary Methamphetamine/Amphetamine Admissions

Of the 1.8 million admissions to substance abuse treatment in 2005, 169,500 admissions were for primary methamphetamine/amphetamine abuse, representing 9% of all admissions. In addition, more than 80,000 admissions were for secondary or tertiary methamphetamine/amphetamine abuse, representing an additional 4% of all admissions. Sixty-six percent of primary methamphetamine/amphetamine admissions reported use of other substances, including marijuana (41%), alcohol (34%), and cocaine (10%).

Demographic Characteristics

In 2005, admissions in which methamphetamine/amphetamine was the primary substance of abuse were, on average, three years younger than admissions in which other substances were primary (31 years versus 34 years). Conversely, primary methamphetamine/amphetamine admissions were an average of three years older than other admissions when they first used their primary substance (21 years versus 18 years). Taken together, these findings indicate that the duration of use of their primary drug before admission to treatment was, on average, six years less for persons admitted to treatment for primary methamphetamine/amphetamine abuse than it was for persons admitted for abuse of other primary substances.

Primary methamphetamine/amphetamine admissions were more likely to be female than admissions for other primary substances (46% versus 31%).

Nearly three-quarters of primary methamphetamine/amphetamine admissions were White (71%) compared with 58% of other admissions. Hispanic admissions also accounted for a higher proportion of primary methamphetamine/amphetamine admissions than of other admissions (18% versus 13%). In contrast, Black admissions accounted for a greater proportion of admissions for other primary substances than of primary methamphetamine/amphetamine admissions (24% versus 3%).

Geographic region: Most primary methamphetamine/amphetamine substance abuse treatment admissions in 2005 were in the West (65%), followed by the Midwest (19%), South (15%), and Northeast (1%). In contrast, the highest proportion of admissions for other primary substances was in the Northeast (34%), followed by the Midwest (24%), South (22%), and West (20%).

In 2005, the criminal justice system was the principal source of referral for 49% of primary methamphetamine/amphetamine substance abuse treatment admissions compared with 34% of admissions in which other substances were primary. Other community referrals also accounted for a higher proportion of primary methamphetamine/amphetamine admissions than of other admissions (17% versus 11%). However, self/individual referrals accounted for a lower proportion of primary methamphetamine/amphetamine admissions than of other admissions (24% versus 35%), as did substance abuse care providers (5% versus 11%).

Table 71.1. Primary Methamphetamine/Amphetamine Admissions, by Race/Ethnicity: 2005

Race/Ethnicity	Primary Methamphetamine/ Amphetamine Admission	Other Substance Abuse Treatment Admissions
White	71%	58%
Black	3%	24%
Hispanic	8%	13%
Other	8%	5%

Source: 2005 SAMHSA Treatment Episode Data Set (TEDS).

Chapter 72

Therapy That Reduces Drug Abuse among Patients with Severe Mental Illness

Comorbidity: Addiction and Other Mental Illnesses

How should comorbid conditions be treated?

A fundamental principle emerging from scientific research is the need to treat comorbid conditions concurrently—which can be a difficult proposition. Patients who have both a drug use disorder and another mental illness often exhibit symptoms that are more persistent, severe, and resistant to treatment compared with patients who have either disorder alone. Nevertheless, steady progress is being made through research on new and existing treatment options for comorbidity and through health services research on implementation of appropriate screening and treatment within a variety of settings.

Medications: Effective medications exist for treating opioid, alcohol, and nicotine addiction and for alleviating the symptoms of many other mental disorders. Most of these medications have not been studied in patients with comorbidities, although some may prove effective for treating comorbid conditions. For example, preliminary results of a recent study point to the potential of using divalproex (trade name:

This chapter includes text from "Comorbidity: Addiction and Other Mental Illnesses," National Institute on Drug Abuse (NIDA), December 2008; and "New Therapy Reduces Drug Abuse among Patients with Severe Mental Illness: Research Findings," *NIDA Notes* Vol. 21, No. 6, National Institute on Drug Abuse (NIDA), June 2008.

Depakote®)—an anticonvulsant commonly used to treat bipolar disorder—to treat patients with comorbid bipolar disorder and primary cocaine dependence. Other evidence suggests that bupropion (trade names: Wellbutrin®, Zyban®), approved for treating depression and nicotine dependence, might also help reduce craving and use of methamphetamine. Most medications have not been well studied in comorbid populations or in populations taking other psychoactive medications. Therefore, more research is needed to fully understand and assess the actions of combined or dually effective medications.

Promising Behavioral Therapies for Patients with Comorbid Conditions

Adolescents

Multisystemic therapy (MST): MST targets key factors (attitudes, family, peer pressure, school and neighborhood culture) associated with serious antisocial behavior in children and adolescents who abuse drugs.

Brief strategic family therapy (BSFT): BSFT targets family interactions that are thought to maintain or exacerbate adolescent drug abuse and other co-occurring problem behaviors. These problem behaviors include conduct problems at home and at school, oppositional behavior, delinquency, associating with antisocial peers, aggressive and violent behavior, and risky sexual behaviors.

Cognitive-behavioral therapy (CBT): CBT is designed to modify harmful beliefs and maladaptive behaviors. CBT is the most effective psychotherapy for children and adolescents with anxiety and mood disorders, and also shows strong efficacy for substance abusers. (CBT is also effective for adult populations suffering from drug use disorders and a range of other psychiatric problems.)

Adults

Therapeutic communities (TCs): TCs focus on the resocialization of the individual and use broad-based community programs as active components of treatment. TCs are particularly well suited to deal with criminal justice inmates, individuals with vocational deficits, women who need special protections from harsh social environments, vulnerable or neglected youth, and homeless individuals. In addition, some evidence suggests the utility of incorporating TCs for adolescents who have been in treatment for substance abuse and related problems.

Assertive community treatment (ACT): ACT programs integrate the behavioral treatment of other severe mental disorders, such as schizophrenia, and co-occurring substance use disorders. ACT is differentiated from other forms of case management through factors such as a smaller caseload size, team management, outreach emphasis, a highly individualized approach, and an assertive approach to maintaining contact with patients.

Dialectical behavior therapy (DBT): DBT is designed specifically to reduce self-harm behaviors (such as self-mutilation and suicidal attempts, thoughts, or urges) and drug abuse. It is one of the few treatments that are effective for individuals who meet the criteria for borderline personality disorder.

Exposure therapy: Exposure therapy is a behavioral treatment for some anxiety disorders (phobias, post-traumatic stress disorder [PTSD]) that involves repeated exposure to or confrontation with a feared situation, object, traumatic event, or memory. This exposure can be real, visualized, or simulated, and always is contained in a controlled therapeutic environment. The goal is to desensitize patients to the triggering stimuli and help them learn to cope, eventually reducing or even eliminating symptoms. Several studies suggest that exposure therapy may be helpful for individuals with comorbid PTSD and cocaine addiction, although retention in treatment is difficult.

Integrated group therapy (IGT): IGT is a new treatment developed specifically for patients with bipolar disorder and drug addiction, designed to address both problems simultaneously.

Behavioral therapies: Behavioral treatment (alone or in combination with medications) is the cornerstone to successful outcomes for many individuals with drug use disorders or other mental illnesses. And while behavior therapies continue to be evaluated for use in comorbid populations, several strategies have shown promise for treating specific comorbid conditions.

New Therapy Reduces Drug Abuse among Patients with Severe Mental Illness

A new intervention enhances prospects for substance abusers whose mental illness complicates the path to recovery. In a recent clinical trial, a six-month course of behavioral treatment for substance abuse in severe and persistent mental illness (BTSAS) reduced drug abuse, boosted treatment-session attendance, and improved the quality of life of outpatients with a wide spectrum of mental disorders.

A Focus on Extra Obstacles

Dr. Alan S. Bellack and colleagues at the University of Maryland School of Medicine in Baltimore designed BTSAS to counter the factors that make recovery from addiction especially difficult for people who have co-occurring severe and persistent mental illness. These factors include frequent failure to meet their own and others' expectations, inconsistent motivation, and social and personal pressure to appear normal.

Table 72.1. Treatment Outcomes

	BTSAS*	STAR**
Drug-free urine samples	59%	25%
Four weeks of abstinence	54%	16%
Multiple 4-week blocks	44%	10%
Eight weeks of abstinence	33%	8%

*BTSAS: Behavioral treatment for substance abuse in severe and persistent mental illness.
**STAR: Supportive treatment for addiction recovery.

BTSAS therapy comprises six integrated components:

- motivational interviews (directive counseling that explores and resolves ambivalence) to increase the desire to stop using drugs;

- contingency contracts linking drug-free urine samples with small financial rewards;

- realistic, short-term, structured goal-setting sessions;

- training in social and drug-refusal skills;

- information on why and how people become addicted to drugs and the dangers of substance use for people with mental illness; and

- relapse-prevention training that inculcates behavioral strategies for coping with cravings, lapses, and high-risk situations.

Twice-weekly sessions begin with urine tests. Patients who have provided drug-free urine samples are praised by the therapists and group members. They also receive financial incentives that start at $1.50 for the first drug-free sample and increase in $0.50 increments for every consecutive one thereafter, up to $3.50. The amount is set back to $1.50 after a drug-positive sample or an absence.

When participants submit drug-positive samples, the group takes a non-accusatory approach by focusing on problem solving to help them achieve future abstinence. Each participant agrees upon a personal goal for drug abuse reduction or abstinence that he or she believes is achievable during the coming week and signs a contract stating that he or she will strive for it. The rest of the session consists of drug abuse education plus training in social skills and relapse-prevention strategies.

Superior Results

Substance abuse is common among the mentally ill. For example, surveys estimate that 48% of those with schizophrenia, 56% with bipolar disorder, and as many as 65% with severe and persistent mental illness have abused substances.

Dr. Bellack's research team recruited 175 patients from community clinics and a Veterans Affairs medical center in Baltimore. All had a dual diagnosis of severe and persistent mental illness and an addiction to cocaine, heroin, or marijuana. Among the participants, 38.3% met the diagnostic criteria for schizophrenia or schizoaffective disorders, 54.9% for major affective disorders, and the remainder for other mental disorders. Cocaine was the predominant drug abused by 68.6% of participants, opiates by 24.6%, and marijuana by 6.8%.

The researchers assigned half the trial participants to BTSAS group therapy and half to a program called Supportive Treatment for Addiction Recovery (STAR), which is the typical treatment at the University of Maryland clinics. Unlike participants in BTSAS, those in STAR do not follow a structured format but instead select their own topics and work at their own pace. Patient interaction with other patients is encouraged but not required as it is with BTSAS. Although urine samples are collected before each session, results are not discussed in the group, and no systematic feedback is provided to the patient.

Assignments to the BTSAS and STAR groups were balanced for gender, psychiatric diagnosis, type of drug dependency, and number of substance use disorders. Treatment groups of four to six participants met twice a week for six months. BTSAS and STAR group sessions were all led by trained therapists and lasted from 60 to 90 minutes. Group meetings were videotaped weekly and then reviewed and assessed by independent reviewers to verify that the therapists were following the programs' parameters correctly.

The BTSAS group fared better than the STAR group on a wide range of treatment-related criteria. For example, more people in the BTSAS group stayed in treatment throughout the six-month trial period (57.4% versus 34.7%). The BTSAS group produced more drug-free urine samples and had longer periods of abstinence. They also had better clinical and general living outcomes than people in the STAR group and reported larger improvements in their ability to perform the activities of daily living.

"It was apparent from watching videotapes of treatment sessions that subjects in BTSAS valued the intervention and were learning important skills for reducing drug use," says Dr. Bellack. "We were very gratified that the data supported our clinical observations." The researchers reported that the extra costs of running the BTSAS program were modest. For the six-month trial, monetary rewards averaged roughly $60 per patient; total per-patient cost, including therapist time, was $372.

Ongoing Refinements

The trial data indicate that patients who remain in BTSAS for at least three sessions are much more likely to finish the six-month program than patients who do not make it through the third session. Because a third of individuals initially recruited for the study left before the third treatment session, the researchers are currently developing new intervention strategies to keep people in the program until they have truly given it a chance. The innovation has two key components: a structured intervention to help patients overcome obstacles to treatment and an intervention to enlist family and friends as partners to connect patients with treatment.

"The BTSAS program will help clinicians make a difference in the lives of a very difficult-to-treat population," says Dr. Dorynne Czechowicz of NIDA's Division of Clinical Neuroscience and Behavioral Research. "One of its key strengths is that it positively affects many aspects of patients' lives. Moreover, as an outpatient treatment, it is well-suited to the situation. Most mentally ill people who abuse drugs live in the community, not in a sheltered facility, and this is where the majority of clinicians must treat them."

Sources

Bellack, A.S., et al. A randomized clinical trial of a new behavioral treatment for drug abuse in people with severe and persistent mental illness. *Archives of General Psychiatry* 63(4):426–432, 2006. [Full Text]

Kinnaman, J.E., et al. Assessment of motivation to change substance use in dually-diagnosed schizophrenia patients. *Addictive Behaviors* 32(9):1798–1813, 2007. [Abstract]

Chapter 73

Drug Abuse Treatment in the Criminal Justice System

Chapter Contents

Section 73.1—Drug Courts 428

Section 73.2—Treating Drug Abuse Offenders
Benefits Public Health and Safety.................... 432

Section 73.1

Drug Courts

This section includes text from "In the Spotlight: Drug Court," U.S. Department of Justice, September 10, 2009; and from "High-Risk Offenders Do Better with Close Judicial Supervision," *Research Findings*, Vol. 22, No. 2, National Institute on Drug Abuse (NIDA), December 2008.

Drug Courts

Drug courts can be defined as "special court calendars or dockets designed to achieve a reduction in recidivism and substance abuse among nonviolent, substance abusing offenders by increasing their likelihood for successful rehabilitation through early, continuous, and intense judicially supervised treatment; mandatory periodic drug testing; and the use of appropriate sanctions and other rehabilitation services" (*Drug Courts: Overview of Growth, Characteristics, and Results*, Government Accountability Office, 1997).

Summary

Drug court participants undergo long-term treatment and counseling, sanctions, incentives, and frequent court appearances. Successful completion of the treatment program results in dismissal of the charges, reduced or set aside sentences, lesser penalties, or a combination of these. Most importantly, graduating participants gain the necessary tools to rebuild their lives. Because the problem of drugs and crime is much too broad for any single agency to tackle alone, drug courts rely upon the daily communication and cooperation of judges, court personnel, probation, and treatment providers.

Drug courts vary somewhat from one jurisdiction to another in terms of structure, scope, and target populations, but they all share three primary goals: (1) to reduce recidivism, (2) to reduce substance abuse among participants, and (3) to rehabilitate participants. Achieving these goals requires a special organizational structure. Specifically, the drug court model includes the following key components:

- Incorporating drug testing into case processing

- Creating a non-adversarial relationship between the defendant and the court

- Identifying defendants in need of treatment and referring them to treatment as soon as possible after arrest

- Providing access to a continuum of treatment and rehabilitation services

- Monitoring abstinence through frequent, mandatory drug testing

- Establishing a coordinated strategy to govern drug court responses to participants' compliance

- Maintaining judicial interaction with each drug court participant

- Monitoring and evaluating program goals and gauging their effectiveness

- Continuing interdisciplinary education to promote effective drug court planning, implementation, and operations

- Forging partnerships among drug courts, public agencies, and community-based organizations to generate local support and enhance drug court effectiveness

While analyses on the effectiveness of drug courts are ongoing, research indicates that drug courts can reduce recidivism and promote other positive outcomes. The magnitude of a court's impact may depend upon how consistently court resources match the needs of the offenders in the drug court program. Drug court participants report that interactions with the judge are one of the most important influences on the experience they have while in the program.

Although the cost-effectiveness of drug courts has been difficult to determine, one definitive cost-benefit evaluation estimated the average investment per program participant was $5,928; the savings were $2,329 in avoided criminal justice system costs and $1,301 in avoided victimization costs over a 30 month period (*Drug Courts: The Second Decade*, National Institute of Justice, 2006).

As of June 2009, there were 2,038 drug courts operating in all 50 states, the District of Columbia, Northern Mariana Islands, Puerto Rico, and Guam. Another 226 drug court programs were in the planning stages. An important force behind the drug court movement was the Violent Crime Control and Law Enforcement Act of 1994, which called for federal support for planning, implementing, and enhancing drug courts for nonviolent drug offenders. Additionally, the fervent support of national leaders raised the status of drug courts.

The drug court model has paved the way for the latest criminal justice innovation—therapeutic jurisprudence. A number of jurisdictions are developing special dockets, modeled after the drug court format. Courts and judges have become more receptive to new approaches, resulting in a proliferation of problem-solving courts, including driving under the influence (DUI) courts, domestic violence courts, and mental health courts.

High-Risk Offenders Do Better with Close Judicial Supervision

Adjusting the frequency of mandatory drug court monitoring sessions according to offenders' risk of lapsing into criminal activity, including drug abuse, can enhance program success rates while conserving resources, according to a recent NIDA-supported study. Researchers found that high-risk drug offenders—those with antisocial personality disorder or prior histories of drug abuse treatment—achieved better outcomes when ordered to attend a judicial status hearing every two weeks, rather than at the four- to six-week intervals that drug courts typically impose. In contrast, lower risk offenders' treatment success was not compromised when courts required them to appear only if they committed serious or repeated infractions of program rules.

"Our research represents a first step in tailoring adaptive supervision interventions to drug-abusing offenders," says Dr. Douglas Marlowe of the Treatment Research Institute and the University of Pennsylvania, Philadelphia. Dr. Marlowe, Dr. David Festinger, and colleagues conducted the study as part of a broader effort to improve the efficacy and cost-effectiveness of drug court interventions by identifying which components of the model work best for various groups of drug offenders.

Drug court frequency can affect treatment outcome: Participants who were considered high-risk provided more drug-free urine samples when they were required to appear in drug court every two weeks rather than according to the standard schedule of every four to six weeks. In contrast, participants who were at lower risk of relapse did comparably well on the standard schedule and when court appearances were scheduled only in response to treatment-rule infractions.

"Adjusting the frequency of court hearings to participants' risk status will make a difference, but there still will be considerable room for improvement in drug court outcomes," Dr. Marlowe notes. For high-risk participants who continue to have drug or alcohol problems, the program needs further tailoring, he explains. Those who are not compliant with the program—for example, those who fail to attend counseling sessions or to deliver urine specimens—might respond to more frequent judicial supervision or to sanctions such as home curfews. In contrast, increasing the scope of treatment services might be more effective with high-risk participants who are compliant with program rules but fail to achieve abstinence because of the severity of their drug addiction or a related difficulty, such as a co-occurring mental disorder, family problems, unemployment, or homelessness. Dr. Marlowe notes that even low-risk drug offenders need more effective interventions. Dr. Marlowe says, "We hope that drug court programs eventually become flexible enough to allow participants doing poorly to be switched to a more intensive track and allow those doing well in an intensive program to move to a lower supervision regimen."

Drug courts add value: Studies have shown that drug courts significantly increase the time drug abusers stay in treatment. An average of 60% of drug court clients complete at least twelve months of treatment, whereas only 10% of probationers and parolees typically remain for a year in community-based drug treatment programs, says Dr. Douglas Marlowe of the University of Pennsylvania, summarizing several research reports. A 1998 review of 13 drug court studies found that drug court clients abuse substances less frequently than comparable probationers (10% of urine tests were positive, compared with 31%). What's more, drug courts reduce re-arrest rates by 8–24%, according to five meta-analyses in 2005 and 2006. Although drug courts tend to be more expensive than other programs, the reduction in recidivism decreases later judicial costs and financial loss to crime victims.

Section 73.2

Treating Drug Abuse Offenders Benefits Public Health and Safety

This section includes text from "Drug Abusing Offenders Not Getting Treatment They Need in Criminal Justice System," National Institute on Drug Abuse (NIDA), January 13, 2009; and from "Principles of Drug Abuse Treatment for Criminal Justice Populations," NIDA, July 22, 2009.

Treating Inmates Has Proven Public Health, Safety, and Economic Benefits

The vast majority of prisoners who could benefit from drug abuse treatment do not receive it, despite two decades of research that demonstrate its effectiveness, according to researchers at the National Institute on Drug Abuse (NIDA), part of the National Institutes of Health. In a report published in the January 2009, *Journal of the American Medical Association*, NIDA scientists note that about half of all prisoners (including some sentenced for non-drug-related offenses) are dependent on drugs, yet less than 20% of inmates suffering from drug abuse or dependence receive formal treatment.

"Treating drug-abusing offenders improves public health and safety," said NIDA Director and report coauthor Dr. Nora D. Volkow. "In addition to the devastating social consequences for individuals and their families, drug abuse exacts serious health effects, including increased risk for infectious diseases such as human immunodeficiency virus (HIV) and hepatitis C; and treatment for addiction can help prevent their spread. Providing drug abusers with treatment also makes it less likely that these abusers will return to the criminal justice system." In fact, most studies indicate that outcomes for those who are legally pressured to enter treatment are as good as or better than outcomes for those who enter treatment without legal pressure, the researchers note.

There are several ways in which drug abuse treatment can be incorporated into the criminal justice system. These include therapeutic alternatives to incarceration, treatment merged with judicial oversight in drug courts, treatments provided in prison and jail, and reentry programs to help offenders transition from incarceration back into the community.

Principles of Drug Abuse Treatment for Criminal Justice Populations

1. **Drug addiction is a brain disease that affects behavior:** Drug addiction has well-recognized cognitive, behavioral, and physiological characteristics that contribute to continued use of drugs despite the harmful consequences. Scientists have also found that chronic drug abuse alters the brain's anatomy and chemistry and that these changes can last for months or years after the individual has stopped using drugs. This transformation may help explain why addicts are at a high risk of relapse to drug abuse even after long periods of abstinence and why they persist in seeking drugs despite deleterious consequences.

2. **Recovery from drug addiction requires effective treatment, followed by management of the problem over time:** Drug addiction is a serious problem that can be treated and managed throughout its course. Effective drug abuse treatment engages participants in a therapeutic process, retains them in treatment for an appropriate length of time, and helps them learn to maintain abstinence over time. Multiple episodes of treatment may be required. Outcomes for drug abusing offenders in the community can be improved by monitoring drug use and by encouraging continued participation in treatment.

3. **Treatment must last long enough to produce stable behavioral changes:** In treatment, the drug abuser is taught to break old patterns of thinking and behaving and to learn new skills for avoiding drug use and criminal behavior. Individuals with severe drug problems and co-occurring disorders typically need longer treatment and more comprehensive services. Early in treatment, the drug abuser begins a therapeutic process of change. In later stages, he or she addresses other problems related to drug abuse and learns how to manage the problem.

4. **Assessment is the first step in treatment:** A history of drug or alcohol use may suggest the need to conduct a comprehensive assessment to determine the nature and extent of an individual's drug problems, establish whether problems exist in

other areas that may affect recovery, and enable the formulation of an appropriate treatment plan. Personality disorders and other mental health problems are prevalent in offender populations; therefore, comprehensive assessments should include mental health evaluations with treatment planning for these problems.

5. **Tailoring services to fit the needs of the individual is an important part of effective drug abuse treatment for criminal justice populations:** Individuals differ in terms of age, gender, ethnicity and culture, problem severity, recovery stage, and level of supervision needed. Individuals also respond differently to different treatment approaches and treatment providers. In general, drug treatment should address issues of motivation, problem solving, and skill-building for resisting drug use and criminal behavior. Lessons aimed at supplanting drug use and criminal activities with constructive activities, and at understanding the consequences of one's behavior are also important to include. Treatment interventions can facilitate the development of healthy interpersonal relationships and improve the participant's ability to interact with family, peers, and others in the community.

6. **Drug use during treatment should be carefully monitored:** Individuals trying to recover from drug addiction may experience a relapse, or return, to drug use. Triggers for drug relapse are varied; common ones include mental stress and associations with peers and social situations linked to drug use. An undetected relapse can progress to serious drug abuse, but detected use can present opportunities for therapeutic intervention. Monitoring drug use through urinalysis or other objective methods, as part of treatment or criminal justice supervision, provides a basis for assessing and providing feedback on the participant's treatment progress.

7. **Treatment should target factors that are associated with criminal behavior:** Criminal thinking is a combination of attitudes and beliefs that support a criminal lifestyle and criminal behavior. These can include feeling entitled to have things one's own way, feeling that one's criminal behavior is justified, failing to be responsible for one's actions, and consistently failing to anticipate or appreciate the consequences of one's behavior. This pattern of thinking often contributes to drug use and

criminal behavior. Treatment that provides specific cognitive skills training to help individuals recognize errors in judgment that lead to drug abuse and criminal behavior may improve outcomes.

8. **Criminal justice supervision should incorporate treatment planning for drug abusing offenders, and treatment providers should be aware of correctional supervision requirements:** The coordination of drug abuse treatment with correctional planning can encourage participation in drug abuse treatment and can help treatment providers incorporate correctional requirements as treatment goals. Treatment providers should collaborate with criminal justice staff to evaluate each individual's treatment plan and ensure that it meets correctional supervision requirements, as well as that person's changing needs, which may include housing and childcare; medical, psychiatric, and social support services; and vocational and employment assistance. For offenders with drug abuse problems, planning should incorporate the transition to community-based treatment and links to appropriate post-release services to improve the success of drug treatment and re-entry. Abstinence requirements may necessitate a rapid clinical response, such as more counseling, targeted intervention, or increased medication, to prevent relapse. Ongoing coordination between treatment providers and courts or parole and probation officers is important in addressing the complex needs of these re-entering individuals.

9. **Continuity of care is essential for drug abusers re-entering the community:** Those who complete prison-based treatment and continue with treatment in the community have the best outcomes. Continuing drug abuse treatment helps the recently released offender deal with problems that become relevant only at re-entry, such as learning to handle situations that could lead to relapse, learning how to live drug-free in the community, and developing a drug-free peer support network. Treatment in prison or jail can begin a process of therapeutic change, resulting in reduced drug use and criminal behavior post-incarceration. Continuing drug treatment in the community is essential to sustaining these gains.

10. **A balance of rewards and sanctions encourages prosocial behavior and treatment participation:** When providing correctional supervision of individuals participating in drug abuse

treatment, it is important to reinforce positive behavior. Generally, less punitive responses are used for early and less serious noncompliance, with increasingly severe sanctions issuing from continued problem behavior. Rewards and sanctions are most likely to have the desired effect when they are perceived as fair and when they swiftly follow the targeted behavior.

11. **Offenders with co-occurring drug abuse and mental health problems often require an integrated treatment approach:** High rates of mental health problems are found both in offender populations and in those with substance abuse problems. Drug abuse treatment can sometimes address depression, anxiety, and other mental health problems. Personality, cognitive, and other serious mental disorders can be difficult to treat and may disrupt drug treatment. The presence of co-occurring disorders may require an integrated approach that combines drug abuse treatment with psychiatric treatment, including the use of medication.

12. **Medications are an important part of treatment for many drug abusing offenders:** Medicines such as methadone and buprenorphine for heroin addiction have been shown to help normalize brain function and should be made available to individuals who could benefit from them. Effective use of medications can also be instrumental in enabling people with co-occurring mental health problems to function successfully in society. Behavioral strategies can increase adherence to medication regimens.

13. **Treatment planning for drug abusing offenders who are living in or re-entering the community** should include strategies to prevent and treat serious, chronic medical conditions, such as human immunodeficiency virus/acquired immunodeficiency syndrome (HIV/AIDS), hepatitis B and C, and tuberculosis (TB). Infectious diseases affect not just the offender, but also the criminal justice system and the wider community. Consistent with federal and state laws, drug-involved offenders should be offered testing for infectious diseases and receive counseling on their health status and on ways to modify risk behaviors.

Chapter 74

Employee Assistance Programs (EAPs) for Substance Abuse

Chapter Contents

Section 74.1—Addressing Workplace
Substance Use Problems 438

Section 74.2—Symptoms and Intervention
Techniques When Employees
Abuse Drugs 442

Section 74.3—Employment Status Is Relevant
to Substance Abuse Treatment
Outcomes 444

Section 74.4—EAPs for Substance Abuse Benefit
Employers and Employees 447

Section 74.1

Addressing Workplace Substance Use Problems

The workplace provides a unique opportunity to address the entire spectrum of substance use problems, both diagnosable abuse or dependence and other problematic use. Most adults with substance use problems are employed, and an estimated 29% of full-time workers engage in binge drinking and 8% engage in heavy drinking; 8% have used illicit drugs in the past month. Substance use problems contribute to reduced productivity, absenteeism, occupational injuries, increased health care costs, worksite disruption, and potential liability as well as other personal and societal harms.

Employee assistance programs (EAPs), which grew out of occupational alcohol programs, have dramatically evolved into a more comprehensive behavioral health resource that is widely available. Given the current level of concern regarding health care costs and productivity—and the awareness that substance use problems are under-recognized and undertreated—it follows that interest in EAPs is stronger than ever. This section describes the contemporary EAP, explores key issues in service delivery, and proposes a research agenda to help drive the future direction of this important behavioral health resource.

EAPs as a Behavioral Health Resource

EAPs are workplace-based programs designed to address substance use and other problems that negatively affect employees' well-being or job performance. About 66% of work sites with 100 or more employees and 90% of Fortune 500 firms have an EAP. Most contemporary EAPs are broad-brush programs that address a wide spectrum of substance use, mental health, work-life balance, and other issues. EAPs typically offer three to eight visits for assessment or short-term counseling or both, with no copayment. Employees may be referred by supervisors for poor job performance related to substance use or other problems, or—more commonly—they may self refer. Services are often extended to family members. In some cases, short-term counseling is sufficient to address a client's needs. In others, the client is assessed, referred to behavioral health treatment outside the EAP, and provided follow-up support as needed.

Contemporary EAPs typically deliver services off site through contracted networks of managed behavioral health care organizations. An EAP can be a separate benefit feature or it can be integrated with behavioral health benefits. Although a utilization rate of 5%–8% has been suggested as a desirable target, reported utilization rates vary widely, partly because of differences in services and segments of the population counted. Often a sizable minority of EAP clients have substance use problems, although they do not always have a substance use diagnosis. EAPs also provide services at the organizational level to improve the work environment and enhance job performance—for example, by developing workplace substance abuse policies, providing consultation to supervisors dealing with problem employees, and implementing drug-free workplace and other health promotion activities.

Key Issues in Contemporary EAPs

Discerning the Effects of EAPs

Many organizations find that EAPs are useful and generate cost savings, which accounts for the near-ubiquity of EAPs in large workplaces. In fact, a substantial body of literature describes the impact of EAPs on outcomes, health care utilization, and direct and indirect costs. Reviews of EAP research, only some of which is specific to substance use problems, indicate that most studies have found improved clinical and work outcomes and positive economic effects measured in a variety of ways. However, the complexities of determining cost-related effects are illustrated by evidence that EAP users' health care costs may actually rise temporarily, possibly because of EAPs' facilitation of needed services.

Reviews have also noted significant methodological limitations in this body of research and a relative dearth of recent studies applicable to current EAP models. Many studies are limited to single cases, lack control or appropriate comparison groups, have threats to validity because of self-selection bias or regression to the mean, or were conducted in program models that are now rare. Thus questions remain regarding how contemporary EAPs affect outcomes and costs.

Implications of Changes in Service Delivery

Some observers postulate that the evolution to a broad-brush approach delivered by external practitioners has diluted EAPs' traditional focus on substance use problems. Providers in managed behavioral health networks may be mental health practitioners with scant workplace-specific substance abuse training, historically a core competency for employee assistance professionals. A lack of close relationships between off-site EAP providers and supervisory personnel may reduce opportunities for early problem identification. However, because stigma and fear of work-related consequences are often even higher for workers with substance use problems than for those with other behavioral health problems, embedding services for substance use problems in broadly configured EAPs may increase acceptability.

Workplace Culture and EAP Promotion

Optimal utilization of EAPs and their effectiveness in addressing substance use problems may depend on how services are promoted. The presence of an EAP is highly correlated with an organization's guidelines against the use of alcohol at work-related functions and the existence of no-smoking policies, suggesting that some workplace cultures more strongly emphasize proactive approaches to employee behavioral health. Strategies to increase utilization through enhanced outreach can be effective. Factors such as employee awareness of the EAP, positive attitudes toward company policy, and belief in EAP confidentiality improve willingness to use EAPs. Supervisor training is also important.

Measuring EAP Performance

Evaluation and comparison of EAP services has been made more difficult by the lack of common performance measures. Performance measures can be used for quality improvement, accountability, and performance-based contracting and can be incorporated into research to yield more comparable evaluations. Following the overall trend in health care, there is a growing movement toward developing and adopting standardized performance measures in the EAP field. This trend will benefit all stakeholders, including purchasers, providers, and ultimately service users.

Where Do EAPs Fit?

Employers continue to offer EAPs as well as a growing number of other health promotion, disease management, and disability programs. Although this expanding menu of health-related initiatives may be designed to encourage access, fragmentation and redundancy of services are potential pitfalls. Employer groups and advocacy organizations have called for increased coordination and integration between EAPs and other programs to enhance quality of care.

A Research Agenda

The evolution of EAPs and the key issues noted give rise to a new agenda for research. Areas for research include descriptive studies of EAP utilization and costs to provide an up-to-date picture of services; investigations of how externally delivered, broad-brush programs address substance use problems, including management consultation for early identification; further studies of EAPs' effects on outcomes and costs, including a focus on productivity and outcomes for work groups; systematic examination of the relationship between EAP activities and other workplace resources; efforts to further identify facilitators of and barriers to EAP utilization; and finally, development, testing, and validation of EAP performance measures.

Methodological approaches to help implement this research agenda include fielding larger-scale studies that encompass multiple work sites and employers; using group level randomization, quasi-experimental designs, and statistical techniques to reduce selection bias, identify causal connections, and control for group differences; capturing a wider range of factors in multiple domains to more accurately measure utilization, outcomes, and costs; and making greater use of standardized instruments when measuring clinical outcomes and productivity.

Section 74.2

Symptoms and Intervention Techniques When Employees Abuse Drugs

This section includes text from "Symptoms and Intervention Techniques," U.S. Department of Labor, March 11, 2009.

If substance abuse is contributing to an employee's poor performance, ignoring or avoiding the issue will not help the situation. An employee's use of alcohol or drugs may be the root of the performance problem; however, substance abuse on the part of someone close to the employee also could be the source. Regardless, abuse of alcohol or other drugs inevitably leads to costly and potentially dangerous consequences in the workplace unless action is taken to confront the issue.

It is important to note that diagnosis of an alcohol or other drug problem is not the job of a supervisor. However, remaining alert to changes in employee performance and working to improve employee productivity is a core component of every supervisor's job. Because substance abuse seriously affects an employee's ability to fulfill his or her responsibilities, supervisors play a key role in keeping a workplace alcohol and drug free.

To carry out this responsibility, a supervisor must clearly understand a company's drug-free workplace policy and have the ability to identify performance problems that may be the result of alcohol and drug abuse. Furthermore, a supervisor should be capable of making appropriate referrals to employees in need of assistance for alcohol- or drug-related problems.

Symptoms

The following performance and behavior problems are common to many employed individuals who abuse alcohol and/or other drugs. It is important to note that if an employee displays these symptoms, it does not necessarily mean he or she has a substance abuse problem.

Performance

- Inconsistent work quality
- Poor concentration
- Lowered productivity
- Increased absenteeism
- Unexplained disappearances from the job site
- Carelessness, mistakes
- Errors in judgment
- Needless risk taking
- Disregard for safety
- Extended lunch periods and early departures

Behavior

- Frequent financial problems
- Avoidance of friends and colleagues
- Blaming others for own problems and shortcomings
- Complaints about problems at home
- Deterioration in personal appearance
- Complaints and excuses of vaguely defined illnesses

Intervention

When an employee's performance deteriorates for whatever reason, his or her supervisor has an obligation to intervene. The supervisor does not need to be an expert on alcohol and drug abuse to do so because the intervention should be focused on the employee's performance problem.

The following principles of intervention may be followed by supervisors who need to confront a staff member about a performance problem that may be related to substance abuse.

Maintain control:

- Stick to the facts as they affect work performance.
- Do not rely on memory; have all supporting documents and records available.

- Do not discuss alcohol or drug use.

Be clear and firm:

- Explain company policy concerning performance.
- Explain company drug-free workplace policy.
- Explain consequences if performance expectations are not met.

Be supportive, but avoid emotional involvement:

- Offer help in resolving performance problems.
- Identify resources for help in addressing personal problems.

Section 74.3

Employment Status Is Relevant to Substance Abuse Treatment Outcomes

Excerpted from "Employment Status and Substance Abuse Treatment Admissions: 2006," Substance Abuse and Mental Health Services Administration (SAMHSA), March 20, 2008.

Employment is among the best predictors of successful substance abuse treatment. It is also considered an important measure of success in substance abuse treatment: increased employment is one of the desired outcomes in the Substance Abuse and Mental Health Services Administration's National Outcome Measures (NOMs) framework. Thus, employment status is relevant both to substance abuse treatment outcomes and policy making.

The employment status of admissions to substance abuse treatment can be examined with the Treatment Episode Data Set (TEDS), an annual compilation of data on the demographic characteristics and substance abuse problems of those admitted to substance abuse treatment, primarily at facilities that receive some public funding. TEDS records represent admissions rather than individuals, as a person may be admitted to treatment more than once during a single year.

This report focuses on substance abuse treatment admissions aged 18 to 64, the age group that is typically expected to be in the labor force. In 2006, 31% of substance abuse treatment admissions aged 18 to 64 were employed, 33% were unemployed, and 36% were not in the labor force (not employed and not looking for work). In comparison, 75% of noninstitutionalized civilians in the United States aged 18 to 64 were employed in 2006, 3% were unemployed, and 22% were not in the labor force.

In 2006, 31 states or jurisdictions reported detailed "not in labor force" status. Among admissions aged 18 to 64 who reported that they were not in the labor force in these states, 22% were disabled, 7% were inmates of institutions, 5% were students, 3% were homemakers, and 2% were retired. The remaining 61% were not in the labor force for other reasons, and will be referred to here as "labor force dropouts."

This report compares substance abuse treatment admissions aged 18 to 64 in five employment status groups: full-time employed, unemployed, and three not-in-labor-force groups—labor force dropouts, disabled, and homemakers. Altogether, these groups comprise over 86% of the admissions in the 31 states reporting detailed not-in-labor-force information in 2006.

Primary Substance of Abuse

In 2006, admissions to substance abuse treatment varied by employment group in their primary substance of abuse. While alcohol was the most frequently reported primary substance for each employment group, admissions who were employed full time were more likely to report alcohol as the primary substance of abuse (58%) than admissions who were homemakers (35%), unemployed (39%), labor force dropouts (39%), or disabled (46%).

On the other hand, admissions who were unemployed, labor force dropouts, or disabled were about twice as likely as admissions who were employed full time to report opiates (21%, 25%, or 19% versus 11%) or cocaine (16%, 20%, or 17% versus 9%) as their primary substance of abuse. Admissions who were homemakers were more likely than other admissions to report primary stimulant abuse (9% versus 4–7% among the other groups).

Frequency of Use

In 2006, substance abuse treatment admissions who were unemployed, labor force dropouts, or disabled were more likely than admissions

445

who were employed full time or who were homemakers to report daily use of the primary substance of abuse. For example, admissions who were labor force dropouts were more than twice as likely as admissions who were employed full time to report daily use of their primary substance in the past month (56% versus 26%). Admissions who were unemployed or labor force dropouts were less likely than admissions who were employed full time or who were homemakers to report no use in the past month. For example, admissions who were unemployed (26%) were less likely than admissions who were employed full time (34%) to report no use of the primary substance in the past month. These overall patterns held true regardless of primary substance of abuse.

Prior Treatment Episodes

In 2006, admissions who were homemakers or who were employed full time were more likely to report entering treatment for the first time (59% and 57%, respectively) than admissions who were unemployed (40%), labor force dropouts (47%), or disabled (41%). Substance abuse treatment admissions who were unemployed or disabled were more likely than other admissions to report five or more prior treatment episodes.

Service Setting

Substance abuse treatment admissions who were unemployed, labor force dropouts, or disabled were more likely than admissions who were employed full time or who were homemakers to be in detoxification service settings and less likely to be in ambulatory treatment in 2006. Admissions who were labor force dropouts were more likely than admissions in any of the other employment groups to be in rehabilitation/residential service settings (31% versus 9–18% among the other groups).

Section 74.4

EAPs for Substance Abuse Benefit Employers and Employees

This section includes text from "Issue Brief #9 for Employers: An EAP That Addresses Substance Abuse Can Save You Money," Substance Abuse and Mental Health Services Administration (SAMHSA), 2008.

Substance use disorders can negatively affect an employer's bottom line by increasing health care costs and reducing productivity. But employers have a simple and cost-effective tool available for addressing these risks: a workplace substance abuse program administered through an employee assistance program (EAP).

Employee assistance programs (EAPs) are designed to help identify and resolve productivity problems affecting employees who are impaired by personal concerns. EAPs come in many different forms, from telephone-based to on-site programs. Face-to-face programs provide more comprehensive services for employees with substance use disorders, including confidential screening, treatment referrals, and follow-up care. Assuring that workers with substance use disorders receive treatment can help employers save money. Intervening early can prevent the need for more intensive treatment and hospitalizations down the road.

Employers See Savings When EAPs Address Substance Abuse

- Eighty percent of federal workers and their family members who received treatment for alcohol or drug problems through the federal occupational health EAP reported improvements in work attendance. A majority also reported improvements in both work performance and social relationships.

- Chevron-Texaco found that from 1990 to 1996, 75% of employees who entered the company EAP with alcohol problems were able to retain their employment, saving the company the cost of recruiting and training new employees.

447

- Gillette Company saw a 75% drop in inpatient substance abuse treatment costs after implementing an EAP.

- A large international holding company found that employees who used an EAP for help with mental health and substance use problems had fewer inpatient medical days than those who only participated in the company's medical insurance plan. In addition, the company saved an average of $426,000 each year on mental health and substance abuse treatment as a result of employees' participation in the EAP.

How Substance Abuse Impacts the Workplace

Substance abuse costs the nation an estimated $276 billion a year. Lost work productivity and excess healthcare expenses account for the majority of those costs. The magnitude of the cost, coupled with the fact that 76% of people with drug or alcohol problems are in the work force, gives employers a major stake in ensuring that employees have access to treatment.

Substance abuse by employees results in higher healthcare expenses for injuries and illnesses; more absenteeism; reductions in job productivity and performance; more workers' compensation and disability claims; and, increased safety, and other, risks for employers.

Conducting random drug testing and firing offending employees can have a short-term impact but may ultimately be more costly because the cost of replacing employees is high and the risk remains that new employees may also abuse drugs or alcohol.

How to Hire an EAP

1. Develop specifications and request proposals from several EAP vendors.

2. Evaluate their capabilities, for example, the range of services they offer, the types of clients they currently serve, their ability to meet your company's specific needs.

3. Include performance standards in your EAP contract so you can measure the effectiveness of your investment.

EAPs Can Reduce Costs Related to Substance Abuse

EAPs address a wide variety of concerns that may negatively affect job performance, including mental health issues, financial and legal problems, career advancement, and other personal problems. EAPs can:

- screen for risky behaviors involving alcohol and drugs;
- educate employees about the health consequences of substance use;
- when necessary, refer employees for appropriate treatment; and
- provide support services that address recovery and the chronic nature of addiction.

Incorporating a substance abuse component into an EAP can help reduce absenteeism, improve employee health and job performance, and reduce medical costs, all of which save employers money.

EAP benefits: Replacing an employee costs from 25% to almost 200% of his or her annual compensation—not to mention the loss of institutional knowledge, service continuity, and coworker productivity and morale that can accompany employee turnover. The Federal Occupational Health agency, in a prospective cost-benefit estimate of employee assistance programs, showed that for every $1 spent on the EAP, the expected savings for the first year would be $1.27, and those savings would rise to $7.21 by the fifth year.

Make an EAP part of your benefits Package : Most EAP providers charge for their services on a per-person basis, and annual fees of $12 to $30 per employee are common. It also is possible to contract with an EAP provider for services used, usually at an hourly rate.

Chapter 75

Individual Rights When in Recovery from Substance Abuse Problems

Federal Non-Discrimination Laws That Protect You

Federal civil rights laws prohibit discrimination in many areas of life against qualified individuals with disabilities. Many people with past and current alcohol problems and past drug use disorders, including those in treatment for these illnesses, are protected from discrimination by:

- The Americans with Disabilities Act (ADA),

- The Rehabilitation Act of 1973,

- The Fair Housing Act (FHA), and

- The Workforce Investment Act (WIA).

Under these federal laws, an individual with a disability is someone who: has a current physical or mental impairment that substantially limits one or more of that person's major life activities, such as caring for one's self, working, and so forth; has a record of such a substantially limiting impairment; or, is regarded as having such an impairment.

Text in this chapter is excerpted from "Know Your Rights," Substance Abuse and Mental Health Services Administration (SAMHSA), 2007.

Whether a particular person has a disability is decided on an individualized, case-by-case basis. Substance use disorders (addiction) are recognized as impairments that can and do, for many individuals, substantially limit the individual's major life activities. For this reason, many courts have found that individuals experiencing or who are in recovery from these conditions are individuals with a disability protected by federal law.

To be protected as an individual with a disability under federal nondiscrimination laws, a person must show that his or her addiction substantially limits (or limited, in the past) major life activities. People wrongly believed to have a substance use disorder (in the past or currently) may also be protected as individuals regarded as having a disability.

People who currently engage in the illegal use of drugs are not protected under these non-discrimination laws, except that individuals may not be denied health services (including drug rehabilitation) based on their current illegal use of drugs if they are otherwise entitled to those services. People whose use of alcohol or drugs poses a direct threat, a significant risk of substantial harm to the health or safety of others, are not protected. Also, people whose use of alcohol or drugs does not significantly impair a major life activity are not protected (unless they show they have a record of or are regarded as having a substance use disorder—addiction—that is substantially limiting).

Discriminating against someone on the basis of his or her disability—for example, just because he has a past drug addiction or she is in an alcohol treatment program—may be illegal discrimination. Discrimination means treating someone less favorably than someone else because he or she has, once had, or is regarded as having a disability.

Acting against a person for reasons other than having a disability is not generally illegal discrimination, even if the disability is related to the cause of the adverse action. For instance, it is not likely to be ruled unlawful discrimination if someone in substance abuse treatment or in recovery is denied a job, services, or benefits because he does not meet essential eligibility requirements; is unable to do the job; creates a direct threat to health or safety by his behavior, even if the behavior is caused by a substance use disorder; or violates rules or commits a crime, including a drug or alcohol-related one, when that misconduct is cause for excluding or disciplining anyone doing it. Since the basis for the negative action in these cases is not (or not solely) the person's disability, these actions do not violate federal non-discrimination laws.

Employment

The Americans with Disabilities Act and the Rehabilitation Act prohibits most employers from refusing to hire, firing, or discriminating in the terms and conditions of employment against any qualified job applicant or employee on the basis of a disability. The ADA applies to all state and local governmental units, and to private employers with 15 or more employees. The Rehabilitation Act applies to federal employers and other public and private employers who receive federal grants, contracts, or aid.

In general, these employers may not deny a job to or fire a person because he or she is in treatment or in recovery from a substance use disorder, unless the person's disorder would prevent safe and competent job performance; must provide reasonable accommodations, when needed, to enable those with a disability to perform their job duties; and must keep confidential any medical-related information they discover about a job applicant or employee, including information about a past or present substance use disorder.

Medical Inquiries and Examinations

As a general rule, employers may not use information they learn about an individual's disability in a discriminatory manner. They may not deny or treat anyone less favorably in the terms and conditions of employment if he or she is qualified to perform the job. Also, employers must maintain the confidentiality of all information they obtain about applicants' and employees' health conditions, including addiction and treatment for substance use disorders.

Before making a job offer, employers may not ask questions about whether a job applicant has or has had a disability, or about the nature or severity of an applicant's disability. Pre-offer medical examinations also are illegal. And questions about whether a job applicant is or has ever abused or been addicted to drugs or alcohol, or if the applicant is being treated by a substance abuse rehabilitation program, or has received such treatment in the past are illegal.

After employment begins, employers may make medical inquiries or require an employee to undergo a medical examination, but only when doing this is job-related and justified by business necessity. Such exams and inquiries may be permitted if the employer has a reasonable belief, based on objective evidence, that an employee has a health (including substance use-related) condition that impairs his or her

453

ability to perform essential job functions, or that poses a direct threat to health or safety.

Workplace Drug Testing

Employers are permitted to test both job applicants and employees for illegal use of drugs, and may refuse to hire—or may fire or discipline—anyone whose test reveals such illegal use. Employers may not fire or refuse to hire any job applicant or employee solely because a drug test reveals the presence of a lawfully used medication (such as methadone). Employers must keep confidential information they discover about an employee's use of lawfully prescribed medications.

Medical Leave

The Family and Medical Leave Act (FMLA) gives many employees the right to take up to 12 weeks of unpaid leave in a 12-month period when needed to receive treatment for a serious health condition—which, under the FMLA, may include substance abuse. The leave must be for treatment; absence because of the employee's use of the substance does not qualify for leave.

The FMLA covers federal, state, and local government employers; public and private elementary and secondary schools; and private employers with 50 or more employees. To be eligible for leave under FMLA, you must have been employed by a covered employer for at least 12 months, worked at least 1,250 hours during the 12 months immediately before the leave, and work at a worksite where there are at least 50 employees or within 75 miles of that site.

Job Training

The Workforce Investment Act (WIA) provides financial assistance for job training and placement services for many people through the One-Stop Career Center system. Section 188 of WIA and the other non-discrimination laws prohibit most job training and placement service providers from denying services to, or discriminating in other ways against, qualified applicants and recipients on the basis of disability—including people with past or current substance use disorders—who otherwise meet the eligibility requirements for these services and are currently not using drugs illegally.

Housing

The Fair Housing Act (FHA) makes discrimination in housing and real estate transactions illegal when it is based on a disability. The FHA protects people with past and current alcohol addiction and past drug addiction—although other federal laws sometimes limit their rights. The FHA does not protect people who currently engage in illegal drug use.

Rights: Landlords and other housing providers may not refuse to rent or sell housing to people in recovery or who have current alcohol disorders, and may not discriminate in other ways against them in housing transactions solely on the basis of their disability. It is also illegal to discriminate against housing providers (such as sober or halfway houses for people in recovery) because they associate with individuals with disabilities.

Limits on public housing eligibility: Federal law limits some people's eligibility for public and other federally assisted housing because of past or current substance use-related conduct. The Quality Housing and Work Responsibility Act requires public housing agencies, Section 8, and other federally assisted housing providers to exclude:

- Any person evicted from public, federally assisted, or Section 8 housing because of drug-related criminal activity (including possession or sale). This bar ordinarily lasts for 3 years after the individual's eviction. A public housing agency can lift or shorten that time period if the individual successfully completes a rehabilitation program.

- Any household with a member who is abusing alcohol or using drugs in a manner that may interfere with the health, safety, or right to peaceful enjoyment of the premises by other residents. Exceptions can be made if the individual demonstrates that he or she is not currently abusing alcohol or using drugs illegally and has successfully completed a rehabilitation program.

- Permits applicants for public housing to be denied admission if a member of the household has engaged in any drug-related criminal activity (or certain other criminal activity) within a reasonable time of the application.

Limits on Rights and Opportunities Due to Drug Convictions

Public assistance and food stamps—Drug Felony Ban: The federal welfare law (the Personal Responsibility and Work Opportunity Act of 1996) imposes a lifetime ban on federal cash assistance and food stamps for anyone convicted of a drug-related felony (including possession or sale) after August 22, 1996. However, states may opt out of or modify this federal rule: 12 states do not impose this ban; 21 other states have modified the ban, and allow people who get treatment, show they are rehabilitated, or meet other requirements to become eligible again.

Education student loans and aid: The Higher Education Act of 1998 makes students convicted of drug offenses (including possession or sale) ineligible for federally funded student loans, grants, or work assistance. Ineligibility lasts for varying lengths of time, depending on the type of drug offense and if it is a repeat offense. This bars students from getting federally funded education loans or aid in college, and in many other educational and training programs. States cannot opt out of or otherwise modify this federal rule.

Driver's licenses: The Department of Transportation (DOT) Appropriation Amendment offers federal financial incentives to states that agree to revoke or suspend, for at least six months, the driver's license of anyone convicted of a drug offense (including not only drug-related driving offenses, but also those involving drug possession or sale). Many states choose not to opt out of this law.

Other Services

The Americans with Disabilities Act requires public accommodations as well as government agencies to comply with its non-discrimination requirements. Public accommodations are private facilities that provide goods or services to the public. They include: schools and universities; hospitals, clinics, and health care providers; social service agencies such as homeless shelters, day care centers, and senior centers.

Private service providers that receive federal grants, contracts, or aid must comply with the same non-discrimination requirements under the Rehabilitation Act and the Workforce Investment Act, when it applies. In offering or providing their goods or services, public accommodations (and other private entities covered by the Rehabilitation Act or WIA) must not discriminate against individuals on the basis of their past, current, or perceived disability. This means they must ensure that individuals with disabilities enjoy the equal opportunity to participate in or benefit from the facility's goods and service and receive goods or services in the most integrated setting possible. Segregating or providing different services to people with disabilities generally is not allowed.

How You Can Protect Your Rights

If you believe you are being or have been discriminated against because of your past or current alcohol disorder or past drug use disorder, you can challenge the violation of your rights in two ways: You may file a complaint with the Office of Civil Rights, or similar office, of the federal agency(s) with power to investigate and remedy violations of the disability discrimination laws. You do not need a lawyer to do this. Filing with the government can be faster and easier than a lawsuit and get you the same remedies. However, the deadline for filing these complaints can be as soon as 180 days after the discriminatory act—or even sooner, with federal employers—so always check. In most (but not all) cases, you also may file a lawsuit in federal or state court, in addition to or instead of filing an administrative complaint. Deadlines for lawsuits vary from 1–3 years following the discriminatory act. You must file employment discrimination claims under the ADA with the U.S. Equal Opportunity Employment Commission (EEOC). You may not file a lawsuit first or instead of filing with the EEOC. If your complaint is upheld, the persons or organizations that discriminated against you may be required to correct their actions and policies, compensate you, or give you other relief.

Chapter 76

Substance Abuse Treatment Statistics

Chapter Contents

Section 76.1—Treatment Received for Substance Abuse......... 460

Section 76.2—Predictors of Substance Abuse
Treatment Completion 468

Section 76.3—Treatment Outcomes for Clients
Discharged from Residential
Substance Abuse Treatment 471

Section 76.1

Treatment Received for Substance Abuse

Text in this section is from "Results from the 2007 National Survey on
Drug Use and Health: National Findings," Substance Abuse and Mental
Health Services Administration (SAMHSA), September 2008.

Past Year Treatment for a Substance Use Problem

Estimates described in this section refer to treatment received for
illicit drug or alcohol use, or for medical problems associated with the
use of illicit drugs or alcohol. This includes treatment received in the
past year at any location, such as a hospital (inpatient), rehabilitation facility (outpatient or inpatient), mental health center, emergency
room, private doctor's office, prison or jail, or a self-help group, such
as Alcoholics Anonymous or Narcotics Anonymous. Persons could report receiving treatment at more than one location. Specialty treatment only includes treatment at a hospital (inpatient), a rehabilitation
facility (inpatient or outpatient), or a mental health center.

Individuals who reported receiving substance use treatment but
were missing information on whether the treatment was specifically
for alcohol use or illicit drug use were not counted in estimates of illicit drug use treatment or in estimates of alcohol use treatment; however, they were counted in estimates for "drug or alcohol use"
treatment.

- In 2007, 3.9 million persons aged 12 or older (1.6% of the population) received some kind of treatment for a problem related
to the use of alcohol or illicit drugs. Of these, 1.4 million received treatment for the use of both alcohol and illicit drugs,
0.8 million received treatment for the use of illicit drugs but not
alcohol, and 1.3 million received treatment for the use of alcohol but not illicit drugs. (Note that estimates by substance
do not sum to the total number of persons receiving treatment
because the total includes persons who reported receiving
treatment but did not report for which substance the treatment was received.)

- The number and the percentage of the population aged 12 or older receiving substance use treatment within the past year remained stable between 2006 and 2007 and between 2002 and 2007 (3.9 million [1.6%] in 2007; 4.0 million [1.6%] in 2006; and 3.5 million [1.5%] in 2002).

- In 2007, among the 3.9 million persons aged 12 or older who received treatment for alcohol or illicit drug use in the past year, 2.2 million persons received treatment at a self-help group, and 1.7 million received treatment at a rehabilitation facility as an outpatient (Figure 76.1). There were 1.0 million persons who received treatment at a rehabilitation facility as an inpatient, 889,000 persons who received treatment at a mental health center as an outpatient, 779,000 at a hospital as an inpatient, 593,000 at a private doctor's office, 523,000 at an emergency department, and 302,000 at a prison or jail. None of these estimates changed significantly between 2006 and 2007 or between 2002 and 2007.

- In 2007, during their most recent treatment in the past year, 2.5 million persons aged 12 or older reported receiving treatment for alcohol use, and 936,000 persons reported receiving treatment for marijuana use (Figure 76.2). Accordingly, estimates on receiving treatment for the use of other drugs were 809,000 persons for cocaine, 558,000 for pain relievers, 335,000 for heroin, 311,000 for stimulants, and 303,000 for hallucinogens. None of these estimates changed significantly between 2006 and 2007, except that the numbers who received treatment for marijuana use and for nonmedical use of stimulants in 2007 were lower than the numbers in 2006 (1.2 million and 535,000 persons, respectively). None of these estimates changed significantly between 2002 and 2007, except that the number who received treatment for the use of pain relievers in 2007 was higher than the number in 2002 (360,000 persons). (Note that respondents could indicate that they received treatment for more than one substance during their most recent treatment.)

Need for and Receipt of Specialty Treatment

Specialty treatment is defined as treatment received at any of the following types of facilities: hospitals (inpatient only), drug or alcohol rehabilitation facilities (inpatient or outpatient), or mental health centers. It does not include treatment at an emergency room, private doctor's office, self-help group, prison or jail, or hospital as an outpatient. An individual is defined as needing treatment for an alcohol or drug use problem if he or she met the *Diagnostic and Statistical Manual of Mental Disorders, 4th Edition (DSM-IV)* (American Psychological Association, 1994) diagnostic criteria for dependence on or abuse of alcohol or illicit drugs in the past 12 months or if he or she received specialty treatment for alcohol use or illicit drug use in the past 12 months.

In this section, an individual needing treatment for an illicit drug use problem is defined as receiving treatment for his or her drug use problem only if he or she reported receiving specialty treatment for drug use in the past year. Thus, an individual who needed treatment for illicit drug use but only received specialty treatment for alcohol

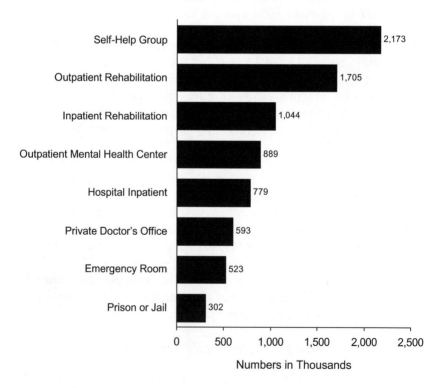

Figure 76.1. *Locations Where Past Year Substance Use Treatment Was Received among Persons Aged 12 or Older: 2007*

use in the past year or who received treatment for illicit drug use only at a facility not classified as a specialty facility was not counted as receiving treatment for drug use. Similarly, an individual who needed treatment for an alcohol use problem was only counted as receiving alcohol use treatment if the treatment was received for alcohol use at a specialty treatment facility. Individuals who reported receiving specialty substance use treatment but were missing information on whether the treatment was specifically for alcohol use or drug use were not counted in estimates of specialty drug use treatment or in estimates of specialty alcohol use treatment; however, they were counted in estimates for "drug or alcohol use" treatment.

In addition to questions about symptoms of substance use problems that are used to classify respondents' need for treatment based on *DSM-IV* criteria, the National Survey on Drug Use and Health

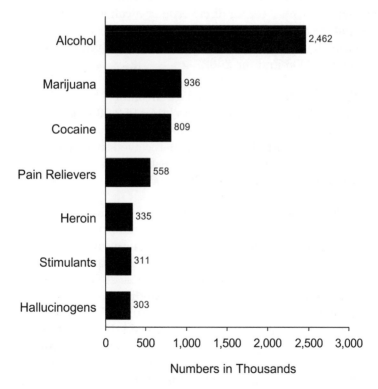

Figure 76.2. *Substances for Which Most Recent Treatment Was Received in the Past Year among Persons Aged 12 or Older: 2007*

(NSDUH) includes questions asking respondents about their perceived need for treatment (for example, whether they felt they needed treatment or counseling for illicit drug use or alcohol use). In this report, estimates for perceived need for treatment are only discussed for persons who were classified as needing treatment (based on *DSM-IV* criteria) but did not receive treatment at a specialty facility. Similarly, estimates for whether a person made an effort to get treatment are only discussed for persons who felt the need for treatment.

Illicit Drug or Alcohol Use Treatment and Treatment Need

- In 2007, 23.2 million persons aged 12 or older needed treatment for an illicit drug or alcohol use problem (9.4% of the persons aged 12 or older). Of these, 2.4 million (1.0% of persons aged 12 or older and 10.4% of those who needed treatment) received treatment at a specialty facility. Thus, 20.8 million persons (8.4% of the population aged 12 or older) needed treatment for an illicit drug or alcohol use problem but did not receive treatment at a specialty substance abuse facility in the past year. These estimates are similar to the estimates for 2006 and for 2002.

- Of the 2.4 million people aged 12 or older who received specialty substance use treatment in 2007, 952,000 received treatment for alcohol use only, 728,000 received treatment for illicit drug use only, and 615,000 persons received treatment for both alcohol and illicit drug use. These estimates are similar to the estimates for 2006 and for 2002.

- In 2007, among persons who received their last or current substance use treatment at a specialty facility in the past year, 53.3% reported using their own savings or earnings as a source of payment for their most recent specialty treatment, 34.9% reported using private health insurance, 26.3% reported using public assistance other than Medicaid, 19.7% reported using Medicare, 19.6% reported using funds from family members, and 18.2% reported using Medicaid. None of these estimates changed significantly between 2006 and 2007 and between 2002 and 2007, except that the 53.3% reported using their own savings or earnings as a source of payment in 2007 was higher than the 42.1% reported in 2006. (Note that persons could report more than one source of payment.)

- Of the 20.8 million persons in 2007 who were classified as needing substance use treatment but not receiving treatment at a specialty facility in the past year, 1.3 million persons (6.4%) reported that they perceived a need for treatment for their illicit drug or alcohol use problem. Of these 1.3 million persons who felt they needed treatment but did not receive treatment in 2007, 380,000 (28.5%) reported that they made an effort to get treatment, and 955,000 (71.5%) reported making no effort to get treatment.

- The number and the percentage of youths aged 12 to 17 who needed treatment for an illicit drug or alcohol use problem remained unchanged between 2006 and 2007; however, there was a significant decrease between 2002 and 2007 (2.0 million youths [7.9%] of the population in 2007; 2.1 million [8.2%] in 2006; and 2.3 million [9.1%] in 2002). Of the 2.0 million youths who needed treatment in 2007, 150,000 received treatment at a specialty facility (about 7.6% of the youths who needed treatment), leaving 1.8 million who needed treatment for a substance use problem but did not receive it at a specialty facility.

- Based on 2004–2007 combined data, five of the most often reported reasons for not receiving illicit drug or alcohol use treatment among persons who needed but did not receive treatment at a specialty facility and perceived a need for treatment included (a) not ready to stop using (38.7%), (b) no health coverage and could not afford cost (31.1%), (c) possible negative effect on job (11.6%), (d) not knowing where to go for treatment (11.6%), and (e) concern that receiving treatment might cause neighbors/community to have negative opinion (11.1%).

Illicit Drug Use Treatment and Treatment Need

- In 2007, the number of persons aged 12 or older needing treatment for an illicit drug use problem was 7.5 million (3.0% of the total population). Of these, 1.3 million (0.5% of the total population, 17.8% of the persons who needed treatment) received treatment at a specialty facility for an illicit drug use problem in the past year. Thus, there were 6.2 million persons (2.5% of the total population) who needed treatment but did not receive treatment at a specialty facility for an illicit drug use problem in 2007. None of these estimates changed significantly between 2006 and 2007 and between 2002 and 2007.

- The number of persons needing treatment for illicit drug use in 2007 (7.5 million) was similar to the number needing treatment in 2002 (7.7 million), 2003 (7.3 million), 2004 (8.1 million), 2005 (7.6 million), and 2006 (7.8 million). Also, the number of persons needing but not receiving specialty treatment in the past year for an illicit drug use problem in 2007 (6.2 million) was similar to the estimates in 2002 (6.3 million), 2003 (6.2 million), 2004 (6.6 million), 2005 (6.3 million), and 2006 (6.2 million).

- Of the 6.2 million people aged 12 or older who needed but did not receive specialty treatment for illicit drug use in 2007, 548,000 (8.9%) reported that they perceived a need for treatment for their illicit drug use problem. Of the 548,000 persons

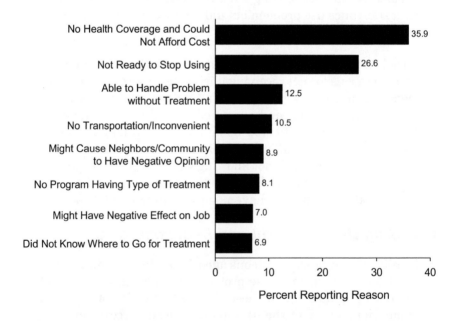

Figure 76.3. *Reasons for Not Receiving Substance Use Treatment among Persons Aged 12 or Older Who Needed and Made an Effort to Get Treatment but Did Not Receive Treatment and Felt They Needed Treatment: 2004-2007 Combined*

who felt a need for treatment in 2007, 205,000 (37.5%) reported that they made an effort and 343,000 (62.5%) reported making no effort to get treatment.

- Among youths aged 12 to 17, there were 1.1 million (4.5%) who needed treatment for an illicit drug use problem in 2007. Of this group, only 111,000 received treatment at a specialty facility (9.9% of youths aged 12 to 17 who needed treatment) leaving 1.0 million youths who needed treatment but did not receive it at a specialty facility.

- Among people aged 12 or older who needed but did not receive illicit drug use treatment and felt they needed treatment (based on 2004–2007 combined data), six of the most often reported reasons for not receiving treatment were (a) no health coverage and could not afford cost (34.3%), (b) not ready to stop using (31.8%), (c) concern that getting treatment might cause neighbors/community to have negative opinion (14.4%), (d) not knowing where to go for treatment (13.5%), (e) being able to handle the problem without treatment (12.7%), and (f) possible negative effect on job (11.7%).

Alcohol Use Treatment and Treatment Need

- In 2007, the number of persons aged 12 or older needing treatment for an alcohol use problem was 19.3 million (7.8% of the population aged 12 or older). Of these, 1.6 million (0.6% of the total population and 8.1% of the people who needed treatment for an alcohol use problem) received alcohol use treatment at a specialty facility. Thus, there were 17.7 million people who needed treatment but did not receive treatment at a specialty facility for an alcohol use problem. None of these estimates changed significantly between 2006 and 2007 and between 2002 and 2007.

- Among the 17.7 million people aged 12 or older who needed but did not receive treatment for an alcohol use problem in 2007, there were 859,000 (4.8%) who felt they needed treatment for their alcohol use problem. The number and the percentage were higher than those reported in 2006 (541,000 persons and 3.0%, respectively), but were similar to those reported in 2002 (761,000 persons and 4.5%, respectively). Of these, 619,000 (72.1%) did not make an effort to get treatment, and 240,000 (27.9%) made an effort but were unable to get treatment in 2007.

• In 2007, there were 1.4 million youths (5.5%) aged 12 to 17 who needed treatment for an alcohol use problem. Of this group, only 82,000 received treatment at a specialty facility (0.3% of all youths and 5.9% of youths who needed treatment) leaving 1.3 million youths who needed but did not receive treatment.

Section 76.2

Predictors of Substance Abuse Treatment Completion

Excerpted from "Predictors of Substance Abuse Treatment Completion or Transfer to Further Treatment by Service Type," Substance Abuse and Mental Health Services Administration (SAMHSA), February 26, 2009. The complete document is available at http://oas.samhsa.gov/2k9/ TXpredictors/TXpredictors.htm.

Among adults who seek treatment for an alcohol or drug abuse problem, many do not complete an entire course of treatment. This finding is a concern given the research showing that length of stay in treatment is one of the strongest predictors of positive treatment outcomes. Identifying factors that predict treatment completion is an important step towards understanding what leads to successful treatment.

The Treatment Episode Data Set (TEDS) is an annual compilation of data on the demographic characteristics and substance abuse problems of those admitted to and discharged from substance abuse treatment. TEDS also collects information on reasons for leaving substance abuse treatment. These include treatment completion, transfer to another substance abuse program or facility within a single episode of treatment, left against professional advice (dropped out), terminated by the facility (discharge was not because the client dropped out, was incarcerated, or any other client reason), and other reasons, such as death. Clients' treatment may be terminated by a facility for a variety of reasons, such as not following facility rules or exhibiting violent behavior.

This report focuses on the 973,000 clients who were discharged from outpatient, intensive outpatient, long-term residential (more than 30 days), and short-term residential (30 days or fewer) treatment in 2005. Specifically, this report examines the proportion of clients discharged who completed treatment or transferred to further treatment and the demographic and substance use characteristics that predict treatment completion and transfer. Because treatment completion and transfer to further treatment represent positive conclusions to a treatment episode, understanding the characteristics of clients who are completing treatment or transferring to further treatment may assist providers to tailor programs that will yield more successful outcomes for their clients.

Treatment Completion and Transfer to Further Treatment, by Treatment Type

In 2005, clients discharged from short-term residential treatment were more likely to complete treatment than clients discharged from long-term residential, outpatient, or intensive outpatient treatment settings (57% versus 38% or less). Clients discharged from intensive outpatient and short-term residential treatment were more likely to transfer to another program or facility than clients discharged from long-term residential and outpatient treatment settings (19% and 17% versus 13% and 12%).

Demographic and Substance Use Characteristics That Predict Treatment Completion or Transfer to Further Treatment

To examine the client characteristics associated with treatment completion or transfer to further treatment, a statistical analysis was conducted. This analysis identifies the likelihood of one group completing treatment or transferring to further treatment compared with another group. The remainder of this report presents the client characteristics that significantly predicted treatment completion or transfer to further treatment for each of the four major service types.

Table 76.1. Reason for Discharge from Outpatient, Intensive Outpatient, Long-Term Residential, and Short-Term Residential Treatment: TEDS 2005

Reason for Discharge	Outpatient	Intensive Outpatient	Short-term Residential	Long-term Residential
Completed	36%	36%	57%	38%
Transferred	12%	19%	17%	13%
Dropped Out	29%	24%	15%	31%
Terminated	11%	13%	7%	9%
Other	12%	8%	4%	9%

Source: 2005 SAMHSA Treatment Episode Data Set (TEDS).

- Significant predictors of treatment completion or transfer among clients who were discharged from outpatient, intensive outpatient, long-term residential, or short-term residential treatment included: alcohol as the primary substance of abuse, less than daily use at admission, being over age 40, having 12 or more years of education, being White, referral to treatment by the criminal justice system, and being employed.

- Among clients who were discharged from intensive outpatient treatment, men were more likely than women to complete treatment or transfer to another program or facility; however, among clients who were discharged from outpatient or long-term residential treatment, women were more likely than men to complete treatment or transfer to another facility.

Identifying factors that predict treatment completion is a critical part of understanding what leads to successful treatment. The TEDS analyses presented here look at the relationship between treatment completion or transfer to further treatment and gender, age at admission, race/ethnicity, primary substance of abuse, frequency of use, referral source, employment status, and education. The results show that the client characteristics that most strongly predicted treatment completion varied depending on the type of treatment (outpatient, intensive outpatient, short-term residential, or long-term residential). The findings underscore the strong positive influence of being employed on the likelihood of completing treatment or transferring to further treatment. These findings provide important insights to treatment providers and policy makers as they work to ensure that treatment is successful for all clients in all service settings.

Section 76.3

Treatment Outcomes for Clients Discharged from Residential Substance Abuse Treatment

Text in this section is from "Treatment Outcomes among Clients Discharged from Residential Substance Abuse Treatment: 2005," Substance Abuse and Mental Health Services Administration (SAMHSA), February 12, 2009.

Treatment completion is an important predictor of improved outcomes, such as long-term abstinence, among clients admitted to treatment for substance abuse and dependence. Type of treatment, drug use patterns, gender, and education are associated with completion and dropout rates. Dropout rates, in turn, are associated with relapse and return to substance use. Understanding the characteristics of clients discharged from short-term and long-term residential services that completed treatment, dropped out of treatment, or were terminated by the facility may lead to improved completion rates. This understanding may also assist in providing appropriate services for clients who are in need of residential services but at a higher risk for failing to complete treatment.

Using data from the Treatment Episode Data Set (TEDS), an annual compilation of data on the demographic characteristics and substance abuse problems of those admitted for substance abuse treatment, this report examines the characteristics of clients discharged from short-term (30 days or fewer) and long-term (more than 30 days) residential treatment. In particular, this report examines those clients who completed treatment, dropped out, or whose treatment was terminated by the facility. Of the 1.37 million client discharges in 2005 who reported a reason for discharge, a total of 601,000 or 44% completed treatment, 343,000 or 25% dropped out of treatment,

471

Table 76.2. Percentage of Discharges from Short-Term and Long-Term Residential Substance Abuse Treatment, by Reason for Discharge: 2005

Reason for Discharge	Short-term Residential	Long-term Residential
Completed Treatment	57%	38%
Dropped Out	15%	31%
Terminated by Facility	7%	9%
Transferred	17%	13%
Other	4%	9%

Source: 2005 SAMHSA Treatment Episode Data Set (TEDS).

Table 76.3. Percentage of Discharges from Short-term and Long-term Residential Substance Abuse Treatment, by Primary Substance of Abuse and Reason for Discharge: 2005

		Reason for Discharge		
Length of Stay	Substance of Abuse	Completed Treatment	Dropped Out	Terminated by Facility
Short-term Residential	Alcohol	66%	12%	5%
	Marijuana	51%	14%	12%
	Cocaine	50%	16%	8%
	Opiates	51%	21%	8%
	Stimulants	46%	19%	9%
Long-term Residential	Alcohol	46%	25%	9%
	Marijuana	36%	29%	13%
	Cocaine	33%	33%	9%
	Opiates	35%	36%	11%
	Stimulants	40%	33%	4%

Source: 2005 SAMHSA Treatment Episode Data Set (TEDS).

and 115,000 or 8% had their treatment terminated by the facility. Of these three groups, nearly 10% (101,281 discharges) were from short-term and almost 9% (91,639 discharges) were from long-term residential treatment.

Treatment Completion, Dropping Out, and Termination by a Facility

In 2005, clients discharged from short-term residential treatment were more likely to complete treatment than clients discharged from long-term residential treatment (57% versus 38%) and less likely to drop out of treatment (15% versus 31%). Similar percentages of clients discharged from short-term residential and long-term residential treatment were terminated by the facility (7% and 9%).

Primary Substance of Abuse

Clients discharged from short-term residential treatment in 2005 were more likely to complete treatment than drop out or be terminated by the facility regardless of the primary substance of abuse. Among clients discharged from short-term residential service settings, treatment completion was highest among those reporting primary alcohol abuse (66%) and lowest among those reporting primary stimulant abuse (46%). The proportion of clients discharged from short-term residential treatment who dropped out of treatment was highest among those reporting primary opiate (21%) or primary stimulant (19%) abuse. The proportion of discharges from short-term residential service settings who were terminated by the facility ranged from 5% of clients reporting primary alcohol abuse to 12% of clients reporting primary marijuana abuse.

Among clients discharged from long-term residential service settings, treatment completion was highest among those reporting primary alcohol abuse (46%); treatment completion was lowest among those reporting primary cocaine abuse (33%) or primary opiate abuse (35%). Clients discharged from long-term residential treatment who reported primary cocaine abuse were equally likely to complete treatment or drop out of treatment (33% each); similarly, clients discharged from long-term residential treatment who reported primary opiate abuse were almost equally likely to complete treatment or drop out of treatment (35% and 36%). Clients discharged from long-term residential treatment who reported primary stimulant abuse were less likely than those who reported other primary substances to be terminated by the facility (4% versus 9–13%).

473

Gender

Among clients discharged from short-term residential treatment in 2005, males were more likely than females to complete treatment (58% versus 52%). However, among clients discharged from long-term residential service settings, males and females were about equally likely to complete treatment (39% and 38%). Similar proportions of male and female clients discharged from short-term and long-term residential service settings dropped out of treatment (short-term—15% and 17%; long-term—31% and 30%) or were terminated by the facility (short-term—7% each; long-term—9% and 8%).

Race/Ethnicity

Clients discharged from short-term residential treatment in 2005 were more likely to complete treatment than drop out or be terminated by the facility regardless of race or ethnicity. A higher proportion of American Indian/Alaska Native and Asian/Pacific Islander short-term residential discharges completed treatment than short-term residential discharges of other races or ethnic groups (63% and 60% versus 57% or lower). The proportions of clients discharged from short-term residential treatment that dropped out of treatment ranged from 14% of Whites to 19% of Hispanics. The proportion of clients discharged from short-term residential treatment who were terminated by the facility was similar across the racial and ethnic groups (ranging from 6% to 8%).

In comparison, a higher proportion of White and American Indian/Alaska Native clients discharged from long-term residential treatment completed treatment than long-term residential discharges of other races or ethnic groups (42% each versus 34% or lower). Similar proportions of Blacks discharged from long-term residential treatment completed or dropped out (34% and 33%), as did Asian/Pacific Islander discharges (28% each). Hispanics were the only group in which a lower proportion completed long-term residential treatment than dropped out of treatment (34% versus 39%). The proportions of long-term residential clients who were terminated by the facility ranged from 6% of Hispanics to 10% of American Indians/Alaska Natives.

Educational Level

Among clients discharged from short-term residential treatment, treatment completion increased from 53% of clients with less than a high school education to 62% of those with some college. The proportion of short-term residential clients who dropped out of treatment decreased as educational level increased, from 18% of clients with less than a high school education to 13% of those with some college. The proportion of clients discharged from short-term residential treatments that were terminated by the facility varied only slightly by educational level (ranging from 6% of those with some college to 8% of those with less than a high school education).

Treatment completion increased as educational level increased among clients discharged from long-term residential treatment, from 35% of those with less than a high school education to 44% of those with some college. Like short-term residential discharges, the proportion of clients discharged from long-term residential treatment who dropped out of treatment decreased as educational level increased (from 36% of clients with less than a high school education to 26% of clients with some college). Long-term residential discharges across the educational levels were equally likely to be terminated by the facility (8% each).

Discussion

In 2005, clients discharged from short-term residential treatment were more likely than clients discharged from long-term residential treatment to complete treatment and less likely to drop out of treatment. In addition, certain client characteristics, such as primary alcohol abuse and higher educational level, were associated with treatment completion regardless of the type of residential treatment received. Understanding the client characteristics associated with treatment completion, dropping out, and termination in various service settings may help program managers and treatment providers design treatment programs that maximize treatment completion rates for specific at-risk populations.

Part V

Drug Abuse Prevention

Chapter 77

Effective Responses to Reducing Drug Abuse

Making the Drug Problem Smaller

A major preoccupation of parents since the 1960s, the problem of illegal drug use has been implicated in everything from urban crime to undermining worker productivity and lowering scholastic achievement test (SAT) scores. In fact, drug abuse can rightly be blamed for worsening social problems such as teen pregnancy, undermining the safety of public housing, polluting Andean watersheds to fostering terrorism in the hemisphere. The good news is that drug use is down, in some cases down sharply, with the use of some drugs at or near historic lows. Drug use among young people has only been lower in three of the past 17 years.

Evidence is building, moreover, that these reductions in drug use, which have largely erased the run-up that began in 1993, are the result of innovations in the way we educate young people about the harms of illegal drugs, provide help to those already embarked on a career of drug use, and interdict the drugs and drug traffickers seeking to compromise the integrity of our borders.

Stopping Use before It Starts

The National Youth Anti-Drug Media Campaign, for example, combines paid and donated advertising to reach young people and their

Text in this chapter is from "Making the Drug Problem Smaller, 2001–2008," Office of National Drug Control Policy, January 2009.

parents to change teen beliefs and intentions toward drug use. The media campaign has been in existence for years, but in its more recent incarnation the campaign has been refocused to take advantage of more sophisticated advertising techniques and best practices, as well as using new technologies in wide use among young people, such as social networking sites and text messaging, and has contributed to increasing youth perceptions of risk and social disapproval of drug use.

The campaign has become adept at responding to new drug threats. When teen abuse of prescription drugs began to rise, the campaign worked with the Partnership for a Drug Free America to launch an unprecedented effort to educate parents about the harms of misuse. After a debut in the Super Bowl (the television event most watched by parents and teens together) and an innovative advertising and marketing blitz, parental awareness of this emerging problem more than doubled, from 31 to 67 percent.

Student drug testing, an approach first popularized for student athletes but then hamstrung by a decade of litigation, has exploded in popularity over the past eight years, with 1,839 school districts currently operating programs, in addition to many private schools. The purpose of random testing is not to catch, punish, or expose students who use drugs, but to prevent drug dependence and to help drug-dependent students become drug-free in a confidential manner.

The psychology behind student drug testing programs is straightforward. They give kids an out, says Flemington, New Jersey school Superintendent Lisa Brady, who started a student drug testing program as principal of Hunterdon High School. "Kids will tell you that the program gives them a reason to say no. They're just kids, after all; they need a crutch. Being able to say, I'm a cheerleader, I'm in the band, I'm a football player, and my school drug tests—it really gives them some tools to be able to say no." Not surprisingly, drug use fell sharply after the program was initiated.

Involving the Community

In addition to outreach efforts like the media campaign and student drug testing programs, the effort to contain drug use among young people has been aided by an upsurge in local community groups. Research confirms that established coalitions significantly reduce drug and alcohol use among young people as compared to areas without coalitions. Community coalitions come in as many shapes and sizes as there are coalitions, but the best among them identify a specific problem and relentlessly target a solution. A little over a decade ago, for instance, a group of parents in Kansas City, Kansas, decided that they had had enough of teenage drinking and drug use and set out to do something about it. What came to be known as the Tri-County Northland Coalition pulled together existing community efforts that were being run out of 15 area school districts. The group targeted keg parties, taking out billboard and newspaper ads to get out the message that parents could be held legally liable for allowing keg parties.

But they did not stop there. The coalition followed up through an initiative with local merchants to tag every keg rented in the tri-county area. Keg tracking, as it is called, links rented kegs back to the person who actually paid for them. If the police come upon a keg party, they can take that keg back to the place where was rented and then find out who rented it. Hotel and motel managers are given a schedule of local proms and asked to warn customers not to rent rooms for underage parties.

Targeting the Workplace

Curbing the use of illegal drugs by young people is key: research demonstrates that people who do not initiate drug use as young people are statistically much less likely to begin using as adults. Reductions in youth drug use over the past eight years mean that some 900,000 fewer young people are taking drugs each month than was the case in 2001. The overwhelming majority of these young people will grow up without ever embarking on a career of drug use and, ultimately, addiction.

As critical as it is to keep drug use from ever starting among young people, drug policy also needs to look to the needs of the addicted, and those whose drug use has not yet led them into addiction. While young people are a distinct group, and the pool of the addicted is relatively small, the category of drug-using individuals whose use has not led to full-blown addiction is larger and includes hard-to-identify individuals, many of whom are in the workforce and who may go years without showing the ill effects of their drug use. These are the people who use drugs and appear not to be suffering any consequences, who spread the contagion of drug use, and yet who surveys repeatedly indicate are highly unlikely to believe they need treatment.

Reaching these individuals is critical, but difficult. Yet it is especially important to intervene with users during this honeymoon phase. A new, national focus on brief interventions has been leveraging the existing medical infrastructure—which already has extensive experience in identifying problem drinkers—to screen for drug use and offer appropriate and often brief interventions. In Chicago, for example, Cook County Hospital emergency room staff as well as doctors and nurses in other areas of the hospital are trained to flag signs of developing drug use and direct users to treatment. Medicaid and Medicare now provide for reimbursement for brief interventions, and eleven states have adopted billing systems that make it easier to obtain reimbursement for such interventions.

For non-violent offenders with substance abuse problems, drug courts present an alternative to incarceration. Drug courts closely monitor these offenders through regular drug testing and channel them to treatment. By the end of 2007 there were over 2,100 drug courts across the country.

Improving Treatment

Drug using individuals whose needs go beyond a brief session with a counselor have new options thanks to an innovative program launched by the President in his 2003 State of the Union address. The Access to Recovery program uses vouchers to expand treatment capacity where it is most needed and allow clients to play a more significant role in the development of their own treatment plan. Access to Recovery also gives clients the option of working with faith-based providers, who have come forward to provide important recovery support services such as childcare, transportation, and mentoring.

Driving Down Use by Reducing Availability

New efforts such as brief interventions appear to be contributing to a reduction in drug use as identified through workplace drug testing—such tests now show the lowest levels of cocaine and methamphetamine use on record. Yet reductions of this magnitude—cocaine positive tests are down 38% in just two years—typically also involve a restriction in supply.

Similar reductions in youthful use of drugs such as ecstasy and lysergic acid diethylamide (LSD)—both of which have dropped by half or more since 2001—were correlated to the disruption of criminal networks used to distribute those drugs. Similarly, the dramatic reduction in workplace cocaine positives in the past two years correlates with reductions in the amount of cocaine exported from Colombia (down 30% from the peak in 2001) and the aggressive campaign being waged by the government of Mexico against traffickers during the past two years.

The growth in seizures and disruption south of the U.S. border has not only driven up seizures of both cocaine and methamphetamine; it has also demonstrably driven up the prices of both drugs, a key condition for cutting down on use. This is in keeping with the strategy of the U.S. government, which is to disrupt the market for illegal drugs and to do so in a way that both reduces the profitability of the drug trade and increases the costs of drugs to consumers. In other words, we seek to inflict on this business what every legal business fears—escalating costs, diminishing profits, and unreliable suppliers. The evidence suggests that reductions in the amount of cocaine exported to the United States have translated into sharply higher cocaine prices.

Chapter 78

Testing for Drugs of Abuse

Chapter Contents

Section 78.1—How Drug Tests Are Done 486

Section 78.2—Why Drug Tests Are Done 488

Section 78.3—Home Use Test for Drugs of Abuse 494

Section 78.1

How Drug Tests Are Done

Formal name: Drugs of abuse screen

Also known as: Drug screen; drug test; substance abuse testing; toxicology screen; tox screen

The Test Sample: What Is Being Tested?

Drugs of abuse testing is the detection of one or more illegal and/or legal substances in the urine, or more rarely, in the blood, saliva, hair, or sweat. It usually involves an initial screening test followed by a second test that identifies and/or confirms the presence of a drug or drugs. Most laboratories use commercially available tests that have been developed and optimized to screen urine for the major drugs of abuse.

For most drugs of abuse testing, results of initial screening testing are compared with a predetermined cut-off. Anything below that cut-off is considered negative; anything above is considered a positive screening result. Within each class of drug that is tested, there may be a variety of chemically similar drugs. Legal substances that are chemically similar to illegal ones can produce a positive screening result. Therefore, screening tests that are positive for one or more classes of drugs are frequently confirmed with a secondary test that identifies the exact substance present using a very sensitive and specific method, such as gas chromatography/mass spectrometry (GC/MS). Some of the most commonly screened drug classes are listed in Table 78.1.

Substances that are not similar to the defined classes can produce false negative results. Some drugs may be difficult to detect with the standardized assays, either because the test is not set up to detect the drug, such as methylenedioxymethamphetamine (MDMA, ecstasy), oxycodone (OxyContin®), or buprenorphine, or because the drug does not remain in the body long enough to be detected, such as gamma-hydroxybutyrate (GHB).

For sports testing of hormones and steroids, each test performed is usually specific for a single substance and may be quantitative. Athletes, especially those at the national and international level, are tested for illegal drugs and are additionally governed by a long list of prohibited substances called performance enhancers.

Groups of drug tests are typically ordered for medical or legal reasons, as part of a drug-free workplace or as part of a sports testing program. People who use these substances ingest, inhale, smoke, or inject them into their bodies. The amounts that are absorbed and the effects that they have depend on the which drugs are taken, how they interact, their purity and strength, the quantity, timing, method of intake, and the individual person's ability to metabolize and excrete them. Some drugs can interfere with the action or metabolism of other medications, have additive effects such as taking two drugs that both depress the central nervous system (CNS), or have competing effects such as taking one drug that depresses the CNS and another that stimulates it. The drugs tested for are not normally found in the body with the exception of some hormones and steroids measured as part of sports testing.

How is the sample collected for testing?

Urine is the most frequently tested sample, but other body samples such as hair, saliva, sweat, and blood also may be used for drug abuse

Table 78.1. Commonly Screened Drug Classes

Drug class screened	Examples of specific drugs identified during confirmation
Amphetamines	Methamphetamine, amphetamine
Barbiturates	Phenobarbital, secobarbital, pentobarbital
Benzodiazepines	Diazepam, lorazepam
Cannibinoids	Marijuana
Cocaine	Cocaine and/or its metabolite (benzoylecgonine)
Opiates	Codeine, morphine, metabolite of heroin
Phencyclidine (PCP)	PCP

screening but not interchangeably with urine. Urine and saliva are collected in clean containers. A blood sample is obtained by inserting a needle into a vein in the arm. Hair is cut close to the scalp to collect a sample. A sweat sample is typically collected by applying a patch to the skin for a specified period of time.

Is any test preparation needed to ensure the quality of the sample?

No test preparation is needed.

Section 78.2

Why Drug Tests Are Done

© 2009 American Association for Clinical Chemistry. Reprinted with permission. For additional information about clinical lab testing, visit the Lab Tests Online website at www.labtestsonline.org.

Medical Screening

Medical screening for drugs of abuse is primarily focused on determining what drugs or combinations of drugs a person may have taken so that he can receive the proper treatment. The overall effect on a particular person depends on the response of his body to the drugs, on the quantity and combination he has taken, and when each was taken. For instance, MDMA is initially a stimulant with associated psychedelic effects, but it also causes central nervous system (CNS) depression as it is metabolized and cleared from the body. In many cases, drugs have been combined and/or taken with ethanol (alcohol). If someone drinks ethanol during this time period, they will have two CNS depressants in their system, a potentially dangerous combination.

Those who may be tested for drugs for medical reasons include the following:

- Someone in the emergency room who is having acute health problems that the doctor thinks may be drug-related: unconsciousness, nausea, delirium, panic, paranoia, increased temperature, chest pain, respiratory failure, seizures, and/or headaches.

- Someone in the emergency room who has been in an accident, when the doctor suspects that drugs and/or alcohol may have been involved.

- A youth or adult who the doctor suspects may be using drugs.

- Those who are being monitored for known drug use. This may include both legal and illegal drug use. It may be general testing or specific for the substance that has been abused.

- Pregnant women thought to be at risk for drug abuse or neonates exhibiting certain characteristic behaviors.

Legal or Forensic Testing

Drug testing for legal purposes is primarily concerned with the detection of illegal or banned drug use in a variety of situations. Sample collection procedures for this type of testing are strictly controlled and documented to maintain a legal chain-of-custody. The donor provides a sample that is sealed and secured with a tamperproof seal in his or her presence. Specific chain-of-custody paperwork then accompanies the sample throughout the testing process; each person who handles and/ or tests the sample provides their signature and the reason for the sample transfer. This creates a permanent record of each step of the process. Examples of legal drug abuse screening include these:

- Court-mandated drug testing usually involves the random monitoring of someone who has been convicted of illegal drug use. Testing may also be ordered in custody cases to rule out drug use by one or both parents.

- Government child protective services may sometimes require extended monitoring of a parent with a known drug problem to ensure that they have not returned to drug use.

- Law enforcement drug testing may be done when someone has an accident that is suspected to be alcohol- or drug-related.

- Forensic testing utilizes a variety of body fluids and tissues that may be tested for numerous drugs during a crime investigation.

The goal may be to determine whether drugs were a contributing factor to an accident or crime, such as a driving under the influence (DUI) or rape. Testing may also be done to determine whether someone died of a drug overdose or drug-related condition.

- Insurance companies may perform drug screening on their applicants. This may include a test for cocaine and a test for nicotine, even though tobacco is a legal substance.

- Schools may have programs that incorporate random drug testing. This may include illegal drugs of abuse, and with competitive sports may include testing for performance-enhancing substances.

Employment Drug Testing

Employment drug testing may be done prior to employment, on a random basis, following an accident, or if the employer has a reasonable suspicion that their employee is using illegal drugs. The major drugs of abuse are tested, and any positives are confirmed by another method. Employment drug testing is commonplace. It is required in some industries, such as those that involve the U.S. Department of Transportation or federal employees, and accepted practice in many other industries.

As with legal or forensic drug testing, the sample collection and testing procedures for employment drug testing are often strictly controlled and documented to maintain a legal chain-of-custody. A sample is obtained (usually a urine sample) from the employee in a container that is secured with a tamperproof seal in his or her presence. Specific chain-of-custody paperwork then accompanies the sample throughout the testing process and documents each person who handles and/or tests the sample. This creates a permanent record of each step of the process.

Sports/Athletic Screening

While conventional drug testing is performed on competitive athletes, the primary focus is on doping—drugs and/or supplements that are taken to promote muscle growth and/or to improve strength and endurance. On a local level, sports testing may be limited, but on a national and international level, it has become highly organized.

The World Anti-Doping Agency (WADA), U.S. Anti-Doping Agency (USADA), and the International Association of Athletics Federations

(IAAF) work together to monitor athlete drug use on a national, international, and Olympic level. WADA has a written code, which establishes uniform drug testing rules and sanctions for all sports and countries, and a substantial list of prohibited substances. Athletes are responsible for any banned substances that are found in their body during testing. Most of the compounds tested are considered positive if they are detected in any quantity while others, such as caffeine, are only prohibited when they are present in large amounts. Some of the substances, such as anabolic steroids (testosterone) and peptide hormones such as erythropoietin, growth hormone, and insulin-like growth factor-1 are banned but are difficult to measure as they are produced by the body. Testing methods must be able to distinguish between endogenous (that produced by the athlete's body) and supplemented compounds.

Screening programs randomly perform out-of-competition drug tests on athletes during the training season to look for anabolic steroids, such as testosterone, that promote increased muscle growth. During competitions, testing is frequently done both randomly and on all winners and includes categories such as: stimulants, narcotics, anabolic agents, and peptide hormones. Sports such as archery, gymnastics, and shooting add additional testing for substances like beta blockers, which are prohibited in these sports because they decrease blood pressure and heart rate.

While professional sports organizations, such as the NFL (National Football League), NHL (National Hockey League), and NBA (National Basketball Association), are not covered by the WADA code, they have programs in place to test their athletes for panels of drugs that combine aspects of sports and employment testing. Those professional athletes who also take part in the Olympics, however, are subject to the same out-of-competition (pre-game) and in-competition testing as other competing athletes.

When is it ordered?

Drug testing is performed whenever a doctor, employer, legal entity, or athletic organization needs to determine whether a person has illegal or banned substances in his body. It may be ordered prior to the start of some new jobs and insurance policies, at random to satisfy workplace and athletic drug testing programs, as mandated when court ordered, as indicated when ordered by a doctor to monitor a known or suspected substance abuse patient, and whenever a person has symptoms that suggest drug use.

What does the test result mean?

If a result is positive during initial drug screening, then it means that the person has a substance in his body that falls into one of the drug classes and is above the established cutoff level. If the sample is confirmed as positive after secondary testing, such as positive for marijuana, then the person has taken this drug. In some cases, this result can be tied to a window of time that the person took the substance and roughly to the quantity, but in most circumstances that information is not necessary. Interpretation of when and how much drug was consumed can be challenging because the concentration of many drugs varies, as does their rate of metabolism from person to person.

If the drug or drugs is not present or is below the established cutoff, then the result is usually reported as not detected or none detected. A negative result does not necessarily mean that the person did not take a drug at some point. The drug may be present below the established cutoff, the drug may have been already metabolized and eliminated from the body, or the test method does not detect the particular drug present in the sample.

Urine testing shows drug use over the last 2–3 days for amphetamines, cocaine, and opiates. Marijuana and its metabolites, cannabinoids, may be detectable for several weeks. Hair samples, which test the root end of the hair, reflect drug use within the last 2–3 months but not the most recent 2–3 weeks—the amount of time it takes for the hair to grow. Saliva detects which drugs have been used in the last 24 hours. Samples of sweat may be collected on an absorbent patch worn for several days to weeks and therefore can indicate drug use at any point during that extended period of time. These other types of samples are often used for specific purposes. For instance, hair samples may be used as an alternative to urine testing for employment or accident drug testing. Sweat testing may be used as a court-ordered monitoring tool in those who have been convicted of drug use, while saliva is often used by the insurance industry to test insurance applicants for drug use. Blood is most frequently used for alcohol testing.

Interpretation of sports testing results for hormones and steroids should be done by someone who is familiar with the test methods. A negative result indicates that there is a normal amount of the substance present in the body. Positive results reflect the presence of the substance above and beyond what is normally produced by the athlete's body. This can be complicated by the fact that each person will have their own normal baseline concentration and will produce varying amounts of hormones and steroids, depending upon the circumstances.

Is there anything else I should know?

Symptoms associated with drug abuse and drug overdose will vary from person to person, from time to time, and do not necessarily reflect drug concentrations in the body.

Ethanol may be measured in both the blood and the breath. This is the basis for the breathalyzer test used by law enforcement.

For some types of testing, such as workplace testing of federal employees, there are many regulations that cover the test from collection through interpretation and reporting of results. It is important for the ordering physician, law enforcement representative, forensic professional, government entity, insurance agent, employer, and sports organization as well as for the person being tested to understand what exactly is included in the testing, how it is done, and how the results may or may not be interpreted. This process is not nearly as simple or straightforward as collecting a sample and requesting drug testing.

Certain prescription and over-the-counter drugs may give a positive screening result. You should declare any medications that you have taken and/or for which you have prescriptions when you have a drug test so that your results can be interpreted correctly. Also, poppy seeds that have not been washed can cause a positive opiate screening result if eaten, for example, with a bagel or muffin. You may want to avoid these foods if you have drug testing done.

Section 78.3

Home Use Test for Drugs of Abuse

"Home Use Tests: Drugs of Abuse," U.S. Food and Drug
Administration (FDA), July 11, 2009.

First Check 12 Drug Test

What does this test do? The First Check 12 Drug Test indicates if one or more prescription or illegal drugs are present in urine. It is currently the only over-the-counter test available designed to detect prescription drugs that are being abused. The test detects the presence of 12 prescription and illegal drugs: marijuana, cocaine, opiates, methamphetamine, amphetamines, PCP, benzodiazepine, barbiturates, methadone, tricyclic antidepressants, ecstasy, and oxycodone.

This test is done in two steps. First, you do a quick at-home test. Second, if the test suggests that drugs may be present, you send the sample to a laboratory for additional testing.

What are prescription drugs of abuse? Prescription drugs of abuse are medicines (for example, Oxycodone or Valium) that are obtained legally with a doctor's prescription, but are being taken for a nonmedical purpose. Nonmedical purposes include taking the medication for longer than your doctor prescribed it for or for a purpose other than what the doctor prescribed it for. Medications are not drugs of abuse if they are taken according to your doctor's instructions.

What type of test is this? This is a qualitative test—you find out if a particular drug may be in the urine, not how much is present.

When should you do this test? You should use this test when you think someone you care about might be abusing prescription or illegal drugs. If you are worried about a specific drug, make sure to check the label to confirm that this test is designed to detect the drug you are looking for.

How accurate is this test? The at-home testing part of this test is fairly sensitive to the presence of drugs in the urine. This means that if drugs are present, you will usually get a preliminary (or presumptive) positive test result. If you get a preliminary positive result, you should send the urine sample to the laboratory for a second test.

It is very important to send the urine sample to the laboratory to confirm a positive at-home result because certain foods, food supplements, beverages, or medicines can affect the results of at-home tests. Laboratory tests are the most reliable way to confirm drugs of abuse.

Note that all amphetamine results should be considered carefully, even those from the laboratory. Some over-the-counter medications cannot be distinguished from illegally abused amphetamines.

Many things can affect the accuracy of this test, including (but not limited to):

- the way you did the test,
- the way you stored the test or urine,
- what the person ate or drank before taking the test, or
- any other prescription or over-the-counter drugs the person may have taken before the test.

Does a positive test mean that you found drugs of abuse? No. Take no serious actions until you get the laboratory's result. Remember that many factors may cause a false positive result in the home test. Remember that a positive test for a prescription drug does not mean that a person is abusing the drug, because there is no way for the test to indicate acceptable levels compared to abusive levels of prescribed drugs.

If the test results are negative, can you be sure that the person you tested did not abuse drugs? No. There are several factors that can make the test results negative even though the person is abusing drugs. First, you may have tested for the wrong drugs. Or, you may not have tested the urine when it contained drugs. It takes time for drugs to appear in the urine after a person takes them, and they do not stay in the urine indefinitely; you may have collected the urine too late or too soon. It is also possible that the chemicals in the test went bad because they were stored incorrectly or they passed their expiration date.

If you get a negative test result, but still suspect that someone is abusing drugs, you can test again at a later time. Talk to your doctor if you need more help deciding what steps to take next.

How soon after a person takes drugs, will they show up in a drug test? And how long after a person takes drugs, will they continue to show up in a drug test? The drug clearance rate tells how soon a person may have a positive test after taking a particular drug. It also tells how long the person may continue to test positive after the last time he or she took the drug. Clearance rates for common drugs of abuse are listed in Table 78.2. These are only guidelines, however, and the times can vary significantly from these estimates based on how long the person has been taking the drug, the amount of drug they use, or the person's metabolism.

How do you do the two-step test? The kit contains a urine collection cup, a plastic lid containing 12 test strips, and an instruction booklet. It also includes a numbered sticker for confidential confirmation testing and packaging for sending samples to the laboratory for confirmation.

You collect a urine sample in the collection cup, and secure the lid onto the cup. The test strips in the lid contain chemicals that react with each possible drug and show a visible result for each drug they detect. Read and follow the directions carefully and exactly. If the test indicates the presence of one or more drugs, you should send the urine sample to the laboratory for confirmation.

Table 78.2. Drug Clearance Rate

Drug	How soon after taking drug will there be a positive drug test?	How long after taking drug will there continue to be a positive drug test?
Marijuana/pot	1–3 hours	1–7 days
Crack (cocaine)	2–6 hours	2–3 days
Heroin (opiates)	2–6 hours	1–3 days
Speed/uppers (amphetamine, methamphetamine)	4–6 hours	2–3 days
Angel dust/PCP	4–6 hours	7–14 days
Ecstacy	2–7 hours	2–4 days
Benzodiazepine	2–7 hours	1–4 days
Barbiturates	2–4 hours	1–3 weeks
Methadone	3–8 hours	1–3 days
Tricyclic antidepressants	8–12 hours	2–7 days
Oxycodone	1–3 hours	1–2 days

Chapter 79

Talking to Your Child about Drugs

Just as you inoculate your kids against illnesses like measles, you can help "immunize" them against drug use by giving them the facts before they're in a risky situation.

When kids don't feel comfortable talking to parents, they're likely to seek answers elsewhere, even if their sources are unreliable. Kids who aren't properly informed are at greater risk of engaging in unsafe behaviors and experimenting with drugs.

Preschool to Age 7

Before you get nervous about talking to young kids, take heart. You've probably already laid the groundwork for a discussion. For instance, whenever you give a fever medication or an antibiotic to your child, you have the opportunity to discuss the benefits and the appropriate and responsible use of those drugs. This is also a time when your child is likely to be very attentive to your behavior and guidance.

Start taking advantage of "teachable moments" now. If you see a character on a billboard or on television with a cigarette, talk about smoking, nicotine addiction, and what smoking does to a person's body.

This can lead into a discussion about other drugs and how they can potentially cause harm.

Keep the tone of these discussions calm and use terms that your child can understand. Be specific about the effects of the drugs: how they make a person feel, the risk of overdose, and the other long-term damage they can cause. To give your kids these facts, you might have to do a little research.

Ages 8 to 12

As your kids grow older, you can begin conversations with them by asking them what they think about drugs. By asking the questions in a nonjudgmental, open-ended way, you're more likely to get an honest response.

Kids this age usually are still willing to talk openly to their parents about touchy subjects. Establishing a dialogue now helps keep the door open as kids get older and are less inclined to share their thoughts and feelings.

Even if your question doesn't immediately result in a discussion, you'll get your kids thinking about the issue. If you show your kids that you're willing to discuss the topic and hear what they have to say, they might be more willing to come to you for help in the future.

News, such as steroid use in professional sports, can be springboards for casual conversations about current events. Use these discussions to give your kids information about the risks of drugs.

Ages 13 to 17

Kids this age are likely to know other kids who use alcohol or drugs, and to have friends who drive. Many are still willing to express their thoughts or concerns with parents about it.

Use these conversations not only to understand your child's thoughts and feelings, but also to talk about the dangers of driving under the influence of drugs or alcohol. Talk about the legal issues—jail time and fines—and the possibility that they or someone else might be killed or seriously injured.

Consider establishing a written or verbal contract on the rules about going out or using the car. You can promise to pick your kids up at any time (even 2:00 a.m.) no questions asked if they call you when the person responsible for driving has been drinking or using drugs.

The contract also can detail other situations: For example, if you find out that someone drank or used drugs in your car while your son or daughter was behind the wheel, you may want to suspend driving privileges for six months. By discussing all of this with your kids from the start, you eliminate surprises and make your expectations clear.

Laying Good Groundwork

No parent, child, or family is immune to the effects of drugs. Some of the best kids can end up in trouble, even when they have made an effort to avoid it and even when they have been given the proper guidance from their parents.

However, certain groups of kids may be more likely to use drugs than others. Kids who have friends who use drugs are likely to try drugs themselves. Those feeling socially isolated for whatever reason may turn to drugs.

So it's important to know your child's friends—and their parents. Be involved in your children's lives. If your child's school runs an anti-drug program, get involved. You might learn something. Pay attention to how your kids are feeling and let them know that you're available and willing to listen in a nonjudgmental way. Recognize when your kids are going through difficult times so that you can provide the support they need or seek additional care if it's needed.

A warm, open family environment—where kids are encouraged to talk about their feelings, where their achievements are praised, and where their self-esteem is bolstered—encourages kids to come forward with their questions and concerns. When censored in their own homes, kids go elsewhere to find support and answers to their most important questions.

Chapter 80

Making Your Home Safe

Your Home

As a parent, you've always made it your goal to safeguard your children from things in your home that could harm them—when they were toddlers, it may have been something as simple as installing electrical outlet covers to keep curious fingers from getting shocked—as they've grown up, asking them to clear a pathway in their room from their bed to the door (in case of fire) may be about the best you can do! But even though you think you have every danger covered, you may inadvertently be ignoring the dangers of drug abuse in your own home.

Drug Risks in Every Room of Your Home

Here's something that may shock you: Every American house is filled with items that, if misused, can actually put your children at risk of drug abuse. Think about it—everything from the prescription and nonprescription items in your medicine cabinet, to the aerosol spray cans and cleaning liquids in the kitchen, to the paint cans in the garage—can all be a potential threat.

By learning how to identify these types of products or paraphernalia, you may be helping to end potential drug use before it even starts. Take a tour of your house and identify items and places in your home that may be putting your children at risk of drug abuse.

This chapter includes "Your Home," Drug Enforcement Administration (DEA), 2009; and "Digital Monitoring," DEA, 2009.

Kitchen cabinets: Teens reported that most of the medications they use to get high are taken from the home such as cough syrup and other over-the-counter drugs.

Under sinks: Common household products such as solvents, glues, paints, and aerosols can be used to get high.

Bathroom medicine cabinet: Powerful painkillers are the most abused drug after marijuana. One in ten teens has used a pain medication to get high.

Family room computer: Having a computer in the family room makes it easier to monitor teens online activities. But do you speak the same language as your teens.

Bedroom computer: The internet is a major source of information on drugs. It also brings drug dealers—such as pill pushers disguised as pharmacies—right into a teen's computer.

Ordinary objects: Pens, lipstick cores, candy dispensers, soda cans can be used to conceal drug use.

Posters of athlete(s) for girls and boys: Many teens feel pressured to change their bodies. Sometimes they use steroids to build body mass and loss weight.

Back pack: In school, teens can be exposed to drug dealing and use. Drugs are easy to hide, and access to medications such as methylphenidate (Concerta® and Ritalin®) makes it easier to share pills with friends.

Remember: Secrecy (for example, spending lots of time isolated in a bedroom) and other behavioral changes can indicate that a teen is using drugs.

Digital Monitoring

Get Smart about Digital Habits and Influences

Today's kids are entrenched in communication. Always connected is no longer just a trend—it's an affordable reality. Technology is easy, accessible, and portable. These kinds of communications are quick and ever-present—and a central influence in your child's life. American teens are more wired now than ever before. According to the latest survey, 93% of all Americans between 12 and 17 years old use the internet (Pew Internet and American Life Project).

For nearly all American teens, constant connectivity keeps the rhythm of everyday life. In fact, the average teen now spends more than 27 hours per month online. And 24% of kids age 10–11 have their own cell phones—that number rises to 38% for the 12 and above age group. Add that to the fact that their online connections travel everywhere they do, and you can see how pervasive digital influences truly are.

You probably already realize that most teens far outpace their parents when it comes to technology. Technology has made it easier for children to communicate about many subjects—including drugs and drug activity. So unless you're wise to their online networks and digital habits, and understand the real meaning of the digital language they share, your child may be relaying information you need to be aware of—right under your nose.

Your child's online profile: If your child is a part of the popular online youth network MySpace, make sure it is your space, too. Learn about risks and what you need to know about the most popular online gathering place for teens, tweens, and young adults.

Messaging: Whether it is instant messaging on the computer or text messaging on the cell phone, kids are in constant communication—without actually saying a word. Make sure you understand the risks in these silent conversations.

Lingo you need to know: You may not LOL (laugh out loud) the next time you glance over your child's shoulder when he's online—because you'll probably find that he's chatting in a different language. Learn how to translate.

Chapter 81

Preventing Adolescent Drug Abuse

Chapter Contents

Section 81.1—Keeping Your Teens Drug-Free 506

Section 81.2—Youth Prevention-Related Measures 510

Section 81.3—Family Dinners Reduce Likelihood That
Teens Will Abuse Drugs 516

Section 81.1

Keeping Your Teens Drug-Free

Text in this section is from "Keeping Your Teens Drug-Free:
A Family Guide," National Youth Anti-Drug Media Campaign,
September 2005.

This section provides ideas and examples of the skills busy parents can use to keep their teens away from marijuana and other illicit drugs. There are opportunities every day to turn ordinary times like driving your child to school, to the mall, or watching television together into teachable moments to let your teen know what's important to you. Many parents put off talking to their kids about drugs or alcohol because of time constraints, but just a little of your time once in a while can make a lifetime of difference. Teens who learn about the risks of drug use from their parents or caregivers are less likely to use drugs. Parents are the most important influence in their kids' lives. Many parents do not realize that they play a crucial role in their teen's decision not to use drugs. Two-thirds of youth ages 13 to 17 say losing their parents' respect and pride is one of the main reasons they do not smoke marijuana or use other drugs.

Teens, Marijuana and Other Drugs

While no one wants to think negatively about their children, it is likely your teen will be exposed to illicit drugs. Nearly a third of 12- to 17-year-olds in the United States (U.S.) have used an illicit drug in their lifetime. Teens today are using drugs at younger and younger ages, when their brains and bodies are still developing. Of all of the illicit drugs, marijuana is the most widely used. If your child is exposed to drugs, he or she will most likely be offered marijuana.

Tell Your Teen What You Expect

It is important that your teen knows what you expect. Make it clear that you do not want any marijuana or any illicit drug use in your house. Tell your teen that there will be consequences for using drugs.

As your teen enters middle school and then high school, your child will be at greater risk of using marijuana and alcohol if you have not made your expectations clear. Teens need to know where you stand. Here are some clear ways you can tell your teens what you expect: "I've been thinking lately that I have never actually told you this: I do not want you using marijuana, alcohol, tobacco, or any drug." "The rule in our house is that nobody uses drugs."

Set rules: Even though your teens are getting older and spending more time without you, it is more important than ever to set rules and expectations. Setting a firm rule of no marijuana or other drug use will help your teen resist pressures to use drugs.

When your teen breaks the rules: Parents need to enforce rules consistently and fairly. When rules are broken, some possible consequences could include: restricting internet use and television, suspending outside activities, such as going to the mall or movies, or disallowing telephone calls.

Risky Situations

Let your teens know that you do not want them in risky situations. Tell them: "I don't want you riding in a car with a driver who's been using marijuana or who's been drinking." "It's my job as a parent to keep you safe, so I'm going to ask you questions about who you're with and what you are doing."

Giving advice on avoiding risky situations: Here are some lines you can give your teens to help them stay away from risky situations: "I like you, but I don't like drugs." "My dad (or mom, grandmother) would ground me if he (or she) knew I was around marijuana." "No, thanks. It's not for me." "I don't do drugs. I could get kicked off the team if anyone found out."

Beware of Messages That Encourage Drug Use

Many parents are concerned about messages on television, in movies and music that encourage or trivialize drug use and that fail to show the harm of using drugs. You can set rules about what your teens watch on television, in the movies they see, or the songs they listen to. If you have a computer at home connected to the internet, you should let your children know that you are in charge of their time online. Teens can find websites that promote drugs, and they can actually buy drugs over the internet.

Stay Involved in Your Teen's Life

Experts say that to create an environment that helps keep your kids away from marijuana and other drugs, you should do the following:

- Get involved in your kids' lives.

- Know what your children are doing—their activities and how they spend their time.

- Know who your teen's friends are.

- Check in with the parents who are hosting the party your teen will be attending.

- Praise and reward good behavior.

Research shows that kids who are not regularly monitored by their parents are four times more likely to use drugs. Before going out, have them tell you who they are going to be spending time with, what they will be doing, when or what time they will be at their expected destination and finally, exactly where they are going to be. Every once in a while, check on your teens to see if they are where they said they would be. It is not pestering, it is parenting.

Lots of teens get in trouble with marijuana, other illicit drugs, or alcohol right after school, from 3–6 p.m. Try to be with your teens then, but if you can't, make sure your child is doing something positive with a trusted adult around: sports, jobs, clubs, after-school programs or faith-based groups. If your teens have to be at home, make sure they are doing homework or chores and not hanging out unsupervised with friends. Remember how important you are in keeping your teens away from marijuana and other drugs.

Catching Your Child with Drugs

If you've caught your child using drugs or holding them for a friend, wait until you are calm to talk to your teen. Then tell your teen it is okay to be honest with you, that you want to know the truth. The following phrases can get good communication going: "I'm really disappointed. You know I do not approve of drug use. I do not approve of your using marijuana, alcohol, or other drugs."

Your child admits to having tried drugs: The idea is to reinforce the rules about marijuana and other drug use while keeping the lines of communication open. "I'm glad you told me, but let me remind you that drugs get in the way of your being healthy and happy. You can lose your driver's license. You can get kicked off the team. You can fail at school." If your child has admitted to using drugs recently, you might want to ask your doctor or counselor for help.

Your child says: Everyone is doing it: You say, "I'm not interested in what other kids are doing. I know I do not want you using marijuana or other drugs."

Your teen's friend or parent tried drugs: You can say, "I do not want you hanging out with kids who smoke marijuana or drink alcohol. You know that when you are around people who use drugs, I am afraid they will try to pressure you to use drugs."

If your teen asks if you ever used drugs: It is important to be honest, but you do not need to include too many details. If you did use drugs, you can say, "When I was young I smoked marijuana because some of my friends did. I thought I needed to in order to fit in. If I had known then about the consequences, I never would have tried marijuana, and I will do everything I can to help keep you away from it."

If you suspect your teen is using drugs, take action. Ask your child directly. Let your teen know you want him or her to be honest with you. If you need help, contact your child's school counselor, pediatrician, or family physician, or call the National Clearinghouse for Alcohol and Drug Information at 800-788-2800 for drug abuse prevention information and a listing of the treatment centers closest to you. You may also visit the website at www.findtreament.samhsa.gov.

Calling on Your Community

You and your family are not alone. You can call on your neighbors to join forces with you. Many parents have organized networking groups in their neighborhoods for talking about how to handle problems. Other parents organize alcohol- and drug-free neighborhood events and parties. Your teen's school has people who can help—guidance counselors, teachers, coaches, and other adults. Many parents also find help in their faith communities, and many belong to other community groups. When parents and teens take the time to talk to each other, their lives can be healthier and more enjoyable, and in the process, you will be doing your part in helping your teens to grow up drug-free.

Section 81.2

Youth Prevention-Related Measures

This section is excerpted from "Results from the 2006 National Survey on Drug Use and Health: National Findings, Chapter 6," Substance Abuse and Mental Health Services Administration (SAMHSA), September 2007.

The National Survey on Drug Use and Health (NSDUH) includes questions for youths aged 12 to 17 about a number of risk and protective factors that may affect the likelihood that they will engage in substance use. Risk factors are individual characteristics and environmental influences associated with an increased vulnerability to the initiation, continuation, or escalation of substance use. Protective factors include individual resilience and other circumstances that appear to reduce the likelihood of substance use. Risk and protective factors include variables that operate at different stages of development and reflect different domains of influence, including the individual, family, peer, school, community, and societal levels. Interventions to prevent substance use generally are designed to ameliorate the influence of risk factors and enhance the effectiveness of protective factors.

This section presents findings for youth prevention-related measures collected in the 2006 NSDUH and compares these with findings from previous years. Included are measures of perceived risk from substance use (cigarettes, alcohol, and illicit drugs), perceived availability of substances, perceived parental disapproval of substance use, feelings about peer substance use, involvement in fighting and delinquent behavior, participation in religious and other activities, exposure to substance use prevention messages and programs, and parental involvement.

Perceptions of Risk

One factor that can influence whether youths will use tobacco, alcohol, or illicit drugs is the extent to which youths believe these substances might cause them harm. NSDUH respondents were asked how much they thought people risk harming themselves physically and in other ways when they use various substances. Response choices for these items were "great risk," "moderate risk," "slight risk," or "no risk."

The percentages of youths reporting binge alcohol use and use of cigarettes and marijuana in the past month were lower among those who perceived great risk in using these substances than among those who did not perceive great risk. For example, in 2006, 6.0% of youths aged 12 to 17 who perceived great risk from "having five or more drinks of an alcoholic beverage once or twice a week" reported binge drinking in the past month (consumption of five or more drinks of an alcoholic beverage on a single occasion on at least one day in the past 30 days); by contrast, past month binge drinking was reported by 13.2% of youths who saw moderate, slight, or no risk from having five or more drinks of an alcoholic beverage once or twice a week. Past month marijuana use was reported by 1.5% of youths who saw great risk in smoking marijuana once a month compared with 9.5% of youths who saw moderate, slight, or no risk.

- The percentage of youths aged 12 to 17 indicating great risk in having four or five drinks nearly every day increased from 62.2% in 2002 to 64.6% in 2006. However, the rates of past month heavy alcohol use among youths aged 12 to 17 were about the same in 2002 (2.5%) and 2006 (2.4%).

- The percentage of youths aged 12 to 17 perceiving great risk in having five or more drinks of an alcoholic beverage once or twice a week was stable between 2002 and 2006 (38.2% in 2002 and 39.4% in 2006) with the exception of a significant increase between 2004 (38.1%) and 2006. The rates of past month binge alcohol use among youths remained unchanged (10.7% in 2002 and 10.3% in 2006).

- The percentage of youths aged 12 to 17 indicating great risk in smoking marijuana once a month increased from 32.4% in 2002 to 34.7% in 2006. The percentage of youths aged 12 to 17 perceiving great risk in smoking marijuana once or twice a week also increased from 51.5% in 2002 to 54.2% in 2006.

- Coincident with the increase in the perceived great risk of marijuana use, the prevalence of lifetime, past year, and past month marijuana use among youths aged 12 to 17 decreased between 2002 and 2006. During this period, lifetime use of marijuana dropped from 20.6% to 17.3%, past year use declined from 15.8% to 13.2%, and past month use fell from 8.2% to 6.7%.

- Between 2002 and 2006, the percentage of youths aged 12 to 17 perceiving great risk declined for the following substance use patterns: trying heroin once or twice (from 58.5% to 57.2%), using heroin once or twice a week (from 82.5% to 81.2%), using cocaine once a month (from 50.5% to 49.0%), and using lysergic acid diethylamide (LSD) once or twice a week (from 76.2% to 74.7%). Over the same period, however, the percentage of youths aged 12 to 17 indicating great risk for using cocaine once or twice a week (79.8% in 2002 and 79.2% in 2006) and for trying LSD once or twice (52.6% in 2002 and 51.6% in 2006) remained unchanged.

Perceived Availability

In 2006, about half (50.1%) of the youths aged 12 to 17 reported that it would be "fairly easy" or "very easy" for them to obtain marijuana if they wanted some. Around one-quarter reported it would be easy to get cocaine (25.9%). One in seven (14.0%) indicated that LSD would be "fairly" or "very" easily available, and 14.4% reported so for heroin. Between 2002 and 2006, the perceived availability of substances decreased among youths aged 12 to 17 for marijuana (from 55.0% to 50.1%), LSD (from 19.4% to 14.0%), and heroin (from 15.8% to 14.4%).

The percentage of youths who reported that illicit drugs would be easy to obtain was associated with age, with perceived availability increasing with age. For example, in 2006, 20.7% of those aged 12 or 13 said it would be fairly or very easy to obtain marijuana compared with 52.9% of those aged 14 or 15 and 73.9% of those aged 16 or 17. In 2006, 15.3% of youths aged 12 to 17 indicated that they had been approached by someone selling drugs in the past month. This was down from the 16.7% reported in 2002.

Perceived Parental Disapproval of Substance Use

Most youths aged 12 to 17 believed their parents would "strongly disapprove" of their using substances. In 2006, 91.4% of youths aged

12 to 17 reported that their parents would strongly disapprove of their smoking one or more packs of cigarettes per day. A majority of youths (90.4%) reported that their parents would strongly disapprove of their trying marijuana or hashish once or twice, and 89.6% reported their parents would strongly disapprove of their having one or two drinks of an alcoholic beverage nearly every day. These rates of perceived parental disapproval in using substances in 2006 were similar to those reported in 2005.

Youths aged 12 to 17 who believed their parents would strongly disapprove of their using a particular substance were less likely to use that substance than were youths who believed their parents would somewhat disapprove or neither approve nor disapprove. For example, in 2006, past month cigarette use was reported by 7.4% of youths who perceived strong parental disapproval of their smoking one or more packs of cigarettes per day compared with 42.1% of youths who believed their parents would not strongly disapprove. Current marijuana use also was much less prevalent among youths who perceived strong parental disapproval for trying marijuana or hashish once or twice than among those who did not (4.6% versus 26.5%, respectively).

Feelings about Peer Substance Use

A majority of youths aged 12 to 17 reported that they disapprove of their peers using substances. In 2006, 89.1% of youths "strongly" or "somewhat" disapproved of their peers smoking one or more packs of cigarettes per day, and 82.8% strongly or somewhat disapproved of peers using marijuana or hashish once a month or more. These rates were higher than those reported in 2005 (88.2% and 81.4%, respectively). In 2006, 81.7% of youths strongly or somewhat disapproved of peers trying marijuana or hashish once or twice, and 86.4% of youths strongly or somewhat disapproved of peers having one or two drinks of an alcoholic beverage nearly every day. Both estimates were similar to those reported in 2005 (80.8% and 85.6%, respectively).

The percentage strongly or somewhat disapproving of peers' substance use generally decreased with age. In 2006, disapproval of peers using marijuana once a month or more, for example, was reported by 92.4% of youths aged 12 or 13, 82.5% of those aged 14 or 15, and 74.0% of those aged 16 or 17.

In 2006, past month marijuana use was reported by 2.5% of youths aged 12 to 17 who strongly or somewhat disapproved of their peers using marijuana once a month or more compared with 26.4% of youths who reported that they neither approve nor disapprove of such behavior from their peers.

Fighting and Delinquent Behavior

In 2006, 22.6% of youths aged 12 to 17 reported that, in the past year, they had gotten into a serious fight at school or at work; 17.0% had taken part in a group-against-group fight; 3.2% had carried a handgun at least once; 3.3% had sold illegal drugs; 4.8% had, at least once, stolen or tried to steal something worth more than $50 (increased from 4.2% in 2005); and 7.9% had, in at least one instance, attacked others with the intent to harm or seriously hurt them.

Youths aged 12 to 17 who had engaged in fighting or other delinquent behaviors were more likely than other youths to have used illicit drugs in the lifetime, past year, and past month. For example, in 2006, past month illicit drug use was reported by 17.3% of youths who had gotten into serious fights at school or work in the past year compared with 7.6% of those who had not engaged in fighting, and by 37.2% of those who had stolen or tried to steal something worth over $50 in the past year compared with 8.4% of those who had not engaged in such theft.

Religious Beliefs and Participation in Activities

In 2006, 31.7% of youths aged 12 to 17 reported that they had attended religious services 25 or more times in the past year; 77.0% expressed agreement with the statement that religious beliefs are a very important part of their lives; 68.3% agreed with the statement that religious beliefs influence how they make decisions in life; and 35.1% agreed with the statement that it is important for their friends to share their religious beliefs. Findings for these measures remained unchanged from 2005 to 2006. Lifetime, past year, and past month use of illicit drugs, cigarettes, and alcohol (including binge alcohol) were lower among youths who agreed with these statements than among those who disagreed. For example, past month illicit drug use was reported by 7.6% of those who agreed that religious beliefs are a very important part of life compared with 17.1% of those who disagreed with that statement.

Exposure to Substance Use Prevention Messages and Programs

In 2006, approximately one in eight youths aged 12 to 17 (11.4%) reported that they had participated in drug, tobacco, or alcohol prevention programs outside of school in the past year. However, the prevalence of past month use of illicit drugs, marijuana, cigarettes, or binge alcohol was not significantly lower among those who participated in these prevention programs outside of school (8.9%, 6.1%, 8.9%, and 9.8%, respectively) than among those who did not (9.9%, 6.7%, 10.6%, and 10.4%, respectively).

In 2006, 79.4% of youths aged 12 to 17 reported having seen or heard drug or alcohol prevention messages from sources outside of school, which declined from 81.1% in 2005. The prevalence of past month use of illicit drugs, marijuana, cigarettes, or binge alcohol was lower among those who reported having such exposure (9.2%, 6.2%, 9.5%, and 10.0%, respectively) than among those who reported having no such exposure (12.0%, 8.5%, 13.8%, and 11.5%, respectively).

In 2006, 59.8% of youths aged 12 to 17 reported that they had talked at least once in the past year with at least one of their parents about the dangers of drug, tobacco, or alcohol use, which was the same as in 2005. Among youths who reported having had such conversations with their parents, rates of past month use of illicit drugs, cigarettes, and alcohol (including binge alcohol) were lower than among youths who did not talk about substance abuse. That is, past month use of illicit drugs was reported by 8.6% of youths who had talked with their parents about drug, tobacco, or alcohol use compared with 11.3% of those who had not. Past month cigarette use was lower among youths who had talked with their parents (9.4%) than among those who had not (11.8%), and past month binge drinking was lower among youths who had talked with their parents (9.3%) than among those who had not (11.8%).

Parental Involvement

Youths aged 12 to 17 were asked a number of questions related to the extent of support, oversight, and control that they perceived their parents exercised over them in the year prior to the survey. In 2006, among youths aged 12 to 17 enrolled in school in the past year, 79.5% reported that in the past year their parents always or sometimes checked on whether or not they had completed their homework, 79.8% reported that their parents always or sometimes provided help with their homework, and 69.1% reported that their parents limited the amount of time that they spent out with friends on school nights. Also in 2006, among youths aged 12 to 17, 87.5% reported that in the past year their parents made them always or sometimes do chores around the house, 39.4% reported that their parents limited the amount of time that they watched television, and 86.6% reported that their parents always or sometimes let them know that they had done a good job. All of these percentages were similar to those reported in 2005. In addition, among youths aged 12 to 17 in 2006, 86.0% reported that their parents let them know they were proud of something they had done, which increased from the 84.8% in 2005.

Section 81.3

Family Dinners Reduce Likelihood That Teens Will Abuse Drugs

Excerpted from "The Importance of Family Dinners IV," September 2007, National Center on Addiction and Substance Abuse (CASA) at Columbia University, http://www.casacolumbia.org. © 2007. All rights reserved. Reprinted with permission.

For more than a decade, the National Center on Addiction and Substance Abuse (CASA) has been conducting a survey of the attitudes of teens and those, like parents, who most influence them. While other surveys measure the extent of substance abuse in the population, the CASA survey seeks to identify factors that increase or diminish the likelihood that teens will smoke, drink, use illegal drugs or abuse prescription drugs. We believe that parents, armed with this knowledge, can help their teens grow up drug free.

This nation's drug problem is all about kids. A child who gets through age 21 without smoking, abusing alcohol, or using illegal drugs is virtually certain never to do so. And no one has more power to prevent kids from using substances than parents. There are no silver bullets; unfortunately, the tragedy of a child's substance abuse can strike any family. But one factor that does more to reduce teens' substance abuse risk than almost any other is parental engagement, and one of the simplest and most effective ways for parents to be engaged in teens' lives is by having frequent family dinners.

This year, 59% of teens report having dinner with their families at least five times a week, the same proportion we have observed in the past several years, and an increase in family dining from the 1996 CASA survey, when the relationship of frequent family dinners to substance abuse risk was first detected.

Family Dinners and Teen Smoking, Drinking, and Drug Use

Frequent family dining is associated with lower rates of teen smoking, drinking, illegal drug use, and prescription drug abuse. Compared to teens who eat dinner frequently with their families (five or more family dinners per week), those who have infrequent family dinners (fewer than three per week) are:

- three and a half times likelier to have abused prescription drugs,
- three and a half times likelier to have used an illegal drug other than marijuana or prescription drugs,
- three times likelier to have used marijuana,
- more than two and a half times likelier to have used tobacco, and
- one and a half times likelier to have used alcohol.

Family Dinners and Current Teen Substance Use

Teens who have frequent family dinners are less likely to currently use marijuana and tobacco, drink alcohol, and get drunk. Compared

Table 81.1. Percent of Teens Who Have Used Alcohol, Tobacco, Marijuana, Other Illegal Drugs or Abused Prescription Drugs (by frequency of family dinners)

	5 to 7 dinners per week	0 to 2 dinners per week
Alcohol	30	47
Tobacco	10	26
Marijuana	8	25
Other illegal drugs	2	7
Prescription drugs	2	7

to teens who eat dinner frequently with their families, those who have infrequent family dinners are:

- more than twice as likely to have used marijuana in the past 30 days,

- almost twice as likely to have drunk alcohol in the past 30 days,

- almost twice as likely to have used tobacco in the past 30 days, and

- more than one and a half times likelier to have gotten drunk in the past 30 days.

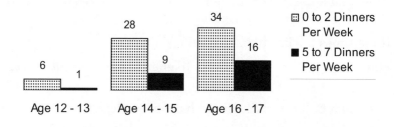

Figure 81.1. *Percent of Teens Who Say They Have Used Marijuana by Age and Frequency of Family Dinners*

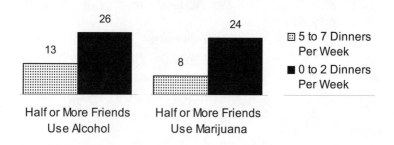

Figure 81.2. *Percent of Teens Who Say Half or More of Their Friends Use Alcohol/Marijuana*

Family Dinners, Age, and Substance Use

The relationship between frequent family dinners and substance use that we observe among all teens is also observed to varying degrees at every age level. The impact of frequent family dinners seems strongest among the youngest children in our survey, and the behavior that appears to be most significantly affected among teens of all ages is marijuana use.

Compared to 12- and 13-year olds who have frequent family dinners, 12- and 13-year olds who have infrequent family dinners are six times likelier to have used marijuana, more than four and a half times likelier to have used tobacco and more than two and a half times likelier to have used alcohol.

Compared to 14- and 15-year olds who have frequent family dinners, 14- and 15-year olds who have infrequent family dinners are three times likelier to have used marijuana and two and a half times likelier to have used tobacco.

Compared to 16- and 17-year olds who have frequent family dinners, 16- and 17-year olds who have infrequent family dinners are more than twice as likely to have used marijuana and almost twice as likely to have used tobacco.

At ages 14 through 17, those teens who have infrequent family dinners are likelier to have used alcohol than those teens who have frequent family dinners.

Family Dinners and Teens with Friends Who Use Substances

Teens who have infrequent family dinners are twice as likely to report that half or more of their friends currently drink beer or other alcoholic beverages, compared to teens who have frequent family dinners.

Chapter 82

Drug Abuse Prevention in Schools

Chapter Contents

Section 82.1—Drug Testing in Schools 522
Section 82.2—Health Education and Services 528

x

Section 82.1

Drug Testing in Schools

"Student Drug-Testing Institute—Frequently Asked Questions,"
U.S. Department of Education, 2008.

The Need for Student Drug Testing

Why do some schools conduct random drug tests?

Random student drug testing is foremost a prevention program. Drug testing is one of several tools that schools can use as part of a comprehensive drug prevention effort. Administrators, faculty, and students at schools that conduct testing view random testing as a deterrent, and it gives students a reason to resist peer pressure to try or use drugs. Drug testing can identify students who have started using drugs so that interventions can occur early, or identify students who already have drug problems, so they can be referred for assessment, counseling, or treatment. Drug abuse not only interferes with a student's ability to learn, but it can also disrupt the teaching environment, affecting other students as well. Each school or school district that wants to start a program needs to involve the entire community in determining whether student drug testing is right for their specific situation.

How many students actually use drugs?

Although drug use among America's youth has declined in recent years, many young people continue to abuse harmful substances. The 2008 Monitoring the Future Survey shows that drug use among school-age youth has been in a state of decline since the 1990s; however, the proportions of 8th- and 12th-grade students indicating any use of an illicit drug in the 12 months prior to the survey showed rather modest increases since the previous year. Nearly half of 12th graders said that they have used drugs in their lifetime, and almost one third said that they use marijuana at least monthly. According to another survey conducted in 2006, an estimated 20.4 million Americans aged

12 or older (8.3% of the population) were current illicit drug users, using within the past month.

Like use of other illicit drugs, steroid usage has seen a decline since usage peaked among male teens in 1999. However, steroid abuse is still a problem for many young people. The 2008 Monitoring the Future data show that 1.2% of 8th graders, 1.4% of 10th graders, and 2.5% of 12th graders reported using steroids at least once in their lifetime. A survey sponsored by the Centers for Disease Control and Prevention (CDC) reported that 3.9% of all high school students surveyed in 2007 reported use of steroid pills/shots without a doctor's prescription at some point in their lives. This figure includes 4.8% of 9th graders, 3.7% of 10th graders, 3.1% of 11th graders, and 3.8% of 12th graders.

Prescription drug abuse is also high and is increasing. The 2008 Monitoring the Future data indicate that 15.4% of 12th graders reported using a prescription drug nonmedically within the past year. Vicodin, an opiate pain reliever, continues to be abused at unacceptably high levels. Many of the drugs used by 12th graders are prescription drugs, or in the case of cough medicine, are available over the counter.

Despite some declines in drug use, much remains to be done. Youth still face a barrage of media messages and peer pressure that promote drug use. Random student drug-testing programs are effective prevention strategies to help adolescents refuse drugs, when offered.

How can schools determine if there is a need for a drug-testing program?

Communities first need to identify their drug problems. This becomes the basis of developing a consensus for student drug testing. Schools must first determine whether there is a need for testing. Such a need can be determined from student drug-use surveys; reports by teachers and other school staff about student drug use; reports about drug use from parents and others in the community; and from discoveries of drugs, drug paraphernalia, or residues at school.

Is student drug testing a stand-alone solution, or do schools need other programs to prevent and reduce drug use?

Drug testing should never be undertaken as a stand-alone response to a drug problem. If testing is done, it should be one component of a comprehensive prevention and intervention program in compliance with local, state, and federal laws, with the common goal of reducing students' use of illegal drugs and misuse of prescription drugs.

What are the benefits of drug testing?

Drug use can turn into abuse and then into addiction, trapping users in a vicious cycle that can ruin lives and destroy families. Studies have shown drug testing to be an effective tool in preventing student drug use. The expectation that they may be randomly tested is enough to make some students stop using drugs—or never start in the first place. School-based drug testing is also an excellent tool for getting students who use drugs the help they need.

According to the 2007 National Survey on Drug Use and Health students who use drugs are statistically more likely to drop out of school, bring guns to school, steal, and be involved in fighting or other delinquent behavior. Drug abuse not only interferes with a student's ability to learn, it also disrupts the orderly environment necessary for all students to succeed. Obviously, reducing the likelihood of these disruptive behaviors benefits everyone involved in a school environment.

Why are teens particularly vulnerable?

Teens are especially vulnerable to drug abuse when the brain and body are still developing. Most teens do not use drugs, but for those that do, it can lead to a wide range of adverse effects on the brain, the body, behavior, and health.

Short term: Even a single use of an intoxicating drug can affect a person's judgment and decision-making—resulting in accidents, poor performance in a school or sports activity, unplanned risky behavior, and the risk of overdosing.

Long term: Repeated drug abuse can lead to serious problems, such as poor academic outcomes, mood changes (depending on the drug: depression, anxiety, paranoia, psychosis), and social or family problems caused or worsened by drugs. Repeated drug use can also lead to the disease of addiction. Studies show that the earlier a teen begins using drugs, the more likely he or she will develop a substance abuse problem or addiction. Conversely, if teens stay away from drugs while in high school, they are less likely to develop a substance abuse problem later in life.

What has research determined about the utility of random drug tests in schools?

There is not very much research in this area and early research shows mixed results. A study published in 2007 found that student athletes who participated in randomized drug testing had overall rates of drug use similar to students who did not take part in the program, and in fact, some indicators of future drug abuse increased among those participating in the drug-testing program.

In another study, Hunterdon Central Regional High School in New Jersey saw significant reductions in 20 of 28 drug use categories after two years of a drug-testing program (for example, cocaine use by seniors dropped from 13% to 4%). A third study, from Ball State University, showed that 73% of high school principals reported a reduction in drug use among students subjected to a drug-testing policy, but only two percent reported an increase. Because of the limited number of studies on this topic, more research is warranted.

Are there any current randomized control studies about the impact of mandatory-random student drug testing on the reduction of student substance use?

Yes, RMC Research is conducting a National Impact Evaluation of Mandatory-Random Student Drug Testing. The four-year study is funded by the U.S. Department of Education's Institute of Education Sciences to assess the effects of school-based mandatory-random drug testing programs. The study population comprises school districts and schools that received grants from the Office of Safe and Drug-Free Schools to implement mandatory-random student drug testing. The study includes the collection of school-level drug testing results and data garnered through student surveys, school-wide record review, and staff interviews. The study, designed as a cluster randomized control trial, is the first of its sort to examine this topic and will contribute to knowledge about the impact of mandatory-random student drug testing on the reduction of student substance use. Preliminary results were expected in November 2009.

Student Drug Testing and Legal Matters

Does the federal government mandate student drug testing?

No. The federal government recognizes drug testing as one tool that local schools can choose as a component of a broad drug prevention effort. Each school or school district that wants to start a program needs to involve the entire community in determining whether student drug testing is right for their specific situation.

What have the courts said?

The Supreme Court of the United States first determined that drug testing of student athletes is constitutional in a June 1995 decision. Voting six to three in *Vernonia School District versus Acton* the court upheld the constitutionality of a policy requiring student athletes to submit to random drug testing.

In June 2002, the U.S. Supreme Court broadened the authority of public schools to test students for illegal drugs. Voting five to four in *Pottawatomie County versus Earls*, the court ruled to allow random drug tests for all middle and high school students participating in competitive extracurricular activities. The ruling greatly expanded the scope of school drug testing.

Just because the U.S. Supreme Court ruled that student drug testing for adolescents in competitive extracurricular activities is constitutional, does that mean it is legal in my city or state?

A school or school district interested in adopting a student drug-testing program should seek legal expertise so that it complies with all federal, state, and local laws. Individual state constitutions and court rulings may dictate different legal thresholds for allowing student drug testing. Communities interested in starting a student drug-testing program should become familiar with the law in their respective states to ensure proper compliance.

The Student Drug-Testing Process

What testing methods are available?

There are several testing methods available for different types of specimens, including urine, hair, oral fluids, and sweat (patch). These methods vary in cost, reliability, drugs detected, and detection period. Schools should determine their needs and choose the method that best suits their requirements, as long as the testing procedures are conducted by a reliable source, such as a certified or nationally accredited drug-testing company or a hospital.

For which drugs can and should students be tested?

Various testing methods normally test for a panel of drugs. Typically, a drug panel tests for marijuana, cocaine, opioids, amphetamines, and PCP. If a school or community has a particular problem with other drugs, such as tobacco, ecstasy (MDMA), gamma hydroxybutyrate (GHB), or steroids, they can include testing for these drugs.

How accurate are drug tests? Is there a possibility a test could give a false positive?

Screening tests are very accurate but not 100% accurate. Usually samples are divided so if an initial test is positive, a confirmation test can be conducted.

Can students beat the tests?

Many drug-using students are aware of techniques that supposedly detoxify their systems or mask their drug use. Popular magazines and internet sites give advice on how to dilute urine samples, and there are even companies that sell drug-free clean urine or products designed to distort test results. A number of techniques and products are focused on urine tests for marijuana, but masking products increasingly are becoming available for tests of hair, oral fluids, and multiple drugs.

Most of these products do not work, are very costly, can be identified in the testing process, and must be readily available at the random time of testing. Moreover, even if the specific drug is successfully masked, the masking product itself can be detected, in which case the student using it would become an obvious candidate for additional screening and attention. In fact, some testing programs consider a test positive if a masking product is detected.

What about alcohol?

Alcohol is a drug and a serious problem among young people. However, alcohol does not remain in the blood long enough for most tests to detect recent use. Breathalyzers and oral fluid tests can detect current use, and can be used to measure impairment. The ethyl glucuronide (EtG) test can be used to detect recent alcohol use; however, the National Institute on Drug Abuse has questioned the reliability of this test. Adolescents with substance abuse problems are often polydrug users (they use more than one drug), so identifying a problem with an illicit or prescription drug may suggest an alcohol problem.

Section 82.2

Health Education and Services

This section includes excerpts from "Alcohol or Other Drug-Use Prevention," School Health Policies and Programs Study (SHPPS) 2006, Centers for Disease Control and Prevention (CDC), 2007.

About School Health Policies and Programs Study (SHPPS) 2006: SHPPS is a national survey periodically conducted to assess school health policies and programs at the state, district, school, and classroom levels. Comprehensive results from SHPPS 2006 are published in the *Journal of School Health*, Volume 77, Number 8, October 2007.

Health Education

During the two years preceding the study:

- 82.0% of states and 71.0% of districts provided funding for staff development or offered staff development on alcohol- or other drug-use prevention to those who teach health education.

- 26.6% of elementary school classes and required middle school and high school health education courses had a teacher who received staff development on alcohol- or other drug-use prevention.

Health Services and Mental Health and Social Services

- The percentage of states that required districts or schools to provide alcohol- or other drug-use treatment services increased from 8.2% in 2000 to 17.6% in 2006, whereas the percentage of

Table 82.1. Percentage of States, Districts, and Schools That Required Teaching Alcohol- or Other Drug-Use Prevention, by School Level

	States	**Districts**	**Schools**
Elementary	76.5	79.0	76.5
Middle	76.5	89.7	84.6
High	82.0	89.3	91.8

districts that required schools to provide these services decreased from 46.2% in 2000 to 33.6% in 2006. Selected changes between 2000 and 2006 are included if they met at least two of three criteria (p is less than .01 from a t-test, a difference greater than ten percentage points, or an increase by at least a factor of two or decrease by at least half). Variables are not included if they did not meet these criteria or if no comparable variable existed in both survey years.

- The percentage of states that required districts or schools to provide alcohol- or other drug-use prevention services in one-on-one or small-group sessions increased from 22.0% in 2000 to 42.0% in 2006.

During the two years preceding the study:

- The percentage of states that provided funding for staff development or offered staff development to school mental health or social services staff on alcohol- or other drug-use prevention services and alcohol- or other drug-use treatment services increased from 82.6% to 93.3%, and from 77.8% to 89.4%, respectively.

- The percentage of school mental health or social services coordinators who served as study respondents who received staff development on alcohol- or other drug-use prevention services decreased from 68.2% in 2000 to 54.9% in 2006.

- The percentage of school health services coordinators who served as study respondents who received staff development on alcohol- or other drug-use treatment services during the two years preceding the study decreased from 49.9% in 2000 to 39.4% in 2006.

Table 82.2. Percentage of states and districts that provided funding for staff development or offered staff development to school nurses during the two years preceding the study

	States	Districts
Alcohol- or other drug-use treatment services	55.3	34.9
Alcohol- or other drug-use prevention services	72.5	44.6

Healthy and Safe School Environment

- Among the 25.2% of districts containing middle schools or high schools that had adopted a student drug-testing policy, 56.1% conducted student drug testing randomly among members of specific groups of students (for example: athletes, students who participate in other extracurricular activities, or student drivers), 63.9% conducted student drug testing when it was suspected that a student was using drugs at school, 37.6% had voluntary drug testing for all students, 3.6% had voluntary drug testing for specific groups of students, and 13.4% used some other unspecified criteria.

- 11.4% of middle schools and 19.5% of high schools conducted drug testing on students.

- The percentage of districts that provided model policies to schools during the two years preceding the study increased from 64.0% in 2000 to 76.2% in 2006 for illegal drug-use prevention and from 64.9% to 75.4% for alcohol-use prevention.

- The percentage of schools that had or participated in a community-based alcohol-use prevention program decreased from 49.6% in 2000 to 38.5% in 2006, and the percentage of schools that had or participated in a community-based illegal drug-use prevention program decreased from 60.0% in 2000 to 46.8% in 2006.

Chapter 83

Keeping the Workplace Drug Free

Chapter Contents

Section 83.1—Drug-Free Workplace Policies 532

Section 83.2—Drug Testing in the Workplace 538

531

Section 83.1

Drug-Free Workplace Policies

Text in this section includes text from "Workplace Resources," National Institute on Drug Abuse (NIDA), July 2008; excerpts from "Frequently Asked Questions," U.S. Department of Labor, March 11, 2009; and "Keeping Your Worksite Drug and Alcohol Free," an undated document from the U.S. Department of Labor.

Workplace Resources

Nearly 75% of all adult illicit drug users are employed, as are most binge and heavy alcohol users. Studies show that when compared with non-substance abusers, substance-abusing employees are more likely to:

- change jobs frequently,

- be late to or absent from work,

- be less productive employees,

- be involved in a workplace accident, and

- file a workers' compensation claim.

Employers who have implemented drug-free workplace programs have important experiences to share.

- Employers with successful drug-free workplace programs report improvements in morale and productivity, and decreases in absenteeism, accidents, downtime, turnover, and theft.

- Employers with longstanding programs report better health status among employees and family members and decreased use of medical benefits by these same groups.

- Some organizations with drug-free workplace programs qualify for incentives, such as decreased costs for workers' compensation and other kinds of insurance.

Questions about Implementing a Drug-Free Workplace Policy

Where can I get help developing a drug-free workplace policy?

The U.S. Department of Labor's (DOL) Working Partners program has a web tool called the Drug-Free Workplace Advisor Policy Builder available online at http://www.dol.gov/elaws/asp/drugfree/drugs/screen1 .asp that helps employers develop customized drug-free workplace policies. If you need to develop a drug-free workplace policy from scratch, this tool guides you through the different components of a comprehensive policy and then generates a policy statement based on your responses to pre-set questions and statements. You can then incorporate your organization's name and logo and further modify the statement if needed. If your organization already has a drug-free workplace policy, you may want to use this tool to ensure it addresses all the issues that it should.

What is required to be certified as a drug-free workplace? Do drug-free workplaces receive a workers' compensation discount?

The U.S. Department of Labor (DOL) does not certify drug-free workplaces, nor does it regulate the area of workplace substance abuse. However, it recognizes that workplace alcohol and drug abuse creates significant safety and health hazards and can lead to decreased productivity and employee morale. Therefore, DOL's Working Partners program encourages employers to develop drug-free workplace programs.

Some states have workers' compensation laws that provide discounts to organizations that have drug-free workplace programs that include certain components, and as part of this process, they may provide drug-free workplace certification. For more information, visit the Working Partners website's listing of state laws that impact drug-free workplace issues or contact your state Department of Labor's Workers' Compensation section.

Keeping Your Worksite Drug and Alcohol Free

When a worker is impaired by the use of drugs or alcohol, he or she threatens the safety and well-being of everyone at a worksite. While it is the responsibility of every employee to work drug free, supervisors can be the first line of defense by taking appropriate action when a worker may be impaired.

Understanding Drug-Free Workplace Policies

Implementing and enforcing a drug-free workplace policy is one important way employers can protect worker safety and health. Though policies may vary from one worksite to the next, prohibitions against drinking alcohol or using illicit drugs during or prior to reporting to work are becoming standard practice in many workplaces.

The goal of these policies is to prevent impairment and improve safety by setting standards and holding workers accountable. Some policies include drug testing, while others do not; and some offer treatment and one or more chances to get help. But no matter how a program is structured, all policies are intended to protect workers and promote safe workplaces.

As a supervisor, it is your job to familiarize yourself with your company's drug-free workplace policy and be able to explain it to others. In addition, you must ensure that your workers understand their responsibility to:

- know your company's drug-free workplace policy;
- follow it and set a good example for others;
- seek help if they or their co-workers need it; and
- notify their supervisor/management if they observe drug or alcohol use or impairment that threatens safety.

Signs That Drug or Alcohol Use Is Becoming a Safety or Health Hazard at Work

Supervisors can play a powerful role in improving workplace safety by intervening and encouraging workers with alcohol or drug problems to seek help. But just how can you tell whether a worker is misusing drugs or alcohol?

Both on and off the job, symptoms of alcohol or drug use may be physical (chills, smell of alcohol, sweating, weight loss, physical deterioration); emotional (increased aggression, anxiety, burnout, denial, depression, paranoia); and/or behavioral (excessive talking, impaired coordination, irritability, lack of energy, limited attention span, poor motivation). While different types of drugs produce different physical symptoms or behaviors, there are numerous ways that misuse affects work behavior—and ultimately job performance and safety. It could be a sign of a drug or alcohol problem if a worker is doing the following:

- Arriving late, leaving early, and/or often absent

- Unreliable and often away from assigned job

- Careless and repeatedly making mistakes

- Argumentative and uncooperative

- Unwilling or unable to follow directions

- Avoiding responsibilities

- Making excuses that are unbelievable or placing blame elsewhere

- Taking unnecessary risks by ignoring safety and health procedures

- Frequently involved in mishaps and accidents or responsible for damage to equipment or property

It is important to note that if an employee displays these signs, it does not necessarily mean he/she has a drug or alcohol problem, but the possibility should not be overlooked.

Supervisor Roles and Responsibilities

Because you have day-to-day responsibility over what goes on in the workplace, you play a critical role in enforcing your employer's drug-free workplace policy. However, you are not expected to perform the role of police officer or counselor. Since it is part of your job to assess employees' job performance to ensure that all necessary tasks are completed in accordance with specifications and deadlines, your primary role in enforcing the policy is to be observant.

When an employee begins to show a consistent pattern of problem behavior, you should take action. Focusing on job performance, even when you think the problem may be caused by drugs or alcohol, allows you to balance both the rights of the individual employee to privacy and fair treatment and the rights of the work group to a safe, secure, and productive environment.

What to Do When You Suspect Drug or Alcohol Misuse

Do not wait until someone gets hurt to address a worker's drug or alcohol misuse. And, no matter how badly you want to shield your workers from disciplinary action, you should not make the problem worse by covering up or making excuses for someone whose use has impaired their job performance. If you suspect a worker has a problem, follow company guidelines which may include these steps:

- Start documenting evidence of declining job performance. List specific incidents (include date and time) and be concrete about what job functions and responsibilities were affected.

- Share this documentation with the appropriate company or union official who is qualified to advise you on how to handle the situation (this could be a shop steward, employee assistance professional, human resources manager, substance abuse program administrator, and so forth).

- Meet with the employee and tell him or her that you are concerned about his or her job performance. Describe specific incidents and problems using your documentation as a guide.

- Ask the employee if he or she has any explanation for the problem. Offer the opportunity to make the connection between alcohol or drug use and performance, but do not accuse the employee—unless you have reasonable suspicion and are going to require a drug test.

- Define what must be done to correct the performance problem and specify the consequences for the employee if the problem is not corrected.

- Refer the employee for professional assistance if he or she has admitted that drug or alcohol use is the root cause of the performance problem. Even if the employee has not admitted he or she has a problem, reconfirm your concern and suggest he or she seek assistance since personal problems—including, but not limited to, alcohol and drug use—are often the root causes of these types of job performance issues.

- Set a time frame for improvement and be willing and able to follow through on your promises about consequences.

There may be instances where there is concrete evidence that a worker is using drugs or alcohol and is impaired by recent use—these should not be ignored. If you directly observe a clear policy violation and/ or unsafe behavior that may pose an imminent threat, company management should be notified. The worker may need to be removed from the site and/or sent for a reasonable suspicion drug test. (Reasonable suspicion is defined as a belief that an employee is using or has used drugs in violation of the employer's policy drawn from specific, objective, and articulated facts and reasonable inferences drawn from those facts in light of experience.) Be sure you know your company's procedures (if any) for having an employee tested and consult with human resources or other designated company management prior to confronting the employee.

Sources of Help

When a worker has a problem with alcohol or drugs, company employee assistance or union member or labor assistance programs are generally the best places to turn for help since they provide confidential services. If these are not available, supervisors might want to consider calling a local drug and alcohol treatment provider who may be able to help determine whether some type of treatment intervention is advisable and, if so, how to get the worker to consider accepting help. Some free and confidential resources include:

Alcoholics Anonymous (AA)
AA World Services, Inc.
P.O. Box 459
New York, NY 10163
Phone: 212-870-3400
Website: http://www.aa.org

Al-Anon
1600 Corporate Landing Pkwy
Virginia Beach, VA 23454
Phone: 757-563-1600
Fax: 757-563-1655
Website: http://www.al-anon.alateen.org
E-mail: wso@al-anon.org

National Council on Alcoholism and Drug Dependence
244 East 58th St., 4th Floor
New York, NY 10022
Toll-Free: 800-NCA-CALL
Phone: 212-269-7797
Fax: 212-269-7510
Website: http://www.ncadd.org
E-mail: national@ncadd.org

Narcotics Anonymous
P.O. Box 9999
Van Nuys, CA 91409
Phone: 818-773-9999
Fax: 818-700-0700
Website: http://www.na.org

Substance Abuse Treatment Locator
Toll-Free: 800-662-HELP
Website: http://dasis3.samhsa.gov

Section 83.2

Drug Testing In the Workplace

Text in this section is from "Frequently Asked Questions,"
U.S. Department of Labor, March 11, 2009.

What does it mean to be a drug-free workplace?

A drug-free workplace is a workplace free of the health, safety, and productivity hazards caused by employees' abuse of alcohol or drugs. To achieve a drug-free workplace, many employers develop drug-free workplace programs. A comprehensive drug-free workplace program generally includes five components—a drug-free workplace policy, supervisor training, employee education, employee assistance, and drug testing.

Can an employer drug test? What are the laws in my state regarding drug testing?

First, it is important to note that the U.S. Department of Labor (DOL) does not regulate the area of workplace drug testing. However, it recognizes that workplace alcohol and drug abuse creates significant safety and health hazards and can lead to decreased productivity and employee morale. Therefore, DOL's Working Partners program encourages employers to develop drug-free workplace programs, which may or may not include drug testing.

Generally, employers have a fair amount of latitude in handling drug testing as they see fit, unless their organization is subject to certain federal laws (such as U.S. Department of Transportation drug-testing regulations). However, there may be state laws that impact how drug testing is implemented. For more information, visit the Working Partners website listing of state laws that impact drug-free workplace issues or contact your state Department of Labor.

DOL strongly recommends that before any drug-testing program is implemented, an employer have a written policy that is shared with all employees and clearly outlines why drug-testing is being implemented, prohibited behaviors, and the consequences for violating the policy. DOL also recommends that if drug testing is used, it be only one component of a comprehensive program that also includes training for supervisors on signs and symptoms of substance abuse, education for employees about the dangers of substance abuse, and some form of assistance or support for employees who may have problems with alcohol and other drugs.

You may obtain more information about drug testing from the Substance Abuse and Mental Health Services Administration (SAMHSA)/Center for Substance Abuse Prevention (CSAP)/Division of Workplace Programs (DWP), or the Drug and Alcohol Testing Industry Association (DATIA).

Can an employer drug test young workers?

As a general rule, if an employer can conduct drug testing, it can conduct drug testing of all employees, regardless of age. DOL's Fair Labor Standards Act (FLSA)—the primary law that sets the rules governing the employment of workers under the age of 18—does not address drug testing. Therefore, the rules on this subject are the same for young workers as they are for adult workers.

In fact, the U.S. Department of Labor (DOL) does not regulate the area of workplace drug testing at all. However, it is important to note that there may be state laws that impact if and how drug testing can be implemented for any employees.

Who pays for a drug test? Does an employee have to be paid for time spent having a drug test?

It is important to note that the U.S. Department of Labor (DOL) does not regulate the area of workplace drug testing. According to the Substance Abuse and Mental Health Services Administration (SAMSHA), an employer normally pays for a drug test. Also, time spent having a required drug test is generally considered hours worked (and thus compensable time) under the Fair Labor Standards Act (FLSA), which is a DOL regulation, for employees covered by the Act. These types of issues are overseen by DOL's Wage and Hour Division. For more guidance, please contact your closest DOL Wage and Hour district office.

What are an employer's notification requirements prior to starting drug testing?

Generally, employers have a fair amount of latitude in handling drug testing as they see fit, unless their organization is subject to certain federal laws (such as U.S. Department of Transportation alcohol and drug testing rules for employees in safety sensitive positions). However, there may be state laws that impact how drug testing can be implemented.

DOL does strongly recommend that before any drug-testing program is implemented, an employer have a written policy that is shared with all employees and clearly outlines why drug testing is being implemented, prohibited behaviors, and the consequences for violating the policy. DOL also recommends that if drug testing is used, it be only one component of a comprehensive drug-free workplace program that also includes training for supervisors on signs and symptoms of substance abuse, education for employees about the dangers of substance abuse and some form of assistance or support for employees who may have problems with alcohol and other drugs.

I take a prescription medication that may affect a drug test. Can I lose my job for taking it? Does my employer have a right to know what medication I am taking?

Because some prescription medications can affect an employee's ability to work safely, employers may have a legitimate interest in addressing them in their drug-free workplace policy. However, employers cannot discriminate in their hiring and firing practices based on an individual's use of prescription medication for legitimate medical purposes. Such discrimination could be a violation of the Americans with Disabilities Act (ADA).

The ADA also prohibits an employer from asking disability-related questions unless they are job related and consistent with business necessity. Therefore, employers should not have a blanket policy requiring all employees to disclose prescription drug use. For more information about this issue, contact the Equal Employment Opportunity Commission (EEOC), which administers the employment provisions of the ADA.

Use of some prescription medications may result in a positive drug test. In this event, a Medical Review Officer (MRO) or other appropriate company personnel may inquire to determine if the employee has a legitimate medical explanation, such as a physician's prescription, for the result.

A drug test result may be considered personal health information. Thus, there may be restrictions on how and whether such information can be shared. This is why employees who take a drug test usually must sign a release in order for their employer to receive the results. For more information about this issue, contact the U.S. Department of Health and Human Services (HHS). This agency administers the Health Insurance Portability and Accountability Act (HIPAA), which dictates under what circumstances and to whom health information may be released.

Does the Drug-Free Workplace Act of 1988 apply to my company?

The Drug-Free Workplace Act of 1988 requires some federal contractors and all federal grantees to agree that they will provide drug-free workplaces as a precondition of receiving a contract or grant from a federal agency. All organizations covered by it are required to take certain steps, such as publishing and providing a drug-free workplace policy statement to all covered employees and establishing a drug-free employee awareness program. There are also notification requirements regarding if an employee is convicted of a criminal drug violation in the workplace. The Drug-Free Workplace Act of 1988 does not require drug testing.

The U.S. Department of Labor (DOL) does not administer the Drug-Free Workplace Act of 1988; however, its Working Partners program's Drug-Free Workplace Advisor assists organizations in determining if they are covered by it and understanding its requirements. This tool also has a policy development section that can help those covered by the Act develop their drug-free workplace policies.

I am an employer and have been asked to provide information about the results of an employee's or ex-employee's drug test. Can I do this?

The result of a drug test may be considered personal health information. Consequently, there may be restrictions on how and whether such information (as well as other information related to an employee's history of alcohol or drug use) can be shared with others. This is why employees who undergo a drug test generally must sign a release (usually at the time of the test) in order for their employer to receive the results.

For more information about issues related to the release of health information, contact the U.S. Department of Health and Human Services (HHS). This agency administers the Health Insurance Portability and Accountability Act (HIPAA), which dictates under what circumstances and to whom health information may be released.

Can an employee who was terminated for violating a drug-free workplace policy collect unemployment insurance?

Some states laws limit the unemployment insurance benefits available to unemployed individuals whose termination was based on the results of a drug test. For more information, visit the Working Partners website available at http://www.dol.gov/workingpartners for a listing of state laws that impact drug-free workplace issues or contact your state Department of Labor's Unemployment Insurance section.

Chapter 84

Religious Involvement Can Be a Protective Factor against Substance Use among Adults

- In 2005, 30.8% of adults aged 18 or older attended religious services 25 or more times in the past year, 78.1% reported that religious beliefs are a very important part of their lives, and 75.1% reported that religious beliefs influence how they make decisions in their lives.

- In 2005, 2.9% of adults who attended religious services 25 or more times in the past year used illicit drugs in the past month compared with 10.1% of those who attended religious services fewer than 25 times.

- Adults who reported that religious beliefs are a very important part of their lives were less likely to use illicit drugs in the past month than those who reported that religious beliefs are not a very important part of their lives (6.1% versus 14.3%).

Public opinion polling has shown that 63% of Americans were members of a church or synagogue in 2006.[1] Religiosity has been identified in other research as an important protective factor against substance use.[2-4] The National Survey on Drug Use and Health (NSDUH) includes questions on religious service attendance and religious beliefs. Respondents are asked to indicate how many times in the past

This chapter is excerpted from "Religious Involvement and Substance Use among Adults (NSDUH Report)," Substance Abuse and Mental Health Services Administration (SAMHSA), March 23, 2007.

12 months they attended religious services, excluding special occasions such as weddings, funerals, or other special events. Respondents also are asked whether their religious beliefs are a very important part of their lives and whether their religious beliefs influence how they make decisions in their lives.[5] NSDUH also includes questions about use of cigarettes, alcohol, and illicit drugs during the month (or 30 days) prior to the interview. Illicit drugs refer to marijuana/hashish, cocaine (including crack), inhalants, hallucinogens, heroin, or prescription-type drugs used nonmedically.[6]

The report examines the relationships between religious service attendance and beliefs and substance use among adults aged 18 or older. All findings are based on data from the 2005 NSDUH.

Religious Involvement among Adults

In 2005, 30.8% of adults aged 18 or older (an estimated 67 million persons) attended religious services 25 or more times in the past year, 78.1% (168 million persons) reported that religious beliefs are a very important part of their lives, and 75.1% (162 million persons) reported that religious beliefs influence how they make decisions in their lives.

Females were more likely than males to report all three types of religious involvement (Table 84.1). The percentages of adults reporting that their religious beliefs are a very important part of their lives and the percentage reporting that religious beliefs influence how they make decisions increased with each age category. For example, 70.6% of young adults aged 18 to 25 reported that religious beliefs are a very important part of their lives compared with 83.7% of older adults aged 65 or older. Adults aged 65 or older were more likely to attend religious services 25 times or more in the past year than adults in all other age groups.

Religious Service Attendance and Substance Use

In 2005, adults aged 18 or older who attended religious services 25 or more times in the past year were less likely to have used cigarettes, alcohol, or illicit drugs in the past month than adults who attended religious services fewer than 25 times in the past year. For example, 2.9% of adults who attended religious services 25 or more times in the past year used illicit drugs in the past month compared with 10.1% of adults who attended religious services fewer than 25 times in the past year.

Table 84.1. Percentages and Standard Errors (SE) of Adults Aged 18 or Older Reporting Religious Involvement, by Age Group and Gender: 2005

Age group/ gender	Attended relig- ious services 25 or more times in the past year		Religious beliefs are a very impor- tant part of their lives*		Religious beliefs influence how they make decisions in their lives*	
	Percent	SE	Percent	SE	Percent	SE
Total	30.8	0.42	78.1	0.32	75.1	0.34
Age						
18–25	21.6	0.43	70.6	0.44	63.5	0.45
26–34	22.6	0.74	75.8	0.69	70.0	0.75
35–64	32.3	0.61	79.1	0.47	77.2	0.48
65 and over	42.8	1.32	83.7	1.01	83.7	1.02
Gender						
Male	26.1	0.54	74.1	0.48	70.5	0.51
Female	35.2	0.54	81.8	0.40	79.2	0.42

*Respondents are asked whether their religious beliefs are a very important part of their lives and whether their religious beliefs influence how they make decisions in their lives. Response options for both questions were (1) strongly disagree, (2) disagree, (3) agree, and (4) strongly agree. For this report, responses of agree/strongly agree were grouped into the "yes" category, and responses of strongly disagree/disagree responses were grouped into the "no" category. Adults with unknown or missing data were excluded from the analysis.

Source: SAMHSA, 2005 NSDUH.

Table 84.2. Percentages of Adults Aged 18 or Older Reporting Past Month Substance Use, by Past Year Religious Service Attendance: 2005

Substance	Attended religious services 25 or more times	Attended religious services fewer than 25 times
Cigarettes	12.4	32.8
Alcohol	45.9	60.5
Illicit drugs	2.9	10.1

Source: SAMHSA, 2005 NSDUH.

Importance of Religious Beliefs and Substance Use

Adults aged 18 or older who reported in 2005 that religious beliefs are a very important part of their lives were less likely to have used cigarettes, alcohol, or illicit drugs in the past month than adults who reported that religious beliefs are not a very important part of their lives. For example, 6.1% of adults who reported that religious beliefs are a very important part of their lives used illicit drugs in the past month compared with 14.3% of adults who reported that religious beliefs are not a very important part of their lives.

Religious Beliefs' Influence on Decisions and Substance Use

Adults aged 18 or older who reported in 2005 that religious beliefs influence how they make decisions in their lives also were less likely to have used cigarettes, alcohol, or illicit drugs in the past month than adults who reported that religious beliefs do not influence how they make decisions. For example, 5.8% of adults who reported that religious beliefs influence how they make decisions in their lives used illicit drugs in the past month compared with 14.0% of adults who reported that religious beliefs do not influence how they make decisions.

Table 84.3. Percentages of Adults Aged 18 or Older Reporting Past Month Substance Use, by Whether or Not Religious Beliefs Influence How They Make Decisions in Their Lives*: 2005

Substance	Religious beliefs influence decisions	Religious beliefs do not influence decisions
Cigarettes	23.2	36.4
Alcohol	52.4	66.9
Illicit drugs	5.8	14.0

*Respondents are asked whether their religious beliefs are a very important part of their lives and whether their religious beliefs influence how they make decisions in their lives. Response options for both questions were (1) strongly disagree, (2) disagree, (3) agree, and (4) strongly agree. For this report, responses of agree/strongly agree were grouped into the "yes" category, and responses of strongly disagree/disagree responses were grouped into the "no" category. Adults with unknown or missing data were excluded from the analysis.

Source: SAMHSA, 2005 NSDUH.

End Notes

1. The Gallup Organization. (2007). *Religion*. Retrieved January 31, 2007, from http://www.galluppoll.com/content/?ci=1690&pg=2.

2. National Center on Addiction and Substance Abuse at Columbia University. (2001, November*). So help me God: Substance abuse, religion and spirituality*. New York: Author. [Available as a PDF at http://www.casacolumbia.org/supportcasa/item.asp ?cID=12&PID=127]

3. Wallace, J. M., Myers, V. L., and Osai, E. R. (2004). *Faith matters: Race / ethnicity, religion and substance use*. Baltimore, MD: The Annie E. Casey Foundation. [Available as a PDF at http:// www.aecf.org/publications/browse.php?filter=21 and http://www .aecf.org/publications/data/1_04_585_faith_matters_report.pdf]

4. Kendler, K. S., Gardner, C. O., and Prescott, C. A. (1997). Religion, psychopathology, and substance use and abuse: A multimeasure, genetic-epidemiologic study. *American Journal of Psychiatry*, 154, 322–329.

5. Response options for both questions were (1) strongly disagree, (2) disagree, (3) agree, and (4) strongly agree. For this report, responses of agree/strongly agree were grouped into the "yes" category, and responses of strongly disagree/disagree responses were grouped into the "no" category.

6. NSDUH measures the nonmedical use of prescription-type pain relievers, sedatives, stimulants, or tranquilizers. Nonmedical use is defined as the use of prescription-type drugs not prescribed for the respondent by a physician or used only for the experience or feeling they caused. Nonmedical use of any prescription-type pain reliever, sedative, stimulant, or tranquilizer does not include over-the-counter drugs. Nonmedical use of stimulants includes methamphetamine use.

Part Six

Additional Help and Information

Chapter 85

Glossary of Terms Related to Drug Abuse

abuser: A person who uses drugs in ways that threaten his health or impair his social or economic functioning.

addiction: The point at which a person's chemical usage causes repeated harmful consequences and the person is unable to stop using the drug of choice. Medically the term implies that withdrawal will take place when the mood-changing chemical is removed from the body.

adulterant: A substance, either a biologically active material such as another drug or an inert material, added to a drug when it is formed into a tablet or capsule.[2]

alcohol: Refers to ethyl alcohol or ethanol.

alcoholism: A treatable illness brought on by harmful dependence upon alcohol which is physically and psychologically addictive. As a disease, alcoholism is primary, chronic, progressive, and fatal.

amphetamines: Synthetic amines (uppers) that act with a pronounced stimulant effect on the central nervous system.

assay: The measurement of the quantity of a chemical component.

Terms in this chapter are from "Glossary of Terms," U.S. Department of Labor, March 12, 2009. Terms marked with a [1] are excerpted from "Comorbidity: Addiction and Other Mental Illnesses," National Institute on Drug Abuse (NIDA), December 2008. Terms marked with a [2] are from "Research Report Series: MDMA (Ecstasy) Abuse," NIDA, March 2006.

barbiturates: A class of drugs used in medicine as hypnotic agents to promote sleep or sedation. Some are also useful in the control of epilepsy. All are central nervous system depressants and are subject to abuse. Depending upon their potency they are classified as schedule I or schedule II drugs.

benzodiazepines: A class of drugs used in medicine as minor tranquilizers which is frequently prescribed to treat anxiety. They are central nervous system depressants and are subject to abuse.

blood alcohol concentration (BAC): The amount of alcohol in the bloodstream measured in percentages. A BAC of 0.10% means that a person has one part alcohol per 1,000 parts blood in the body.

cannabinoids: The psychoactive substances found in the common hemp plant, or Cannabis sativa. Most of the psychological effects are produced by delta-9-tetrahydrocannabinol.

chemical dependency: A harmful dependence on mood-changing chemicals.

cocaine: An alkaloid, methyl benzoylecgonine, obtained from the leaves of the coca tree (Erythroxylum sp.). It is a central nervous system stimulant that produces euphoric excitement; abuse and dependence constitute a major drug problem.

comorbidity: The occurrence of two disorders or illnesses in the same person, either at the same time (co-occurring comorbid conditions) or with a time difference between the initial occurrence of one and the initial occurrence of the other (sequentially comorbid conditions).[1]

depressants: Drugs that reduce the activity of the nervous system (alcohol, downers, and narcotics).

designer drugs: Illegal drugs are defined in terms of their chemical formulas. To circumvent these legal restrictions, underground chemists modify the molecular structure of certain illegal drugs to produce analogs known as designer drugs. Many of the so-called designer drugs are related to amphetamines and have mild stimulant properties but are mostly euphoriants. They can produce severe neurochemical damage to the brain.

dual diagnosis/mentally ill chemical abuser (MICA): Other terms used to describe the comorbidity of a drug use disorder and another mental illness.[1]

dopamine: A neurotransmitter present in regions of the brain that regulate movement, emotion, motivation, and the feeling of pleasure.[2]

downers: Barbiturates, minor tranquilizers, and related depressants.

drug: A drug is any chemical substance that alters mood, perception, or consciousness.

drug abuse: Pathological use of a prescribed or other chemical substance.

employee assistance program (EAP): A program designed to assist employees with drug abuse, or other problems, by mean of counseling, treatment, or referral to more specific centers.

enabling: Allowing irresponsible and destructive behavior patterns to continue by taking responsibility for others, not allowing them to face the consequences of their own actions.

ethyl alcohol: Ethanol is the member of the alcohol series of chemicals which is used in alcoholic beverages. It is less toxic than other members of this series, but it is a central nervous system depressant and has a high abuse potential.

habituation (psychological dependence): The result of repeated consumption of a drug which produces psychological but no physical dependence. The psychological dependence produces a desire (not a compulsion) to continue taking drugs for the sense of improved well-being.

hallucinogens: Drugs that stimulate the nervous system and produce varied changes in perception and mood.

hashish: The concentrated resin of the marijuana plant.

heroin: A semisynthetic derivative of morphine originally used as an analgesic and cough depressant. In harmful doses it induces euphoria; tends to make the user think he or she is removed from reality, tension, and pressures.

hyperthermia: A potentially dangerous rise in body temperature.[2]

inhalants: Inhalants include a variety of psychoactive substances which are inhaled as gases or volatile liquids. Many are readily available in most households and are inexpensive. They include paint thinner, glue, gasoline, and other products that are not considered to be drugs.

lysergic acid diethylamide (LSD): LSD distorts perception of time and space, and creates illusions and hallucinations. It comes in liquid form and most often is swallowed after being placed on a sugar cube or blotting paper. LSD increases blood pressure, heart rate, and blood sugar. Nausea, chills, flushes, irregular breathing, sweating, and trembling occur.

marijuana: Marijuana is prepared by crushing the dried flowering cannabis top and leaves into a tea-like substance, which is usually rolled into a cigarette (a joint) and smoked. The effects are felt within minutes. The user may experience a distorted sense of time and distance, suffer reduced attention span, and loss of memory. Higher doses also cause impaired judgment, slowed reaction time, limited motor skills, confusion of time sense, and short-term memory loss.

mental disorder: A mental condition marked primarily by sufficient disorganization of personality, mind, and emotions to seriously impair the normal psychological or behavioral functioning of the individual. Addiction is a mental disorder.[1]

methadone: A synthetic opiate with action similar to that of morphine and heroin except that withdrawal is more prolonged and less severe. It is used in methadone maintenance programs as a substitute for heroin in the treatment of addicts.

methamphetamine: An addictive stimulant that is closely related to amphetamine, but has longer lasting and more toxic effects on the central nervous system. It has a high potential for abuse and addiction.

methaqualone: A hypnotic drug unrelated to the barbiturates but used as a sedative and sleeping aid. It is also known by its trade name Quaalude.

narcotics: A class of depressant drugs derived from opium or related chemically to compounds in opium. Regular use leads to addiction.

neurotransmitter: A chemical that acts as a messenger to carry signals or information from one nerve cell to another.[2]

norepinephrine: A neurotransmitter present in regions of the brain that affect heart rate and blood pressure.[2]

opiates: Drugs derived from opium such as morphine and codeine, together with the semisynthetic congeners such as heroin.

phencyclidine (PCP): Phencyclidine, also known as PCP or angel dust, is a synthetic (or manufactured) substance that is chemically related to ketamine, which is widely used in anesthesia. Intoxication may result in blurred vision, diminished sensation, muscular rigidity, muteness, confusion, anxious amnesia, distortion of body image, thought disorder, auditory hallucinations, and variable motor depression or stimulation, which may include aggressive or bizarre behavior.

physical dependence: Occurs when a person cannot function normally without the repeated use of a drug. If the drug is withdrawn, the person has severe physical and psychic disturbances.

psychoactive drugs: Drugs that affect the mind, especially mood, thought, or perception.

psychological dependence: (See habituation)

psychosis: A serious mental disorder (such as schizophrenia) characterized by defective or lost contact with reality. Symptoms often include hallucinations or delusions.[1]

schedule I drugs: Drugs in schedule I of the Controlled Substances Act are those substances that have a high potential for abuse, no currently acceptable medical use in treatment, and which lack any accepted safe use under medical supervision.

schedule II drugs: Drugs in schedule II of the Controlled Substances Act are those substances that have a high potential for abuse with severe liability to cause psychic or physical dependence, but have some approved medical use.

self-medication: The use of a substance to lessen the negative effects of stress, anxiety, or other mental disorders (or side effects of their pharmacotherapy). Self-medication may lead to addiction and other drug- or alcohol-related problems.[1]

serotonin: A neurotransmitter present in widespread parts of the brain that is involved in sleep, movement, and emotions.[2]

steroids: A large family of pharmaceutical drugs related to the adrenal hormone cortisone.

stimulants: Drugs that increase the activity of the nervous system, causing wakefulness.

THC: Delta-9-tetrahydrocannabinol, the most active cannabinoid.

Chapter 86

Glossary of Street Terms for Drugs of Abuse

The ability to understand current drug-related street terms is an invaluable tool for law enforcement, public health, and other criminal justice professionals who work with the public. This chapter contains a sample of the over 2,300 street terms that refer to specific drug types or drug activity. The complete listing is available at http://www.streetdrugs.org/pdf/street_terms.pdf.

Alphabetical Listing

All terms are cross-referenced where possible. A single term or similar terms may refer to various drugs or have different meanings, reflecting geographic and demographic variations in slang. All known meanings and spellings are included. No attempt was made to determine which usage is most frequent or widespread. Different definitions for a single term are separated by semi-colons (;). The use of commas (,) and the connective "and" indicates that the term refers to the use of the specified drugs in combination.

African woodbine—Marijuana cigarette

Agonies—Withdrawal symptoms

Air blast—Inhalants

Airhead—Marijuana user

Excerpted from "Street Terms: Drugs and the Drug Trade," Office of National Drug Control Policy, February 2004.

Airplane—Marijuana

Al Capone—Heroin

Alice B. Toklas—Marijuana brownie

All lit up—Under the influence of drugs

All star—User of multiple drugs

Amoeba—Phencyclidine (PCP)

Amp—Amphetamine; marijuana dipped in formaldehyde or embalming fluid, sometimes laced with PCP and smoked

Amp head—LSD user

Amp joint—Marijuana cigarette laced with some form of narcotic

Amped—High on amphetamines

AMT—Dimethyltryptamine

Anadrol—Oral steroids

Angel—PCP

Angel dust—PCP

Angie—Cocaine

Animal tranquilizer—PCP

Antifreeze—Heroin

Apache—Fentanyl

Apple jacks—Crack cocaine

Arnolds—Steroids

Artillery—Equipment for injecting drugs

Ashes—Marijuana

Aspirin—Powder cocaine

Assassin of Youth—Marijuana

Astro turf—Marijuana

Atom bomb—Marijuana mixed with heroin

Aunt Hazel—Heroin

Aunt Mary—Marijuana

Aunt Nora—Cocaine

Aurora borealis—PCP

Author—Doctor who writes illegal prescriptions

Baby habit—Occasional use of drugs

Baby T—Crack Cocaine

Back breakers—Lysergic acid diethylamide (LSD) and strychnine

Badrock—Crack cocaine

Bagging—Using inhalants

Baker—Person who smokes marijuana

Bale—Marijuana

Ball—Crack cocaine; Mexican black tar heroin

Banana split—Combination of 2C-B (Nexus) with other illicit substances, particularly LSD

Banano—Marijuana or tobacco cigarettes laced with cocaine

Bang—Inhalants; to inject a drug

Banging—Under the influence of drugs

Barbies—Depressants

Barbs—Cocaine

Base—Cocaine; crack

Baseball—Crack cocaine

Bash—Marijuana

Batman—Cocaine; heroin

Battery acid—LSD

Bazooka—Cocaine; crack; crack and tobacco combined in a joint; coca paste and marijuana

Beam—Cocaine

Beam me up Scotty—PCP and crack

Beast—Heroin; LSD

Bed bugs—Fellow addicts

Beemers—Crack Cocaine

Belladonna—PCP

Belushi—Combination of cocaine and heroin

Bender—Drug party

Bennie—Amphetamine

Big man—Drug supplier

Bing—Enough drug for one injection

Bingers—Crack addicts

Bingo—To inject a drug

Birdie powder—Cocaine; heroin

Biscuit—50 rocks of crack

Black beauties—Amphetamine; depressants

Black dust—PCP

Black gold—High potency marijuana

Black mollies—Amphetamine

Black pearl—Heroin

Blanket—Marijuana cigarette

Blast—Cocaine; smoke crack; marijuana;

Block busters—Depressants

Blotter acid—LSD; PCP

Blue—Crack cocaine; depressants; OxyContin®

Blue devil—Depressants

Blunt—Marijuana inside a cigar; cocaine and marijuana inside a cigar

Bolo—Crack cocaine

Bolt—Amphetamine; isobutyl nitrite

Bonita (Spanish)—Heroin

Book—100 dosage units of LSD

Boom—Marijuana

Bopper—Crack cocaine

Boppers—Amyl nitrite

Brain pills—Amphetamines

Brick—Crack cocaine; cocaine; marijuana; one kilogram of marijuana

Broccoli—Marijuana

Bromo—Nexus

Brown bombers—LSD

Brown crystal—Heroin

Brown sugar—Heroin

Brownies—Amphetamine

Bubble gum—Cocaine; crack cocaine; marijuana from Tennessee

Bumblebees—Amphetamine

Butter—Marijuana; crack

Buzz bomb—Nitrous oxide

Cactus—Mescaline

Cadillac—Cocaine; PCP

Cakes—Round discs of crack

Candy sugar—Powder cocaine

Casper—Crack cocaine

Casper the ghost—Crack cocaine

Cat—Methcathinone

Cat valium—Ketamine

Catnip—Marijuana cigarette

Chalk—Crack cocaine; amphetamine; methamphetamine

Charley—Heroin

Charlie—Cocaine

Cheap basing—Crack

Cheese—Heroin

Chemical—Crack cocaine

Chemo—Marijuana

Cherry meth—Gamma hydroxybutyrate (GHB)

Chief—LSD; mescaline

China girl—Fentanyl

China White—Heroin; fentanyl; synthetic heroin

Chinese molasses—Opium

Chinese red—Heroin

Chinese tobacco—Opium

Chip—Heroin

Chocolate—Marijuana; opium; amphetamine

Circles—Rohypnol

Clear—Methamphetamine

Climb—Marijuana cigarette

Cloud—Crack cocaine

Coconut—Cocaine

Coffee—LSD

Coke—Cocaine; crack cocaine

Cola—Cocaine

Colas—Marijuana

Conductor—LSD

Contact lens—LSD

Cookies—Crack cocaine

Coolie—Cigarette laced with cocaine

Cotton—Currency; OxyContin®

Courage pills—Heroin; depressants

Crazy coke—PCP

Crying weed—Marijuana

Crystal—Cocaine; amphetamine; methamphetamine; PCP

Crystal joint—PCP

Crystal meth—Methamphetamine

Crystal tea—LSD

Dance fever—Fentanyl

Demolish—Crack

Dep-testosterone—Injectable steroids

Detroit pink—PCP

Devil drug—Crack cocaine

Dew—Marijuana

Diamonds—Amphetamines; methylenedioxymethamphetamine (MDMA)

Dice—Crack cocaine

Diesel—Heroin

Diet pills—Amphetamine

Dip—Crack cocaine

Dipper—PCP

Dirt—Heroin

DOA—Crack; heroin; PCP

Dope—Marijuana; heroin; any other drug

Down—Codeine cough syrup

Downer—Depressants

Dr. Feel Good—Heroin

Dragon rock—Mixture of heroin and crack

Duji—Heroin

Dynamite—Cocaine mixed with heroin

E-bombs—MDMA (methylenedioxymethamphetamine)

Ecstasy—Methylenedioxymethamphetamine (MDMA)

Elephant—Marijuana; PCP

Elvis—LSD

Embalming fluid—PCP

Eye opener—Crack; amphetamine

Fast white lady—Powder cocaine

Finger—Marijuana cigarette

Fives—Amphetamine

Fizzies—Methadone

Flea powder—Low purity heroin

Florida snow—Cocaine

Flower—Marijuana

Forget me drug—Rohypnol

Friend—Fentanyl

Fries—Crack cocaine

Fuel—Marijuana mixed with insecticides; PCP

Galloping horse—Heroin

Geek—Crack mixed with marijuana

GHB—Gamma hydroxybutyrate

Ghost—LSD

Giggle weed—Marijuana

Girlfriend—Cocaine

Glo—Crack cocaine

God's drug—Morphine

God's flesh—LSD; psilocybin/psilocin

God's medicine—Opium

Gold—Marijuana; crack cocaine; heroin

Golden dragon—LSD

Golden eagle—4-methylthioamphetamine

Golden girl—Heroin

Golf ball—Crack cocaine

Gong—Marijuana; opium

Good—PCP; heroin

Good and plenty—Heroin

Goodfellas—Fentanyl

Goody-goody—Marijuana

Goofers—Depressants

Goofy's—LSD

Goon—PCP

Goop—Gamma hydroxybutyrate (GHB)

Gorilla biscuits—PCP

Gorilla pills—Depressants

Grass—Marijuana

Gravel—Crack cocaine

Greens—Marijuana

Gym candy—Steroids

Hamburger helper—Crack cocaine

Hardware—Isobutyl nitrite; inhalants

He-man—Fentanyl

Hillbilly heroin—OxyContin®

Hippie crack—Inhalants

Hocus—Marijuana; opium

Hog—PCP

Honey oil—Ketamine; inhalants

Hot stick—Marijuana cigarette

Hotcakes—Crack cocaine

Huff—Inhalants

Idiot pills—Depressants

Indian boy—Marijuana

Indian hay—Marijuana from India

Indian hemp—Marijuana

Instant Zen—LSD

Jackpot—Fentanyl

Jam—Cocaine; amphetamine

Jane—Marijuana

Jellies—Depressants; MDMA in gel caps

Jelly—Cocaine

Joint—Marijuana cigarette

Jolly bean—Amphetamine

Jolly green—Marijuana

Joy powder—Cocaine; heroin

Joy smoke—Marijuana

Juice—PCP; steroids

Junk—Cocaine; heroin

Junkie—Addict

Kangaroo—Crack

Kansas Grass—Marijuana

Kate bush—Marijuana

Kibbles and Bits—Small crumbs of crack

Kicker—OxyContin®

Kiddie dope—Prescription drugs

Killer—Marijuana; PCP

King Kong pills—Depressants

Kit kat—Ketamine

Kryptonite—Crack cocaine; marijuana

Krystal—PCP

La Rocha—Rohypnol

Lace—Cocaine and marijuana

Lactone—GBL

Lady—Cocaine

Lean—Codeine cough syrup

Lethal weapon—PCP

Lightning—Amphetamine

Liquid ecstasy—Gamma hydroxybutyrate (GHB)

Locker room—Isobutyl nitrite; inhalants

Log—Marijuana cigarette; PCP

Loony toons—LSD

Lucy in the sky with diamonds—LSD

M&M—Depressants

M.J.—Marijuana

Magic—PCP

Meth—Methamphetamine

Mickey Finn—Depressants

Mickey's—Depressant; LSD

Mojo—Cocaine; heroin

Moon—Mescaline

Moon gas—Inhalants

Moonrock—Crack mixed with heroin

Mother's little helper—Depressants

Murder 8—Fentanyl

Nice and easy—Heroin

One way—LSD; heroin

Orange barrels—LSD

Orange crystal—PCP

Oxy—OxyContin®

Oz—Inhalants

Paper acid—LSD

Parabolin—Oral steroids; veterinary steroid

Paradise—Cocaine

Paradise white—Cocaine

Parsley—Marijuana; PCP

Paste—Crack cocaine

Peace pill—PCP

Peace tablets—LSD

Pep pills—Amphetamine

Peter Pan—PCP

Peyote—Mescaline

Pluto—Heroin

Pocket rocket—Marijuana; marijuana cigarette

Poison—Heroin; fentanyl

Pony—Crack cocaine

Poor man's pot—Inhalants

Pot—Marijuana

Potato—LSD

Potato chips—Crack cut with benzocaine

Predator—Heroin

Product—Crack cocaine

Proviron—Oral steroids

Puffy—PCP

Pumpers—Steroids

Queen Ann's lace—Marijuana

Quicksilver—Isobutyl nitrite; inhalants

R-2—Rohypnol

Rambo—Heroin

Recycle—LSD

Reefer—Marijuana

Rhythm—Amphetamine

Roach—Butt of marijuana cigarette

Roach-2—Rohypnol

Road dope—Amphetamine

Rock(s)—Cocaine; crack cocaine

Rocket fuel—PCP

Roofies—Rohypnol

Rooster—Crack cocaine

Ruffles—Rohypnol

Rugs—Marijuana

Rush hour—Heroin

Rush snappers—Isobutyl nitrite

Scoop—Gamma hydroxybutyrate (GHB)

Scootie—Methamphetamine

Scorpion—Cocaine

Scott—Heroin

Seven-Up—Crack cocaine

Shake—Marijuana; powder cocaine

Sheet rocking—Crack and LSD

Shoot—Heroin

Shoot the breeze—Nitrous oxide

Silly putty—Psilocybin/psilocin

Skag—Heroin

Skee—Opium

Sketch—Methamphetamine

Sleep—Gamma hydroxybutyrate (GHB)

Sleet—Crack Cocaine

Sleigh ride—Cocaine

Slick superspeed—Methcathinone

Smack—Heroin

Snow—Cocaine; heroin; amphetamine

Soft—Powder cocaine

Softballs—Depressants

Soles—Hashish

Soma—PCP

South parks—Lysergic acid diethylamide

Space cadet—Crack dipped in PCP

Spaceball—PCP used with crack

Spackle—Methamphetamine

Sparkle plenty—Amphetamine

Speckled birds—Methamphetamine

Spectrum—Nexus

Speed—Crack cocaine; amphetamine; methamphetamine

Spider—Heroin

Stack—Marijuana

Stackers—Steroids

Star dust—PCP

Stink weed—Marijuana

Stones—Crack cocaine

Strawberries—Depressants

Strawberry fields—LSD

Studio fuel—Cocaine

Sugar—Cocaine; crack cocaine; heroin; LSD

Superman—LSD

Surfer—PCP

Sweet dreams—Heroin

Tardust—Cocaine

Tension—Crack cocaine

Tex-mex—Marijuana

Texas shoe shine—Inhalants

Thrust—Isobutyl nitrite; inhalants

Tic tac—PCP

TNT—Fentanyl

Tom and Jerries—Methylenedioxymethamphetamine (MDMA)

Toonies—Nexus

Tootsie roll—Heroin

Top gun—Crack cocaine

Topi—Mescaline

Tops—Peyote

Toxy—Opium

Toys—Opium

Trash—Methamphetamine

Trauma—Marijuana

Triple crowns—Methylenedioxymethamphetamine (MDMA)

Truck drivers—Amphetamine

Tweety birds—Methylenedioxymethamphetamine (MDMA)

Twinkie—Crack cocaine

Uncle Milty—Depressants

Uppers—Amphetamine

Venus—Nexus

Vita-G—Gamma hydroxybutyrate (GHB)

Vitamin K—Ketamine

Vitamin R—Ritalin (methylphenidate)

Vodka acid—LSD

Wac—PCP on marijuana

Wedding bells—LSD

Weed—Marijuana; PCP

Weight trainers—Steroids

West coast—Methylphenidate (Ritalin®)

Whippets—Nitrous oxide

White—Heroin; amphetamine

White ball—Crack cocaine

White boy—Heroin; powder cocaine

White diamonds –Methylenedioxymethamphetamine (MDMA)

White dragon—Powder cocaine; heroin

White dust—LSD

White lightning—LSD

White tornado—Crack cocaine

White-haired lady—Marijuana

Whiteout—Inhalants; isobutyl nitrite

Whiz bang—Cocaine; heroin and cocaine

Wigits—Methylenedioxymethamphetamine (MDMA)

Window glass—LSD

Window pane—LSD; crack cocaine

Wings—Cocaine; heroin

Wolfies—Rohypnol

Work—Methamphetamine

Working man's cocaine—Methamphetamine

Worm—PCP

X-pills—Methylenedioxymethamphetamine (MDMA)

Yellow—LSD; depressants

Yellow fever—PCP

Yellow jackets—Depressants; methamphetamine

Yellow powder—Methamphetamine

Yellow submarine—Marijuana

Zen—LSD

Zero—Opium

Zip—Cocaine

Zombie weed—PCP

Zoom—Marijuana laced with PCP; PCP

Chapter 87

Directory of State Substance Abuse Agencies

Alabama
Substance Abuse Services Div.
P.O. Box 301410
100 N. Union St.
Montgomery, AL 36130
Toll-Free: 800-367-0955
Phone: 334-242-3961
Fax: 334-242-0759
Website: http://
www.mh.alabama.gov

Alaska
Div. of Behavioral Health
Dept. of Health and Social
Services
350 Main St., Suite 214
P.O. Box 110620
Juneau, AK 99811
Phone: 907-465-3370
Fax: 907-465-2668
Website: http://
www.hss.state.ak.us

American Samoa
American Samoa Government
Dept. of Human and Social
Services
P.O. Box 997534
Pago Pago, AS 96799
Phone: 684-633-2609
Fax: 684-633-7449

Arizona
Div. of Behavioral Health
Services
Dept. of Health Services
150 N. 18th Ave.
Phoenix, AZ 85007
Phone: 602-542-1025
Fax: 602-542-0883
Website: http://www.azdhs.gov

Excerpted from "Facility Locator," Substance Abuse and Mental Health Services Administration (SAMHSA). All contact information was verified as current in November 2009.

Arkansas

Office of Alcohol and Drug
Abuse Prevention
Div. of Behavioral Health
Services
305 S. Palm St.
Little Rock, AR 72205
Phone: 501-686-9866
Fax: 501-686-9035
Website: http://
www.arkansas.gov/dhs/dmhs/
alco_drug_abuse_prevention.htm

California

Dept. of Alcohol and Drug
Programs
1700 K Street
Sacramento, CA 95811
Toll-Free: 800-879-2772
Fax: 916-323-1270
Website: http://www.adp.ca.gov/
default.asp
E-mail:
ResourceCenter@adp.ca.gov

Colorado

Div. of Behavioral Health
Dept. of Human Services
3824 W. Princeton Circle
Denver, CO 80236
Phone: 303-866-7400
Fax: 303-866-7481
Website: http://
www.cdhs.state.co.us/adad

Connecticut

Dept. of Mental Health and
Addiction Services
410 Capitol Ave.
P.O. Box 341431
Hartford, CT 06134
Toll-Free: 800-446-7348
Toll-Free TTY: 888-621-3551
Phone: 860-418-7000
Website: http://www.ct.gov/dmhas

Delaware

Alcohol and Drug Services
Div. of Substance Abuse and MH
1901 N. DuPont Hwy., Main Bldg.
New Castle, DE 19720
Phone: 302-255-9399
Fax: 302-255-4428
Website: http://www.dhss
.delaware.gov/dsamh/index.html
E-mail: DHSSInfo@state.de.us

District of Columbia

Addiction, Prevention, and
Recovery Administration
1300 First St., NE
Washington, DC 20002
Phone: 202-727-8857
Fax: 202-442-9433
Website: http://
www.dchealth.dc.gov/doh

Florida

Substance Abuse Program Office
Dept. of Children and Families
1317 Winewood Blvd.
Building 6, 3rd Floor
Tallahassee, FL 32399
Phone: 850-414-9064
Fax: 850-922-4996
Website: http://www.dcf.state
.fl.us/mentalhealth/sa

Georgia
Addictive Diseases Program
Two Peachtree St., NW
22nd Fl., Suite 22-273
Atlanta, GA 30303
Toll-Free: 800-715-4225
Phone: 404-657-2331
Fax: 404-657-2256
Website: http://
mhddad.dhr.georgia.gov

Guam
Drug and Alcohol Treatment
Services
Dept. of Mental Health and
Substance Abuse
790 Governor Carlos Camacho Rd
Tamuning, GU 96913
Phone: 671-647-5330
Fax: 671-649-6948

Hawaii
Alcohol and Drug Abuse Division
Dept. of Health
601 Kamokila Blvd., Rm. 360
Kapolei, HI 96707
Phone: 808-692-7506
Fax: 808-692-7521
Website: http://hawaii.gov/
health/substance-abuse

Idaho
Div. of Behavioral Health
Dept. of Health and Welfare
450 W. State St., 3rd Fl.
P.O. Box 83720
Boise, ID 83720-0036
Toll-Free: 800-926-2588
Phone: 208-334-5935
Fax: 208-332-7305
Website: http://
healthandwelfare.idaho.gov

Illinois
Div. of Alcoholism and
Substance Abuse
Dept. of Human Services
401 S. Clinton St.
Chicago, IL 60607
Toll-Free: 800-843-6154
Toll-Free TTY: 800-447-6404
Website: http://www.dhs.state.il.
us/page.aspx?item=29725

Indiana
Div. of Mental Health and
Addiction
Family and Social Services
Administration
402 W. Washington St., Rm. W353
Indianapolis, IN 46204
Toll-Free: 800-457-8283
Phone: 317-232-7895
Fax: 317-233-3472
Website: http://www.in.gov/fssa/
dmha/index.htm

Iowa
Div. of Behavioral Health
Dept. of Public Health
Lucas State Office Bldg.
321 East 12th St.
Des Moines, IA 50319-0075
Toll-Free: 866-227-9878
Phone: 515-281-7689
Fax: 515-281-4535
Website: http://
www.idph.state.ia.us/bh/
substance_abuse.asp

Kansas

Addiction and Prevention
Services
Dept. of Social and Rehab
Services
915 Harrison St.
Topeka, KS 66612
Phone: 785-296-3959
TTY: 785-296-1491
Fax: 785-296.2173
Website: http://www.srskansas
.org/hcp/AAPSHome.htm

Kentucky

Div. of Mental Health and
Substance Abuse
Dept. for MH/MR Services
100 Fair Oaks Lane, 4E-D
Frankfort, KY 40621
Phone: 502-564-4456
Fax: 502-564-9010
Website: http://mhmr.ky.gov/
mhsas/

Louisiana

Office for Addictive Disorders
The Bienville Bldg.
628 N. 4th Street
P.O. Box 2790, Bin 18
Baton Rouge, LA 70821
Toll-Free: 877-664-2248
Phone: 225-342-6717
Fax: 225-342-3875
Website: http://www.dhh
.louisiana.gov/offices/?ID=23

Maine

Maine Office of Substance Abuse
41 Anthony Ave.
#11 State House Station
Augusta, ME 04333
Toll-Free (ME only): 800-499-0027
Toll-Free TTY: 800-606-0215
Phone: 207-287-2595
Fax: 207-287-8910
Website: http://www.maine.gov/
dhhs/osa
E-mail: osa.ircosa@maine.gov

Maryland

Alcohol and Drug Abuse
Administration
Dept. of Health and Mental
Hygiene
55 Wade Ave.
Catonsville, MD 21228
Phone: 410-402-8600
Fax: 410-402-8601
Website: http://maryland-adaa
.org/ka/index.cfm
E-mail:
adaainfo@dhmh.state.md.us

Massachusetts

Bureau of Substance Abuse
Services
Dept. of Public Health
250 Washington St.
Boston, MA 02108
Toll-Free: 800-327-5050
Toll-Free TTY: 888-448-8321
Website: http://www.mass.gov/
dph/bsas

Michigan
Bureau of Substance Abuse and
Addiction Services
320 S. Walnut
Lansing, MI 48913
Phone: 517-373-4700
TTY: 571-373-3573
Fax: 517-335-2121
Website: http://
www.michigan.gov/mdch-bsaas
E-mail: MDCH-BSAAS
@michigan.gov

Minnesota
Alcohol and Drug Abuse Division
Dept. of Human Services
P.O. Box 64977
Saint Paul, MN 55164
Phone: 651-431-2460
Fax: 651-431-7449
Website: http://
www.dhs.state.mn.us (click
Disabilities, then Alcohol and
Drug Abuse)
E-mail: dhs.adad@state.mn.us

Mississippi
Bureau of Alcohol and Drug
Abuse
Dept. of Mental Health
1101 Robert E Lee Bldg.
239 N. Lamar St.
Jackson, MS 39201
Toll-Free: 877-210-8513
Phone: 601-359-1288
Fax: 601-359-6295
TDD: 601-359-6230
Website: http://www.dmh.state
.ms.us/substance_abuse.htm

Missouri
Div. of Alcohol and Drug Abuse
Missouri Dept. of Mental Health
1706 East Elm St.
P.O. Box 687
Jefferson City, MO 65102
Toll-Free: 800-364-9687
Phone: 573-751-4122
TTY: 573-526-1201
Fax: 573-751-8224
Website: http://www.dmh
.missouri.gov/ada/adaindex.htm
E-mail: dmhmail@dmh.mo.gov

Montana
Addictive and Mental Disorders
Division
Dept. of PH and HS
555 Fuller Ave.
P.O. Box 202905
Helena, MT 59620
Phone: 406-444-3964
Fax: 406-444-9389
Website: http://
www.dphhs.mt.gov/amdd

Nebraska
DHHS Division of Behavioral
Health
P.O. Box 98925
Lincoln, NE 68509
Substance Abuse Hotline:
402-473-3818
Phone: 402-471-7818
Fax: 402-471-7859
Website: http://www.dhhs.ne
.gov/sua/suaindex.htm
E-mail:
BHDivision@dhhs.ne.gov

Nevada
DHHS Mental Health and
Developmental Services
4126 Technology Way. 2nd Floor
Carson City, NV 89706
Phone: 775-684-5943
Fax: 775-684-5964
Website: http://mhds.state.nv.us

New Hampshire
DHHS Bureau of Drug and
Alcohol Services
105 Pleasant St.
Concord, NH 03301
Phone: 603-271-6110
Fax: 603-271-6105
Website: http://
www.dhhs.state.nh.us/dhhs/
atod/a1-treatment

New Jersey
Div. of Addiction Services
P.O. Box 1004
Williamstown, NJ 08094
NJ Addictions Hotline:
800-238-2333
Website: http://
www.njdrughotline.org/
E-mail: contact
@addictionshotlineofnj.org

New Mexico
Behavioral Health Services Div.
Dept. of Health
37 Plaza la Prensa
P.O. Box 2348
Santa Fe, NM 87504
Toll-Free: 800-396-3221
Phone: 505-476-9275
Fax: 505-476-9277
Website: http://
www.bhc.state.nm.us

New York
Office of Alcoholism and
Substance Abuse Services
1450 Western Ave.
Albany, NY 12203
Phone: 518-473-3460
Website: http://www.oasas.state
.ny.us/index.cfm
E-mail: communications@oasas
.state.ny.us

North Carolina
Community Policy Management
Div. of MH/DD/SA Services
325 N. Salisbury St., Suite 679-C
3007 Mail Service Center
Raleigh, NC 27699
Toll-Free: 800-662-7030
Phone: 919-733-4670
Fax: 919-733-4556
Website: http://
www.dhhs.state.nc.us/mhddsas
E-mail: contactdmh@ncmail.net

North Dakota
Div. of MH and SA Services
Dept. of Human Services
1237 W. Divide Ave., Suite 1C
Bismarck, ND 58501
Toll-Free (ND only): 800-755-2719
Phone: 701-328-8920
Fax: 701-328-8969
Website: http://www.nd.gov/dhs/
services/mentalhealth
E-mail: dhsmhsas@nd.gov

Ohio

Dept. of Alcohol and Drug
Addiction Services
280 N. High St., 12th Fl.
Columbus, OH 43215
Toll-Free: 800-788-7254
Phone: 614-466-3445
Fax: 614-752-8645
Website: http://
www.ada.ohio.gov/public
E-mail: info@ada.ohio.gov

Oklahoma

ODMHSAS
1200 NE 13th St.
P.O. Box 53277
Oklahoma City, OK 73152
Toll-Free: 800-522-9054
Phone: 405-522-3908
TDD: 405-522-3851
Fax: 405-522-0650
Website: http://www.odmhsas.org

Oregon

Addictions and Mental Health Div.
Dept. of Human Services
500 Summer St. NE E86
Salem, OR 97301
Phone: 503-945-5763
Fax: 503-378-8467
Website: http://www.oregon.gov/
DHS/addiction/index.shtml
E-mail: oadap.info@state.or.us

Pennsylvania

Bureau of Drug and Alcohol
Programs
Pennsylvania Dept. of Health
02 Kline Plaza
Harrisburg, PA 17104
Toll-Free: 877-724-3258
Phone: 717-783-8200

Puerto Rico

Mental Health and Anti-
Addiction Services
Administration
P.O. Box 21414
San Juan, PR 00928
Toll-Free 800-981-0023
Phone: 787-764-3795 x1229
Fax: 787-765-5888
Website: http://www.gobierno.pr/
assmca/inicio

Rhode Island

Div. of Behavioral Health
14 Harrington Rd.
Cranston, RI 02920
Phone: 401-462-4680
Fax: 401-462-6078
Website: http://
www.mhrh.ri.gov/SA

South Carolina

SC Dept. of Alcohol and Other
Drug Abuse Services
101 Executive Ctr. Dr., Suite 215
Columbia, SC 29210
Phone: 803-896-5555
Fax: 803-896-5557
Website: http://
www.daodas.state.sc.us

South Dakota

DHS Div. of Alcohol and Drug
Abuse
E. Hwy. 34, Hillsview Plaza
500 E. Capitol
Pierre, SD 57501
Phone: 605-773-3123
Fax: 605-773-7076
Website: http://dhs.sd.gov
E-mail:
infodada@dhs.state.sd.us

Tennessee

Dept. of Mental Health and DD
TN Dept. of Health
Cordell Hull Bldg., 1st Fl
425 Fifth Ave. N.
Nashville, TN 37243
Toll-Free Crisis: 800-809-9957
Phone: 615-741-3111
Website: http://
health.state.tn.us/index.htm
E-mail: tn.health@tn.gov

Texas

DSHS Substance Abuse Services
P. O. Box 149347
Austin, TX 78714
Toll-Free: 866-378-8440
Phone: 512-206-5000
Fax: 512-206-5714
Website: http://www.dshs.state
.tx.us/sa/default.shtm
E-mail: contact@dshs.state.tx.us

Utah

Div. of Substance Abuse and
Mental Health
Utah Dept. of Human Services
120 N. 200 W. Rm. 209
Salt Lake City, UT 84103
Phone: 801-538-3939
Fax: 801-538-9892
Website: http://
www.dsamh.utah.gov
E-mail:
dsamhwebmaster@utah.gov

Vermont

Alcohol and Drug Abuse
Programs
Dept. of Health
108 Cherry St.
Burlington, VT 05402
Toll-Free (VT only):
800-464-4343
Phone: 802-863-7200
Fax: 802-865-7754
Website: http://healthvermont
.gov/adap/adap.aspx
E-mail: vtadap@vdh.state.vt.us

Virginia

Office of Substance Abuse
Services
Dept. of MH, MR and SAS
P.O. Box 1797
Richmond, VA 23218
Phone: 804-786-3906
Fax: 804-786-4320
Website: http://www.dbhds
.virginia.gov/OSAS-default.htm

Virgin Islands

Div. of MH, Alcoholism, and
Drug Dependency Services
Dept. of Health
Barbel Plaza, 2nd Fl.
Christiansted, VI 00820
Phone: 340-774-4888
Fax: 340-774-4701

Washington

Div. of Alcohol and Substance
Abuse
Dept. of Social and Health
Services
P.O. Box 45130
Olympia, WA 98504
Toll-Free (WA only):
800-562-1240
Phone: 877-301-4557
Fax: 360-586-0341
Website: http://
www.dshs.wa.gov/DASA
E-mail:
DASAInformation@dshs.wa.gov

West Virginia

Bureau for Behavioral Health
and Health Facilities
350 Capitol St., Rm. 350
Charleston, WV 25301
Phone: 304-558-0627
Fax: 304-558-1008
Website: http://www.wvdhhr.org/
bhhf/ada.asp
E-mail: obhs@wvdhhr.org

Wisconsin

Bureau of Prevention,
Treatment, and Recovery
1 W. Wilson St.
P.O. Box 7851
Madison, WI 53707
Phone: 608-266-2717
Toll-Free TTY: 888-701-1251
Fax: 608-266-1533
Website: http://dhs.wisconsin
.gov/substabuse/INDEX.HTM

Wyoming

Mental Health and Substance
Abuse Services Division
6101 Yellowstone Rd.
Suite 220
Cheyenne, WY 82002
Toll-Free: 800-535-4006
Phone: 307-777-6494
Fax: 307-777-5849
Website: http://wdh.state.wy.us/
mhsa/index.html

Chapter 88

Directory of Organizations with Information about Drug Abuse

Government Organizations

Center for Substance Abuse Treatment (SAMHSA)
Toll-Free: 800-662-4357
Toll-Free TDD: 800-487-4889
Phone: 240-276-2750
Website: http://csat.samhsa.gov
Substance Abuse Treatment Facility Locator: http://www.findtreatment.samhsa.gov

Centers for Disease Control and Prevention (CDC)
1600 Clifton Rd.
Atlanta, GA 30333
Toll-Free: 800-CDC-INFO (232-4636)
Toll-Free TTY: 888-232-6348
Website: http://www.cdc.gov
E-mail: cdcinfo@cdc.gov

Division of Workplace Programs (SAMHSA)
Toll-Free: 800-843-4971
Website: http://www.workplace.samhsa.gov

Drug Enforcement Administration (DEA)
Office of Diversion Control
8701 Morrissette Dr.
Mailstop: AES
Springfield, VA 22152
Toll-Free: 800-882-9539
Phone: 202-307-1000
Website: http://www.justice.gov/dea
E-mail ODE@usdoj.gov

Resources in this chapter were compiled from several sources deemed reliable; all contact information was verified and updated in November 2009.

Drug Policy Information Clearinghouse

Office of National Drug Control Policy
P.O. Box 6000
Rockville, MD 20849
Toll-Free: 800-666-3332
Fax: 301-519-5212
Website: http://
www.whitehousedrugpolicy.gov/
about/clearingh.html

Health Information Network (SAMHSA)

P.O. Box 2345
Rockville, MD 20847
Toll-Free: 877-726-4727
Toll-Free TTY: 800-487-4889
Fax: 240-221-4292
Website: http://www.samhsa.gov/
shin
E-mail: SHIN@samhsa.hhs.gov

National Criminal Justice Reference Service (NCJRS)

P.O. Box 6000
Rockville, MD 20849
Toll-Free: 800-851-3420
Toll-Free TTY: 877-712-9279
Phone: 301-519-5500 (international callers)
Fax: 301-519-5212
Website: http://www.ncjrs.gov

National Drug Intelligence Center

U.S. Department of Justice
Robert F. Kennedy Bldg.
Rm. 1335
950 Pennsylvania Ave., NW
Washington, DC 20530
Phone: 202-532-4040
Website: http://www.justice.gov/
ndic
E-mail:
NDIC.Contacts@usdoj.gov

National Institute on Alcohol Abuse and Alcoholism (NIAAA)

5635 Fishers Ln., MSC 9304
Bethesda, MD 20892
Phone: 301-443-3860
Website: http://
www.niaaa.nih.gov
E-mail: niaaaweb-
r@exchange.nih.gov

National Institute on Drug Abuse (NIDA)

6001 Executive Blvd., Rm. 5213
Bethesda, MD 20892
Phone: 301-443-1124
Fax: 301-443-7397
Websites: http://www.nida.nih
.gov; and
http://www.drugabuse.gov
E-mail:
information@nida.nih.gov

National Institute on Drug Abuse (NIDA) Sponsored Websites

http://www.backtoschool
.drugabuse.gov
http://www.clubdrugs.gov
http://www.hiv.drugabuse.gov
http://www.inhalants.drugabuse
.gov
http://www.marijuana-info.org
http://www.researchstudies
.drugabuse.gov
http://www.smoking.drugabuse
.gov
http://www.steroidabuse.gov
http://www.teens.drugabuse.gov

National Mental Health Information Center

Substance Abuse and Mental
Health Services Administration
P.O. Box 2345
Washington, DC 20847
Toll-Free: 800-789-2647
Toll-Free TDD: 866-889-2647
Phone: 240-221-4021
Fax: 240-221-4295
Website: http://
mentalhealth.samhsa.gov
E-mail: info@mentalhealth.org

Office of Applied Studies (OAS) (SAMHSA)

Phone: 240-276-1212
Website: http://www.oas.samhsa
.gov
E-mail: oaspubs@samhsa.hhs.gov

Office of National Drug Control Policy (ONDCP)

Drug Policy Information Clear-
inghouse
P.O. Box 6000
Rockville, MD 20849
Toll Free: 800-666-3332
Fax: 301-519-5212
Website: http://
www.whitehousedrugpolicy.gov
E-mail: ondcp@ncjrs.gov

ONDCP Sponsored Websites

Above the Influence: http://
www.abovetheinfluence.com
MethResources.gov: http://
www.methresources.gov
National Youth Anti-Media
Campaign: http://www
.whitehousedrugpolicy.gov/
mediacampaign
Pushing Back: http://
pushingback.com

Safe and Drug-Free Schools

400 Maryland Ave. SW
Washington, DC 20202
Toll-Free: 800-872-5327
Toll-Free TTY: 800-437-0833
Phone: 202-260-3954
Fax: 202-401-0689
Website: http://www.ed.gov/
offices/OESE/SDFS
E-mail: safeschl@ed.gov

Substance Abuse and Mental Health Services Administration (SAMHSA)
1 Choke Cherry Rd.
Rockville, MD 20857
Phone: 240-276-2130
Website: http://www.samhsa.gov

U.S. Department of Labor
Working Partners' Drug-Free Workplace Advisor Policy Builder
Website: http://www.dol.gov/elaws/asp/drugfree/drugs/screen1.asp

U.S. Food and Drug Administration (FDA)
10903 New Hampshire Ave.
Silver Spring, MD 20993
Toll-Free: 888-INFO-FDA (463-6332)
Website: http://www.fda.gov

Private Organizations

Alcoholics Anonymous (AA)
AA World Services, Inc.
P.O. Box 459
New York, NY 10163
Phone: 212-870-3400
Website: http://www.aa.org

Al-Anon
1600 Corporate Landing Pkwy.
Virginia Beach, VA 23454
Phone: 757-563-1600
Fax: 757-563-1655
Website: http://www.al-anon.alateen.org
E-mail: wso@al-anon.org

Center of Alcohol Studies
Rutgers, the State University of New Jersey
607 Allison Rd.
Piscataway, NJ 08854
Phone: 732-445-2190
Fax: 732-445-5300
Website: http://www.alcoholstudies.rutgers.edu

Co-Anon Family Groups World Services
P.O. Box 12722
Tuscon, AZ 85732
Toll-Free National Referral Line: 800-347-8998
Toll-Free: 800-898-9985
Phone: 520-513-5028
Website: http://www.co-anon.org
E-mail: info@co-anon.org

Cocaine Anonymous World Services
P.O. Box 492000
Los Angeles, CA 90049
Phone: 310-559-5833
Fax: 310-559-2554
Website: http://www.ca.org
E-mail: cawso@ca.org

Do It Now Foundation (Drug Information)
P.O. Box 27568
Tempe, AZ 85285
Phone: 480-736-0599
Fax: 480-736-0771
Website: http://www.doitnow.org
E-mail: email@doitnow.org

Higher Education Center for Alcohol and Other Drug Abuse and Violence Prevention
Education Development Center, Inc.
55 Chapel St.
Newton, MA 02458
Toll-Free: 800-676-1730
Fax: 617-928-1537
Website: http://www.higheredcenter.org
E-mail: HigherEdCtr@edc.org

NAADAC–The Association for Addiction Professionals
1001 N. Fairfax St. Suite 201
Alexandria, VA 22314
Toll-Free: 800-548-0497
Fax: 800-377-1136
Website: http://www.naadac.org
E-mail: naadac@naadac.org

Narcotics Anonymous
P.O. Box 9999
Van Nuys, CA 91409
Phone: 818-773-9999
Fax: 818-700-0700
Website: http://www.na.org

National Association for Children of Alcoholics
11426 Rockville Pike, Suite 301
Rockville, MD 20852
Toll-Free: 888-55-4COAS (2627)
Phone: 301-468-0985
Fax: 301-468-0987
Website: http://www.nacoa.net
E-mail: nacoa@nacoa.org

National Association of Addiction Treatment Providers
313 W. Liberty St.
Suite 129
Lancaster, PA 17603
Phone: 717-392-8480
Fax: 717-392-8481
Website: http://www.naatp.org
E-mail: rhunsicker@naatp.org

National Center on Addiction and Substance Abuse at Columbia University (CASA)
633 Third Ave., 19th Fl.
New York, NY 10017
Phone: 212-841-5200
Fax: 212-956-8020
Website: http://www.casacolumbia.org

National Council on Alcoholism and Drug Dependence
244 East 58th St., 4th Fl.
New York, NY 10022
Toll-Free Hopeline:
800-NCA-CALL (622-2255)
Phone: 212-269-7797
Fax: 212-269-7510
Website: http://www.ncadd.org
E-mail: national@ncadd.org

National Parents Resource Institute for Drug Education (PRIDE)
PRIDE Youth Programs
4 W. Oak St.
Fremont, MI 49412
Toll Free: 800-668-9277
Phone: 231-924-1662
Fax: 231-924-5663
Website: http://
www.prideyouthprograms.org
E-mail:
info@pridyouthprograms.org

Nemours Foundation
1600 Rockland Rd.
Wilmington, DE 19803
Phone: 302-651-4000
Website: http://
www.kidshealth.org
E-mail: info@kidshealth.org

Partnership for a Drug-Free America
405 Lexington Ave.
Suite 1601
New York, NY 10174
Phone: 212-922-1560
Fax: 212-922-1570
Website: http://
www.drugfreeamerica.org

Students Against Destructive Decisions (SADD)
255 Main Street
Marlborough, MA 01752
Toll Free: 877-SADD-INC
(7233-462)
Fax: 508-481-5759
Website: http://www.sadd.org
E-mail: info@sadd.org

Index

Index

Page numbers followed by 'n' indicate a footnote. Page numbers in *italics* indicate a table or illustration.

A

AA *see* Alcoholics Anonymous
abuser, defined 551
Abyssinian tea (slang) 189
acamprosate 392
acetaminophen, oxycodone use 217–19
Actiq (fentanyl) 161–62
A.D.A.M., Inc., drug abuse first aid publication 375n
Adderall 228
addiction
  club drugs 314–15
  defined 551
  influential factors 251–57
  marijuana 205–6
  methamphetamine 214
  overview 245–49
  questionnaire 305–8
  treatment approaches 389–94
  various viewpoints 379–81
ADHD *see* attention deficit hyperactivity disorder
"Adolescent Admission Reporting Inhalants: 2006" (SAMHSA) 323n

adolescents
  comorbidity 344
  dextromethorphan 145–47
  drug abuse prevention 506–19
  drugged driving 109
  drug use signs 366–72
  gang activity 105–6
  marijuana 202
  substance use disorders 65–71
"Adolescents at Risk for Substance Use Disorders" (NIAAA) 65n
adulterant, defined 551
African salad (slang) 189
African woodbine (slang) 557
age factor
  hallucinogens 317
  OTC medications misuse *271*
  pain reliever abuse 278–81
  prescription drug abuse 275–77
  self-help groups *412*
  substance abuse 351–53
  substance abuse mortality
    rates 16–18
  substance abuse statistics 4–9, *5*, *6*, *8*
  substance first-time use 45–51
  suicidal thoughts *358*
  various viewpoints 379
  workplace substance abuse 97–98
agonies (slang) 557

589

AIDS (acquired immune deficiency
   syndrome), substance abuse 334–39
air blast (slang) 557
airhead (slang) 557
airplane (slang) 558
Alabama, substance abuse agency
   contact information 571
Al-Anon, contact information 537,
   584
Alaska, substance abuse agency
   contact information 571
Al Capone (slang) 558
alcohol, defined 551
"Alcohol Abuse Makes Prescription
   Drug Abuse More Likely" (NIDA)
   302n
Alcoholics Anonymous (AA),
   contact information 537, 584
alcoholism, defined 551
"Alcohol or Other Drug-Use
   Prevention" (CDC) 528n
alcohol use
   addiction treatment 392–93
   adolescent substance use *74*
   cocaine 143
   medical consequences 310–11
   motor vehicle accidents 108
   polydrug use 298–302
   pregnancy 55–57
   prescription drug abuse 302–4
   signs and symptoms 367
   treatment statistics 467–68
   use statistics *296*
   women *90*
Alice B. Toklas (slang) 558
all lit up (slang) 558
all star (slang) 558
"Alpha-Methyltryptamine"
   (DEA) 235n
alpha-methyltryptamine (AMT),
   overview 235–37
alprazolam 153–54, *283*
American Association for Clinical
   Chemistry, drug tests
   publications 486n, 488n
American Samoa, substance abuse
   agency contact information 571
Americans with Disabilities Act
   (ADA; 1990) 451, 453, 540

"Am I an Addict?" (Narcotics
   Anonymous) 305n
amidone (slang) 207
amoeba (slang) 558
amp (slang) 558
amped (slang) 558
amp head (slang) 558
amphetamines
   adolescent substance use *74*
   defined 551
   drug screens *487*
   effects *265*
   medical consequences 311
amp joint (slang) 558
AMT *see* alpha-methyltryptamine
AMT (slang) 558
amyl nitrate
   effects *265*
   medical consequences 324
Amytal *289*
Anabolic Steroid Control Acts
   (1990; 2004) 121–22, 179
anabolic steroids
   effects *265*
   overview 119–22
   see also steroids
"Anabolic Steroids" (DEA) 119n
"Anabolic Steroids: Hidden
   Dangers" (DEA) 119n
anadrol (slang) 558
angel (slang) 558
angel dust (slang) 221, 555, 558
angie (slang) 558
animal tranquilizer (slang) 558
Anti-Drug Abuse Act (1986) 26
antifreeze (slang) 558
Apache (slang) 161, 558
apple jacks (slang) 558
Arizona, substance abuse
   agency contact information 571
Arkansas, substance abuse agency
   contact information 572
Arnolds (slang) 119, 558
arrests, minority substance
   abuse 95–96
   see also criminal justice
      system; inmates
artillery (slang) 558
ashes (slang) 558

aspirin (slang) 558
assassin of youth (slang) 558
assay, defined 551
assertive community treatment,
  described 421
astro turf (slang) 558
Atarax *283*
Ativan (lorazepam) 153–54, *283*
atom bomb (slang) 558
attention deficit hyperactivity
  disorder (ADHD)
  comorbidity 344–45
  described 67
  medications overview 225–30
A2 (slang) 131
Aunt Hazel (slang) 558
Aunt Mary (slang) 558
Aunt Nora (slang) 558
aurora borealis (slang) 558
author (slang) 558
Ava (slang) 181
Ayahuasca 149

B

baby food (slang) 185
baby habit (slang) 558
baby T (slang) 558
BAC *see* blood alcohol concentration
back breakers (slang) 559
badrock (slang) 559
bagging (slang) 559
baker (slang) 559
bale (slang) 559
ball (slang) 559
banana split (slang) 559
banano (slang) 559
bang (slang) 559
banging (slang) 559
barbies (slang) 559
barbiturates
  defined 552
  drug screens *487*
  sedative abuse *289*
barbs (slang) 559
base (slang) 559
baseball (slang) 559
bash (slang) 559

basing, described 140
batman (slang) 559
battery acid (slang) 559
bazooka (slang) 559
beam (slang) 559
beam me up Scotty (slang) 559
beast (slang) 559
beautiful (slang) 123
bed bugs (slang) 559
beemers (slang) 559
"Behavior" (DEA) 366n
behavioral therapy
  drug addictions 393–94
  mental disorders 420–21
Bellack, Alan S. 422–24
belladonna (slang) 559
Belushi (slang) 559
bender (slang) 559
bennie (slang) 559
benzene 324
benzodiazepines
  defined 552
  effects *264*
  overview 153–54
"Benzodiazepines" (DEA) 153n
biak (slang) 193
big man (slang) 559
bing (slang) 559
bingo (slang) 559
birdie powder (slang) 559
biscuit (slang) 560
black beauties (slang) 560
black dust (slang) 560
black gold (slang) 560
black mollies (slang) 560
black pearl (slang) 560
black tar heroin 171
blanket (slang) 560
blast (slang) 560
block busters (slang) 560
blood alcohol concentration
  (BAC), defined 552
blotter acid (slang) 560
blue (slang) 560
blue devil (slang) 560
blue mystic (slang) 123
blunt (slang) 202, 560
boat (slang) 221
boldenone 119

bolo (slang) 560
bolt (slang) 560
bong 201
bonita (slang) 560
book (slang) 560
boom (slang) 201, 560
bopper (slang) 560
boppers (slang) 560
brain pills (slang) 560
brains
  comorbidity 343–44
  inhalants 323–27
  medications 259–62
brick (slang) 560
brief strategic family therapy,
  described 420
broccoli (slang) 560
bromo (slang) 560
brown bombers (slang) 560
brown crystal (slang) 560
brownies (slang) 560
brown sugar (slang) 171, 560
bubble gum (slang) 560
bumblebees (slang) 560
Buprenex 127–28
buprenorphine
  described 174, 392
  overview 127–29
"Buprenorphine" (DEA) 127n
bupropion 392
bushman's tea (slang) 189
BuSpar *283*
Butisol *289*
butter (slang) 560
butyl nitrate
  effects *265*
  medical consequences 324
buzz bomb (slang) 560
BZP (slang) 131

C

cactus (slang) 560
Cadillac (slang) 560
cakes (slang) 561
California, substance abuse agency
  contact information 572
cancer, marijuana 203

candy sugar (slang) 561
cannabinoids, defined 552
cannabis, effects *265*
  see also marijuana
CASA *see* National Center on
  Addiction and Substance Abuse
cash (slang) 161
Casper (slang) 561
Casper the ghost (slang) 561
cat (slang) 561
catnip (slang) 561
cat valium (slang) 185, 561
CCC (slang) 145
CDC *see* Centers for Disease
  Control and Prevention
Center for Substance Abuse
  Treatment, contact information 581
Center of Alcohol Studies, contact
  information 584
Centers for Disease Control
  and Prevention (CDC)
  contact information 581
  publications
    drug overdoses 15n
    health education 528n
    syringe exchange programs 337n
chalk (slang) 41, 561
Charley (slang) 561
Charlie (slang) 561
chat (slang) 189
cheap basing (slang) 561
cheese (slang) 561
chemical (slang) 561
chemical dependency, defined 552
chemo (slang) 561
cherry meth (slang) 561
chief (slang) 561
children
  drug discussions 497–99
  human growth hormone 177
  interventions 383–87
  methamphetamine 12
  stress, substance abuse 256
  substance abuse 54–64
children of alcoholics
  adolescents 66
  described 62–64
China girl (slang) 561
china girl (slang) 161

China white (slang) 561
china white (slang) 161
Chinese molasses (slang) 561
Chinese red (slang) 561
Chinese tobacco (slang) 561
chip (slang) 561
chloral hydrate *289*
chlorinated hydrocarbons 324
chocolate (slang) 561
chocolate chip cookies (slang) 207
chronic (slang) 201
cigarette smoke *see* environmental
  tobacco smoke; tobacco use
circles (slang) 561
cleaning fluids *see* inhalants
clear (slang) 561
clen (slang) 135
"Clenbuterol" (DEA) 135n
clenbuterol, overview 135–37
climb (slang) 561
clonazepam 153–54
cloud (slang) 561
club drugs, medical
  consequences 313–16
CMEA *see* Combat
  Methamphetamine Epidemic Act
Co-Anon Family Groups World
  Services, contact information 584
cocaethylene 143
cocaine
  adolescents *81*
  adolescent substance use *74*
  benzodiazepines 154
  defined 552
  drug screens *487*
  effects *264*
  first-time use statistics *47*, *48*, 49
  medical consequences 311
  minority substance abuse *94*
  overview 139–43
  paraphernalia 373
  pregnancy 58
  signs and symptoms 367
  use statistics *5*, *6*, *8*, *296*
  women *88*, *90*
"Cocaine" (DEA) 139n
Cocaine Anonymous World Services,
  contact information 584
coconut (slang) 561

codeine
  drug screens *487*
  effects *264*
coffee (slang) 561
cognitive behavioral therapy,
  described 420
coke (slang) 139, 561
cola (slang) 561
colas (slang) 561
Colliver, James 304
Colorado, substance abuse agency
  contact information 572
"The Combat Meth Act of 2005:
  Questions and Answers" (DEA) 41n
"Combat Methamphetamine Act of
  2005" (DEA) 41n
Combat Methamphetamine Epidemic
  Act (CMEA; 2005) 41–43
combination drugs *see* comorbidity;
  dual diagnosis; multiple substance
  abuse; polydrug use
"Community-Based Treatment
  Benefits Methamphetamine
  Abusers" (NIDA) 415n
comorbidity
  defined 552
  drug abuse treatment 419–25
  overview 341–45
  see also dual diagnosis;
    multiple substance abuse
"Comorbidity: Addiction and Other
  Mental Illnesses" (NIDA) 341n,
  419n, 551n
Comprehensive Crime Control Act
  (1984) 25–26
Comprehensive Drug Abuse
  Prevention and Control Act
  (1970) 21
Concerta 225, 228
conduct disorder, described 67
conductor (slang) 561
"Congress Passes Ryan Haight
  Online Pharmacy Consumer
  Protection Act" (DEA) 21n
Connecticut, substance abuse
  agency contact information 572
contact lens (slang) 561
controlled substance analogue,
  described 26

controlled substances
  prescriptions 30–33
  record keeping
    requirements 26–27
Controlled Substances Act (CSA;
  1970)
  amendments 33, 121–22
  overview 21–28
Convention on Psychotropic
  Substances (1971) 26
"Co-Occurrence of Substance Use
  Behaviors in Youth" (DOJ) 101n
cookies (slang) 562
coolie (slang) 562
Coricidin 145
cotton (slang) 562
cough medicines, misuse
  overview 269–71
courage pills (slang) 562
crack (slang) 139
"Crack and Cocaine" (NIDA) 139n
crack cocaine *see* cocaine
crank (slang) 41
cravings, addiction 247
crazy coke (slang) 562
criminal justice system
  drug abuse treatment 428–36
  drug addiction treatment 394
  drug use 101–6
  methamphetamine
    treatment options 418
  see also arrests; inmates
crying weed (slang) 562
crystal (slang) 41, 562
crystal joint (slang) 562
crystal meth (slang) 562
crystal tea (slang) 562
Cylert *286*

D

Dalmane *289*
dance fever (slang) 161, 562
DAWN *see* Drug Abuse Warning
  Network
DEA *see* Drug Enforcement
  Administration
death rates *see* mortality rates

Delaware, substance abuse agency
  contact information 572
delirium tremens (DT),
  withdrawal 402
delta-9-tetrahydrocannabinol
  (THC)
  defined 555
  described 37, 38–39, 201
  drugged driving 108–10
demolish (slang) 562
Department of Justice (DOJ)
  see US Department of Justice
Department of Labor (DOL)
  see US Department of Labor
dependence, described 348
  see also addiction; physical
    dependence; psychological
    dependence
depressants
  defined 552
  effects *264*
  signs and symptoms 368
depression
  adolescents 80, 82–86
  inhalants 326–27
  substance abuse 355–62
dep-testosterone (slang) 562
designer drugs, defined 552
Desoxyn *286*
"Detailed Signs and Symptoms"
  (National Youth Anti-Drug
  Media Campaign) 366n
detoxification
  heroin 173–75
  methadone 208
  overview 395–99
  see also withdrawal
"Detoxification and Substance
  Abuse Treatment: A Treatment
  Protocol TIP 45" (SAMHSA) 395n
Detroit pink (slang) 562
devil drug (slang) 562
dew (slang) 562
Dexedrine *286*
Dextroamphetamine *286*
"Dextromethorphan" (DEA) 145n
dextromethorphan (DXM)
  misuse overview 269–71
  overview 145–47

dialectical behavior therapy, described 421
diamonds (slang) 562
diazepam 153–54, *283*
　drug screens *487*
dice (slang) 562
Didrex *286*
diesel (slang) 562
diet pills (slang) 562
diet pills, stimulant abuse *286*
"Digital Monitoring" (DEA) 501n
dip (slang) 562
dipper (slang) 562
dirt (slang) 562
District of Columbia (Washington, DC), substance abuse agency contact information 572
disulfiram 392
diviner's sage (slang) 231
divinorin A, overview 231–33
Division of Workplace Programs, contact information 581
"D-Lysergic Acid Diethylamide" (DEA) 197n
DMT *see* N,N-dimethyltryptamine
DOA (slang) 562
Dr. Feel Good (slang) 562
Do It Now Foundation, contact information 584
DOJ *see* US Department of Justice
DOL *see* US Department of Labor
Dolophine 207
"Don't Put Your Health in the Hands of Crooks: Illegal Online Pharmacies: (FBI) 33n
dopamine
　cocaine 141–42
　defined 553
　drug abuse 247
　medications 261
dope (slang) 171, 562
down (slang) 562
downers (slang)
　defined 553
　described 562
　overview 153–54
dragon (slang) 171
dragon rock (slang) 562

drug abuse
　defined 553
　effects 263–67, *264–65*
　first aid 375–78
　influential factors 251–57
　medical consequences overview 309–12
　overview 245–49
　reduction methods 479–83
　see also substance abuse
"Drug Abuse First Aid" (A.D.A.M., Inc.) 375n
Drug Abuse Warning Network (DAWN) 88, 359–61
"Drug Abusing Offenders Not Getting Treatment They Need in Criminal Justice System" (NIDA) 432n
drug courts, overview 428–31
"Drug Endangered Children" (CASA) 59n
drug endangered children, overview 59–64
Drug Endangered Children Act (2007) 60
Drug Enforcement Administration (DEA)
　contact information 581
　publications
　　alpha-methyltryptamine 235n
　　anabolic steroids 119n
　　benzodiazepines 153n
　　buprenorphine 127n
　　clenbuterol 135n
　　cocaine 139n
　　dextromethorphan 145n
　　drug paraphernalia 372n
　　drug use behavior 366n
　　fentanyl 161n
　　5-methoxy-N,N-diisopropyl-tryptamine 165n
　　4-bromo-2,5-dimethoxy-phenethylamine 239n
　　4-iodo-2,5-dimethoxy-phenethylamine 115n
　　gamma hydroxybutyric acid 167n
　　home safety 501n
　　human growth hormone 177n

Drug Enforcement Administration
(DEA), continued
  publications, continued
    kava 181n
    ketamine 185n
    kratom 193n
    LSD 197n
    medical marijuana 36n
    methadone 207n
    methamphetamine 41n
    methylphenidate 225n
    N-benzylpiperazine 131n
    "N,N-dimethyltryptamine 149n
    online pharmacies 21n
    oxycodone 217n
    phencyclidine 221n
    prescriptions 30n
    Salvia divinorum 231n
    2,5-dimethoxy-4-(n)-propyl-
      thiophenethylamine 123n
drugged driving
  marijuana 204–5
  overview 107–12
drug overdose, first aid 375–78
drug paraphernalia, overview
  372–74
Drug Policy Information
  Clearinghouse, contact
  information 582
"Drugs, Brains, and Behavior:
  The Science of Addiction (Part I)"
  (NIDA) 251n
"Drugs, Brains, and Behavior:
  The Science of Addiction (Part III)"
  (NIDA) 259n
"Drugs, Brains, and Behavior:
  The Science of Addiction (Part IV)"
  (NIDA) 309n
drugs, defined 553
"Drugs and Gangs Fast Facts:
  Questions and Answers" (DOJ)
  101n
"Drugs of Abuse" (DOJ) 21n
"Drugs of Abuse/Uses and
  Effects" (DOJ) 263n
drug tests
  home use tests 494–96
  overview 486–93
"Drug Use and Crime" (DOJ) 101n

dual diagnosis
  defined 552
  overview 341–45
  see also comorbidity; multiple
    substance abuse; polydrug use
duji (slang) 562
Duragesic (fentanyl) 161–63
dynamite (slang) 562

E

EAP *see* employee assistance
  programs
easy lay (slang) 167
E-bombs (slang) 562
ecstasy (MDMA)
  adolescent substance use *74*
  described 48, 562
  effects *265*
  first-time use statistics 50
  medical consequences 311,
    317–22
  minority substance abuse *94*
  overview 155–59
  paraphernalia 373
  phencyclidine 222
  signs and symptoms 368
  use statistics *318*
  women *88*
education levels, residential
  substance abuse treatment
  facilities 474–75
elephant (slang) 563
Elvis (slang) 563
embalming fluid (slang) 563
employee assistance
  programs (EAP)
  defined 553
  overview 438–41
  substance abuse 447–49
"Employment Status Abuse
  Treatment Admissions: 2006"
  (SAMHSA) 444n
enabling, defined 553
environmental factors
  addiction 248
  adolescent substance use 68–70
  children of substance abusers 63

environmental tobacco smoke (ETS)
  children 60–61
  drug addiction 310
ephedrine, described 41–42
Equanil *283*
Eskatrol *286*
ethnic factors
  methamphetamine treatment
    options *418*
  OTC medications misuse *271*
  residential substance abuse
    treatment facilities 474
  self-help groups *412*
  substance abuse 93–96
  substance abuse mortality rates 17
ethyl alcohol, defined 553
executive cognitive dysfunction,
  described 67
exposure therapy, described 421
eye opener (slang) 563

F

"Facility Locator" (SAMHSA) 571n
FAE *see* fetal alcohol effects
Fair Housing Act (FHA) 451, 455
Fair Labor Standards Act (FLSA) 539
Family and Medical Leave Act
  (FMLA) 454
family issues
  adolescent depression 86
  adolescents drug abuse
    prevention 506–19
  adolescent substance use 69–71
  children, drug discussions 497–99
  home safety 501–3
  parental substance abuse 60–64
  prisoners 102
  substance abuse 60–64
  see also adolescents; children
"Family Matters: Substance Abuse
  and The American Family" (CASA)
  54n, 59n
family therapy, mental disorders 420
FAS *see* fetal alcohol syndrome
FASD *see* fetal alcohol spectrum
  disorder
fast white lady (slang) 563

FBI *see* Federal Bureau of
  Investigation
FDA *see* US Food and Drug
  Administration
Federal Bureau of Investigation
  (FBI), online pharmacies
  publication 33n
fentanyl
  overview 161–63
  substance abuse
    mortality rates 17
"Fentanyl" (DEA) 161n
Fentora (fentanyl) 161
fetal alcohol effects (FAE),
  described 56
fetal alcohol spectrum disorder
  (FASD), described 55–56
fetal alcohol syndrome (FAS),
  described 56
financial considerations
  drug abuse 11–13, 245
  drug courts 429
finger (slang) 563
fire (slang) 41
first aid, drug abuse 375–78
"5-Methoxy-N,N-Diisopropyl-
  tryptamine" (DEA) 165n
5-methoxy-N,N-
  diisopropyltryptamine,
  overview 165–66
fives (slang) 563
fizzies (slang) 207, 563
flea powder (slang) 563
Flexeril *283*
Florida, substance abuse agency
  contact information 572
Florida snow (slang) 563
flower (slang) 563
flunitrazepam 154
Focalin 225
Food, Drug, and Cosmetic Act 36, 39
Food and Drug Administration
  (FDA) *see* US Food and Drug
  Administration
forget me drug (slang) 563
"4-Bromo-2,5-Dimethoxy-
  phenethylamine" (DEA) 239n
4-bromo-2,5-dimethoxy-
  phenethylamine, overview 239–41

"4-Iodo-2,5-Dimethoxy-
  phenethylamine" (DEA) 115n
4-iodo-2,5-dimethoxyphenethylamine,
  overview 115–17
foxy (slang) 165
foxy methoxy (slang) 165
free basing, described 140
"Frequently Asked Questions"
  (DOL) 532n, 538n
friend (slang) 161, 563
fries (slang) 563
fry (slang) 221
fuel (slang) 563

G

galloping horse (slang) 563
Galson, Steven K. 386
gamma butyrolactone (GBL) 168–69
"Gamma Hydroxybutyric Acid" (DEA)
  167n
gamma hydroxybutyric acid (GHB)
  effects *264*
  medical consequences 313–16
  overview 167–69
gang activity, drug use 104–6
gangster (slang) 201
gat (slang) 189
GBL *see* gamma butyrolactone
gear (slang) 119
geek (slang) 563
gender factor
  adolescent depression 85
  adolescent substance use 67, 78
  drugged driving 108
  hallucinogens 317
  OTC medications misuse *271*
  residential substance abuse
    treatment facilities 474
  substance abuse mortality rates 17
  various viewpoints 380
"General Questions and Answers"
  (DEA) 30n
"General Workplace Impact" (DOL)
  97n
genes
  Asp40 255
  COMT 254–55

genetics *see* heredity
Genotropin 177
Georgia, substance abuse agency
  contact information 573
Georgia home boy (slang) 167
GHB *see* gamma hydroxybutyric acid
GHB (slang) 167–69, 563
ghost (slang) 563
giggle weed (slang) 563
girlfriend (slang) 563
glo (slang) 563
"Glossary of Terms" (DOL) 551n
glue *see* inhalants
glutamate, drug abuse 247
God (slang) 185
God's drug (slang) 563
God's flesh (slang) 563
God's medicine (slang) 563
gold (slang) 563
golden dragon (slang) 563
golden eagle (slang) 563
golden girl (slang) 563
golf ball (slang) 563
gong (slang) 563
good (slang) 563
good and plenty (slang) 563
goodfella (slang) 161
goodfellas (slang) 563
goody-goody (slang) 564
goofers (slang) 564
goofy's (slang) 564
goon (slang) 564
goop (slang) 167, 564
gorilla biscuits (slang) 564
gorilla pills (slang) 564
graba (slang) 189
grass (slang) 201, 564
gravel (slang) 564
greens (slang) 564
group therapy, described 421
Guam, substance abuse agency
  contact information 573
gym candy (slang) 119, 564

H

habituation, defined 553
Halcion *289*

hallucinations, withdrawal 402
hallucinogens
  adolescents *81*
  alpha-methyltryptamine 235–36
  defined 553
  described 3
  effects *265*
  first-time use statistics *47*, *48*, 49–50
  5-methoxy-N,N-diisopropyl-
    tryptamine 165–66
  4-bromo-2,5-dimethoxy-
    phenethylamine 239–40
  4-iodo-2,5-dimethoxy-
    phenethylamine 115–17
  lysergic acid diethylamide 197–99
  medical consequences 317–22
  N,N-dimethyltryptamine 149
  Salvia divinorum 231–32
  signs and symptoms 368
  2,5-dimethoxy-4-(n)-propylthio-
    phenethylamine 123–24
  use statistics *5*, *6*, *8*, *296*
  women *90*
"Hallucinogens: LSD, Peyote,
  Psilocybin, and PCP" (NIDA) 317n
hamburger helper (slang) 564
hardware (slang) 564
hashish
  defined 553
  described 201
  effects *265*
hash oil 201
Hawaii, substance abuse agency
  contact information 573
health education
  school drug policies 528–30
Health Information Network,
  contact information 582
Health Insurance Portability and
  Accountability Act (HIPAA) 541–42
heart attack, withdrawal 402
he-man (slang) 564
hepatitis, substance abuse 336–37
herb (slang) 201
heredity
  addiction 248, 254–55
  children of substance abusers 63
  comorbidity 343
  substance use disorders 66

heroin
  adolescents *81*
  adolescent substance use *74*
  defined 553
  effects *264*
  first-time use statistics *48*, 49
  medical consequences 311–12
  minority substance abuse *94*
  overview 171–75
  use statistics *5*, *6*, *8*, *296*
  women *88*, *90*
"Heroin" (NIDA) 171n
hexane 324
hGH *see* human growth hormone
Higher Education Act (1998) 456
Higher Education Center for Alcohol
  and Other Drug Abuse and Violence
  Prevention, contact information 585
"High-Risk Offenders Do Better with
  Close Judicial Supervision" (NIDA)
  428n
hillbilly heroin (slang) 217, 564
Hilton, Thomas 416
hippie crack (slang) 564
HIV (human immunodeficiency
  virus), substance abuse 334–39
hocus (slang) 564
hog (slang) 564
"Home Use Tests: Drugs of Abuse"
  (FDA) 494n
honey oil (slang) 564
Horgan, Constance M. 438n
hotcakes (slang) 564
hot stick (slang) 564
"How Drug Tests Are Done"
  (American Association for Clinical
  Chemistry) 486n
"How Young Adults Obtain
  Prescription Pain Relievers for
  Nonmedical Use" (SAMHSA) 278n
Hser, Yih-Ing 415
huff (slang) 564
"Human Growth Hormone" (DEA) 177n
human growth hormone (hGH),
  overview 177–80
Humatrope 177
hydrocodone
  effects *264*
  prescription drug abuse 274

hydromorphone, effects *264*
hyperthermia, defined 553

I

i (slang) 115
ice (slang) 41
Idaho, substance abuse agency
    contact information 573
idiot pills (slang) 564
"If Your Child Is Using: How to Step
    In and Help" (Partnership for Drug-
    Free America) 383n
illicit drug use *see* drug abuse;
    substance abuse
Illinois, substance abuse agency
    contact information 573
immune system, marijuana 204
"The Importance of Family Dinners
    IV" (CASA) 516n
income levels, self-help groups *412*
"Increase in Fatal Poisonings
    Involving Opioid Analgesics in the
    United States, 1999-2006" (CDC) 15n
Indiana, substance abuse agency
    contact information 573
Indian boy (slang) 564
Indian hay (slang) 564
Indian hemp (slang) 564
infectious diseases
    drug abuse 310
    substance abuse 334–39
inhalants
    abuse signs and symptoms 368, 369
    adolescents *81*
    adolescent substance use *74*
    defined 553
    described 3–4
    effects *265*
    first-time use statistics *47, 48*, 50
    medical consequences 311, 323–27
    minority substance abuse *94*
    paraphernalia 374
    use statistics *5, 6, 8, 296*
    women *88, 90*
"Inhalant Use and Major Depressive
    Episode among Youths Aged 12 to
    17: 2004 to 2006" (SAMHSA) 323n

injection drug users, syringe
    exchange programs 337–39
inmates
    drug abuse treatment 432–36
    drug use 101–6
    substance abuse 13
    women 90–91
    see also arrests; criminal justice
        system
instant zen (slang) 564
integrated group therapy, described 421
interventions
    detoxification 395
    middle schools 383–87
    workplace substance use 442–44
"In the Spotlight: Drug Court" (DOJ)
    428n
intoxicating pepper (slang) 181
Ionamin *286*
Iowa, substance abuse agency
    contact information 573
"Issue Brief #9 for Employers: An
    EAP That Addresses Substance
    Abuse Can Save You Money"
    (SAMHSA) 447n

J

jackpot (slang) 161, 564
jam (slang) 564
Jane (slang) 564
jellies (slang) 564
jelly (slang) 564
jet (slang) 185
joint (slang) 201, 564
jolly bean (slang) 564
jolly green (slang) 565
joy powder (slang) 565
joy smoke (slang) 565
juice (slang) 119, 565
junk (slang) 565
junkie (slang) 565

K

K (slang) 185
kakuam (slang) 193
kangaroo (slang) 565

Kansas, substance abuse agency
  contact information 574
Kansas grass (slang) 565
kat (slang) 189
kate bush (slang) 565
"Kava" (DEA) 181n
kava, overview 181–83
kawa kawa (slang) 181
"Keeping Your Teens Drug-Free:
  A Family Guide" (National Youth
  Anti-Drug Media Campaign) 506n
"Keeping Your Worksite Drug and
  Alcohol Free" (DOL) 532n
Kentucky, substance abuse agency
  contact information 574
Ketajet 185
Ketalar 185
ketamine
  described 555
  medical consequences 313–16
"Ketamine" (DEA) 185n
Ketamine Hydrochloride Injection 185
Ketaset 185
Ketavet 185
ketum (slang) 193
kew (slang) 181
khat, overview 189–91
"Khat Fast Facts" (DOJ) 189n
K-hole (slang) 185
kibbles and bits (slang) 565
kicker (slang) 217, 565
kiddie dope (slang) 565
killer (slang) 565
killer joints (slang) 221
King Kong pills (slang) 565
kit kat (slang) 185, 565
k-land (slang) 185
Klonopin (clonazepam) 153–54, *283*
"Know Your Rights" (SAMHSA) 451n
"Kratom (*Mitragyna speciosa Korth*)"
  (DEA) 193n
kratom, overview 193–95
kryptonite (slang) 565
krystal (slang) 565

L

lace (slang) 565
lactone (slang) 565

lady (slang) 565
la rocha (slang) 565
Law Library of Congress, online
  pharmacies publication 33n
lean (slang) 565
least restrictive care 398–99
legal E (slang) 131
legal X (slang) 131
lethal weapon (slang) 565
Librium *283*
LifeRing Secular Recovery 410
limbic system, medications 259–60
Limbitrol *283*
liquid ecstasy (slang) 167, 565
liquid X (slang) 167
locker room (slang) 565
log (slang) 565
lollipop (slang) 161
loony toons (slang) 565
lorazepam 153–54, *283*
  drug screens *487*
Louisiana, substance abuse
  agency contact information 574
lovelies (slang) 221
LSD *see* lysergic acid diethylamide
Lucy in the sky with diamonds
  (slang) 565
lung disorders, marijuana 203
lysergic acid diethylamide (LSD)
  adolescent substance use *74*
  defined 554
  effects *265*
  first-time use statistics *48*
  medical consequences 311,
    317–22
  overview 197–99
  signs and symptoms 368
  use statistics *318*

M

magic (slang) 565
magic mint (slang) 231
Maine, substance abuse agency
  contact information 574
major depressive episode
  see depression

"Making the Drug Problem Smaller, 2001-2008" (Office of National Drug Control Policy) 479n

Manske, Richard 149

Maria Pastora (slang) 231

marijuana
adolescent depression 83–86
adolescents *81*
adolescent substance use *74*
defined 554
drugged driving 108–10
drug screens *487*
effects *265*
first-time use statistics *47*, 47–49, *48*
medical consequences 311, 329–32
minority substance abuse *94*
overview 201–6
paraphernalia 374
pregnancy 57
signs and symptoms 368–69
use statistics *5*, *6*, *8*, *296*
various viewpoints 380
women *88*, *90*
see also medical marijuana

"Marijuana: Facts for Teens" (NIDA) 201n

Marinol 37, 38–40

Marlowe, Douglas 430–31

Mary Jane (slang) 201

Maryland, substance abuse agency contact information 574

Massachusetts, substance abuse agency contact information 574

Matrix Model 215

Mazanor *286*

McCabe, Sean Esteban 302, 304

McCann, Bernard 438n

MDMA see ecstasy

medical marijuana
described 204
overview 36–40
see also marijuana

"Medical Marijuana Reality Check" (Office of National Drug Control Policy) 36n

"Medical Marijuana: The Facts" (DEA) 36n

medications
addiction treatment 391–92
comorbidity 419–20
see also over-the-counter medications; prescription medications

Melemis, Steven M. 401n

mental disorders
comorbidity 342–43
defined 554
drug abuse treatment 419–25
drug addiction 309

mental health, marijuana 330

mental health problems, inmates 103

mental illness, marijuana use 84–85

mentally ill chemical abuser (MICA), defined 552

Meprobamate *283*

Merrick, Elizabeth S. Levy 438n

mescaline 123

Metadate 225

methadone
benzodiazepines 154
defined 554
described 173, 392
overview 207–11
substance abuse mortality rates 17, 18

"Methadone" (DEA) 207n

"Methadone Diversion, Abuse, and Misuse: Deaths Increasing at Alarming Rate" (DOJ) 207n

Methadose 207

methamphetamine
adolescent substance use *74*
defined 554
described 4
drug endangered children 59–60
effects *265*
first-time use statistics 51
medical consequences 311
minority substance abuse *94*
overview 213–16
regulation 41–43
stimulant abuse *286*
treatment options 415–18
women *88*, *90*

methaqualone *289*, 554

Methedrine *286*
methylene chloride 324
Methylin 225
methylphenidate
    effects *265*
    overview 225–30
    stimulant abuse *286*
"Methylphenidate" (DEA) 225n
methyltestosterone 119
mibolerone 119
MICA *see* mentally ill
    chemical abuser
Michigan, substance abuse
    agency contact information 575
Mickey Finn (slang) 565
Mickey's (slang) 566
microdots (slang) 199
military service, substance
    use 348–50
Miltown *283*
Minnesota, substance abuse
    agency contact information 575
Minnesota Twin Family Study 68
"Minorities and Drugs: Facts and
    Figures" (Office of National Drug
    Control Policy) 93n
miraa (slang) 189
Mississippi, substance abuse
    agency contact information 575
Missouri, substance abuse agency
    contact information 575
M.J. (slang) 565
M&M (slang) 565
mojo (slang) 566
Monitoring the Future Survey
    anabolic steroids 120
    club drugs 316
    gamma hydroxybutyric acid 168
    methylphenidate 226
    parenting practices 69
    prescription drug abuse 275
Montana, substance abuse agency
    contact information 575
moon (slang) 566
moon gas (slang) 566
moonrock (slang) 566
morphine
    drug screens *487*
    effects *264*

mortality rates
    minority substance
        abuse 94
    substance abuse 15–19
mother's little helper (slang) 566
motor vehicle accidents,
    drugged driving 107–12
multiple substance abuse
    alcohol use 294–97
    benzodiazepines 154
    ecstasy 156
    marijuana 204
    medical consequences 312
multisystemic therapy,
    described 420
munchies (slang) 202
murder 8 (slang) 161, 566
mutual support groups
    see support groups

N

NAADAC - The Association
    for Addiction Professionals,
    contact information 585
nail (slang) 201
naltrexone
    alcohol abuse 255, 392
    described 174
nandrolone decanoate 119
narcotics
    abuse signs and symptoms 369
    defined 19, 554
    effects *264*
    substance abuse
        mortality rates 17
Narcotics Anonymous,
    contact information 538, 585
Narcotics Anonymous World
    Services, addiction
    questionnaire publication
    305n
National Association for
    Children of Alcoholics,
    contact information 585
National Association of
    Addiction Treatment Providers,
    contact information 585

National Center on Addiction
and Substance Abuse (CASA)
contact information 585
publications
drug endangered children 59n
family dinners 516n
parental substance abuse 54n
National Council on Alcoholism and
Drug Dependence, contact
information 537, 585
National Criminal Justice Reference
Service, contact information 582
National Drug Intelligence Center,
contact information 582
"National Drug Threat Assessment
2009" (DOJ) 11n
National Institute on Alcohol Abuse
and Alcoholism (NIAAA)
contact information 582
publications
adolescent substance abuse 65n
simultaneous polydrug use 298n
National Institute on Drug Abuse
(NIDA)
contact information 582
publications
addiction 245n, 251n, 259n
adolescent substance abuse 74n
alcohol abuse 302n
club drugs 313n
cocaine 139n
comorbidity 341n, 419n
drug abuse 245n
drug addictions medical
consequences 309n
drug addiction treatment 389n
drugged driving 107n
ecstasy 155n
glossary 551n
hallucinogens 317n
heroin 171n
HIV/AIDS 334n
inhalants 323n
inmate addiction treatment 432n
interventions 383n
marijuana 201n, 329n
mental illnesses 419n
methamphetamine 213n, 415n
prescription drug abuse 274n

National Institute on Drug Abuse
(NIDA), continued
publications, continued
stimulant ADHD
medications 225n
stress 251n
workplace substance abuse 532n
sponsored websites 583
National Mental Health Information
Center, contact information 583
National Parents Resource Institute
for Drug Education, contact
information 586
National Youth Anti-Drug Media
Campaign, publications
adolescent drug use
prevention 506n
drug use signs 366n
"N-Benzylpiperazine" (DEA) 131n
N-benzylpiperazine, overview 131–33
Nebraska, substance abuse agency
contact information 575
needle exchange programs
see syringe exchange programs
Nemours Foundation
children, drugs publication 497n
contact information 586
neurotransmitters
defined 554
drug abuse 246–47
medications 260
stress 256
Nevada, substance abuse agency
contact information 576
New Hampshire, substance abuse
agency contact information 576
New Jersey, substance abuse agency
contact information 576
New Mexico, substance abuse
agency contact information 576
"New Therapy Reduces Drug Abuse
among Patients with Severe Mental
Illness: Research Findings" (NIDA)
419n
New York state, substance abuse
agency contact information 576
NIAAA *see* National Institute on
Alcohol Abuse and Alcoholism
nice and easy (slang) 566

nicotine *see* environmental
tobacco smoke; tobacco use
NIDA *see* National Institute
on Drug Abuse
"NIDA Frequently Asked
Questions" (NIDA) 245n
"NIDA InfoFacts: Club Drugs
(GHB, Ketamine, and
Rohypnol)" (NIDA) 313n
"NIDA InfoFacts: Drug Abuse
and the link to HIV/AIDS and
Other Infectious Diseases"
(NIDA) 334n
"NIDA InfoFacts: Drugged
Driving" (NIDA) 107n
"NIDA InfoFacts: Inhalants"
(NIDA) 323n
"NIDA InfoFacts: Marijuana"
(NIDA) 329n
"NIDA InfoFacts: Methamphetamine"
(NIDA) 213n
"NIDA InfoFacts: Stimulant
ADHD Medications -
Methylphenidate and
Amphetamines" (NIDA) 225n
"NIDA Launches Drug Use
Screening Tools for Physicians"
(NIDA) 383n
"NIDA NewsScan: Middle School
Interventions Reduce Nonmedical
Use of Prescription Drugs" (NIDA)
383n
nitrous oxide
described 324
effects *265*
N,N-dimethyltryptamine (DMT),
overview 149–51
"N,N-Dimethyltryptamine (DMT)"
(DEA) 149n
"Nonmedical Stimulant Use, Other
Drug Use, Delinquent Behaviors,
and Depression among Adolescents"
(SAMHSA) 80n
Norditropin 177
norepinephrine, defined 554
North Carolina, substance abuse
agency contact information 576
North Dakota, substance abuse
agency contact information 576

"The NSDUH Report: Misuse of
Over-the-Counter Cough and Cold
Medications among Persons Aged
12 to 25" (SAMHSA) 269n
Nutropin 177

O

oat (slang) 189
Obedrin-LA *286*
OC (slang) 217
Office of Applied Studies,
contact information 583
Office of National Drug Control
Policy
contact information 583
publications
adolescent drug abuse 75n
adolescent marijuana use 83n
medical marijuana 36n
minorities, drugs 93n
reducing drug abuse 479n
street terms (slang) 557n
women, drugs 87n
sponsored websites 583
Ohio, substance abuse agency
contact information 577
Oklahoma, substance abuse
agency contact information 577
one way (slang) 566
online prescription medications,
legislation 27–28, 33–36
opiates
defined 554
pregnancy 57
prescription drug abuse 274–75
women *90*
opioids
addiction treatment 392–93
defined 19
substance abuse mortality
rates 16–18
oppositional defiant disorder,
described 67
orange barrels (slang) 566
orange crystal (slang) 566
Oregon, substance abuse agency
contact information 577

overdose, first aid 375–78
over-the-counter medications,
    misuse overview 269–71
oxandrolone 119
oxy (slang) 217, 566
oxycodone
    effects *264*
    overview 217–19
    prescription drug abuse 274
"Oxycodone" (DEA) 217n
OxyContin
    adolescents 78
    overview 217–19
oxycotton (slang) 217
Oz (slang) 566

P

pain medications
    adolescents 76–77, *81*
    described 3
    first-time use statistics *47*, *48*, 50
    prescription drug abuse 275
    substance abuse 278–81
    use statistics 7, *296*
paper acid (slang) 566
parabolin (slang) 566
paradise (slang) 566
paradise white (slang) 566
parents
    adolescent depression 86
    adolescent substance abuse 515–16
    adolescent substance use 69–71
    prisoners 102
    substance abuse 60–64
    see also children of alcoholics
parsley (slang) 566
Partnership for a Drug-Free America
    contact information 586
    interventions publication 383n
paste (slang) 566
"Patterns in Nonmedical Use of
    Specific Prescription Drugs:
    Chapter 3" (SAMHSA) 282n,
    285n, 288n
PAWS *see* post-acute withdrawal
PCP *see* phencyclidine
PCP (slang) 221

peace pill (slang) 566
peace tablets (slang) 566
peer pressure, adolescent
    substance abuse 70, 513–14
Pennsylvania, substance abuse
    agency contact information 577
pentobarbital, drug screens *487*
pep pills (slang) 566
Percodan 217
perc-o-pop (slang) 161
Personal Responsibility and Work
    Opportunity Act (1996) 456
Peter Pan (slang) 566
peyote (slang) 566
peyote, medical consequences 317–22
phencyclidine (PCP)
    abuse signs and symptoms 369
    defined 555
    drug screens *487*
    first-time use statistics *48*
    medical consequences 317–22
    overview 221–23
    use statistics *318*
    women *90*
"Phencyclidine (Street Names: PCP,
    Angel Dust, Supergrass, Boat, Tic
    Tac, Zoom, Shermans)" (DEA) 221n
phenobarbital, drug screens *487*
phenobarbital, sedative abuse *289*
phenylpropanolamine, described
    41–42
physical dependence, defined 555
Placidyl *289*
Plegine *286*
Pluto (slang) 566
pocket rocket (slang) 566
poison (slang) 566
poisoning deaths
    defined 19
    methadone 207, 210–11
    substance abuse 15–19
polydrug use
    cocaine 143
    ketamine 187
    overview 298–302
    see also comorbidity; dual diagnosis;
        multiple substance abuse
pony (slang) 566
poor man's PCP (slang) 145

poor man's pot (slang) 566
"Post-Acute Withdrawal" (Melemis) 401n
post-acute withdrawal (PAWS) 403–5
posttraumatic stress disorder (PTSD), substance abuse 256–57
pot (slang) 201, 566
potato (slang) 566
potato chips (slang) 566
potential for abuse, described 22–23
predator (slang) 566
"Predictors of Substance Abuse Treatment Completion or Transfer to Further Treatment by Service Type" (SAMHSA) 468n
pregnancy
    alcohol use 55–57
    cocaine 58
    drug abuse 310
    marijuana 57, 205
    methadone 174
    opiates 57
    substance abuse 89
    tobacco use 54–55
Preludin *286*
prescription medications
    abuse signs and symptoms 369
    adolescents 75–79
    alcohol use 302–4
    controlled substances 30–33
    described 4, 30–33
    drug abuse consequences 312
    drugged driving 110–11
    online pharmacies 33–36
    pain reliever abuse 280–81
    scientific research overview 274–77
    sedative abuse 288–91
    stimulant abuse 285–87
    tranquilizer abuse 282–84
"Primary Methamphetamine/ Amphetamine Admissions to Substance Abuse Treatment: 2005" (SAMHSA) 415n
product (slang) 566
proviron (slang) 567
pseudoephedrine, described 41–42
psilocybin, medical consequences 317–22

psychiatric disorders, children of substance abusers 62–64
psychoactive drugs, defined 555
psychological dependence, defined 553
psychological dysregulation, adolescents 66–68
psychosis, defined 555
psychotherapeutics
    described 4
    first-time use statistics 50–51
    use statistics *5, 6, 8*
PTSD *see* posttraumatic stress disorder
Puerto Rico, substance abuse agency contact information 577
puffy (slang) 567
pumpers (slang) 119, 567
purple (slang) 185

Q

qat (slang) 189
Quaalude *289*
Queen Anne's lace (slang) 567
quicksilver (slang) 567

R

R-2 (slang) 567
racial factor
    methamphetamine treatment options *418*
    OTC medications misuse *271*
    residential substance abuse treatment facilities 474
    self-help groups *412*
    substance abuse 93–96
rambo (slang) 567
recidivism, drug courts 428
record keeping requirements, controlled substances 26–27
recovery programs, individual rights 451–57
    see also detoxification; support groups; withdrawal
recycle (slang) 567

reefer (slang) 567

regulation
  marijuana 36, 39
  methamphetamine 41–43

Rehabilitation Act (1973) 451, 457

religion
  adolescent substance abuse 514
  substance use prevention 543–47

"Religious Involvement and
  Substance Use among Adults
  (NSDUH Report)" (SAMHSA) 543n

"Research Report Series: MDMA
  (Ecstasy) Abuse" (NIDA) 155n, 551n

residential substance abuse
  treatment facilities, overview
  471–75

respiratory illness, environmental
  tobacco smoke 61

Restoril (temazepam) 153–54, *289*

"Results from the 2006 National
  Survey on Drug Use and Health:
  National Findings, Chapter 6"
  (SAMHSA) 510n

"Results from the 2007 National
  Survey on Drug Use and Health:
  National Findings, Chapter 5:
  Initiation of Substance Abuse"
  (SAMHSA) 45n

"Results from the 2007 National
  Survey on Drug Use and Health:
  National Findings" (SAMHSA) 3n,
  460n

"Revisiting Employee Assistance
  Programs and Substance Use
  Programs in the Workplace: Key
  Issues and a Research Agenda"
  (Merrick, et al.) 438n

Rhode Island, substance abuse
  agency contact information 577

rhythm (slang) 567

Ritalin
  nonmedical use *286*
  overview 225–30
  prescription drug abuse 276

roach (slang) 567

roach-2 (slang) 567

road dope (slang) 567

Robitussin 145

robo (slang) 145

rock (slang) 139, 567

rocket fuel (slang) 567

Rohypnol *283*, 313–16

roids (slang) 119

roofies (slang) 567

rooster (slang) 567

ruffles (slang) 567

rugs (slang) 567

rush hour (slang) 567

rush snappers (slang) 567

Ryan Haight Online Pharmacy
  Consumer Protection Act
  (2007) 27–28, 33–36

S

Safe and Drug-Free Schools,
  contact information 583

sage of the seers (slang) 231

Saizen 177

sakau (slang) 181

Sally-D (slang) 231

salvia (slang) 231

Salvia divinorum
  medical consequences 317–18
  overview 231–33

"*Salvia divinorum* and Salvinorin A"
  (DEA) 231n

salvinorin A, overview 231–33

SAMHSA *see* Substance Abuse
  and Mental Health Services
  Administration

Samoa *see* American Samoa

Sanorex *286*

Save Our Selves 409–10

schedule I drugs
  cathinone 190
  defined 555
  described 24
  5-methoxy-N,N-diisopropyl-
    tryptamine 166
  gamma hydroxybutyric
    acid 167–69
  lysergic acid diethylamide 199
  N-benzylpiperazine 133
  N,N-dimethyltryptamine 149, 151
  2,5-dimethoxy-4-(n)-propyl-
    thiophenethylamine 125

schedule II drugs
  cocaine 141
  defined 555
  described 24
  fentanyl 163
  methadone 209
  methamphetamine 213
  methylphenidate 227
  oxycodone 217, 219
  phencyclidine 223
  prescriptions 31–32
schedule III drugs
  anabolic steroids 121–22
  buprenorphine 129
  described 24
  ketamine 187
  prescriptions 31–32
  Xyrem 167–69
schedule IV drugs
  benzodiazepines 153–54
  cathine 190
  described 25
  prescriptions 31–32
schedule V drugs
  described 25
  prescriptions 31–32
school settings
  drug tests 522–28
  health education 528–30
"Scientific Research on Prescription
  Drug Abuse, Before the
  Subcommittee on the Judiciary and
  Caucus on International Narcotics
  Control" (NIDA) 274n
scoop (slang) 567
scootie (slang) 567
scorpion (slang) 567
scott (slang) 567
secobarbital, drug screens *487*
Secular Organization for Sobriety
  409–10
sedatives
  adolescents *81*
  first-time use statistics *47*, *48*
  prescription drug abuse 288–91
  use statistics *296*
  women *90*
seizures, withdrawal 402
self-help groups *see* support groups

self-medication, defined 555
Serax *283*
serious psychological distress (SPD),
  overview 348–53
"Serious Psychological Distress and
  Substance Use Disorder among
  Veterans" (SAMHSA) 348n
"Serious Psychological Distress and
  Substance Use Disorder among
  Young Adult Males" (SAMHSA)
  351n
Serostim 177
serotonin, defined 555
seven-up (slang) 567
shake (slang) 567
sheet rocking (slang) 567
shermans (slang) 221
shoot (slang) 567
shoot the breeze (slang) 567
side effects
  anabolic steroids 121–22
  drug addiction 309–12
  ecstasy 156–58
  heroin 172–73
  khat 190
  marijuana 203–4
  methamphetamine use 214–15
  phencyclidine use 222
SIDS *see* sudden infant death
  syndrome
"Signs and Symptoms of Teen
  Drinking and Drug Use" (National
  Youth Anti-Drug Media Campaign)
  366n
silly putty (slang) 567
simultaneous polydrug use
  see polydrug use
Single Convention on Narcotic
  Drugs (1961) 26
sinsemilla 201
skag (slang) 567
skee (slang) 567
sketch (slang) 567
skittles (slang) 145
sleep (slang) 568
sleet (slang) 568
sleigh ride (slang) 568
slick superspeed (slang) 568
smack (slang) 568

SMART Recovery 409
smoked marijuana *see* marijuana; medical marijuana
snow (slang) 139, 568
soft (slang) 568
softballs (slang) 568
soles (slang) 568
Soma *283*
soma (slang) 568
Somali tea (slang) 189
"Some Medications and Driving Don't Mix" (FDA) 107n
Sopor *289*
South Carolina, substance abuse agency contact information 577
South Dakota, substance abuse agency contact information 577
South parks (slang) 568
spaceball (slang) 568
space cadet (slang) 568
spackle (slang) 568
Sparkle Plenty (slang) 568
special K (slang) 185
special la coke (slang) 185
speckled birds (slang) 568
spectrum (slang) 568
speed (slang) 41, 568
spider (slang) 568
spirals (slang) 235
sports activities, drug screens 490–91
spray paints *see* inhalants
stack (slang) 568
stackers (slang) 119, 568
star dust (slang) 568
statistics
  adolescent depression 82–83, 84
  adolescent substance abuse 511–12
  adolescent substance use *74*, 74–82
  cocaine use 143
  dextromethorphan use 147
  drug-related crime 101–3
  ecstasy use 156
  gang activity 105–6
  heroin use 175
  methadone deaths 207, 210–11
  methamphetamine use 215–16
  methylphenidate use 226–27
  minority substance abuse 93–96

statistics, continued
  oxycodone use 218–19
  pain reliever abuse 278–81
  polydrug use 298–302
  prescription drug abuse 274–77
  Salvia divinorum use 232
  self-help groups *412*
  substance abuse 4–9, 351–53
  substance abuse mortality rates 15–18
  substance abuse treatment completion 468–75
  substance abuse treatment overview 460–68
  substance first-time use 45–51
  suicides 355–59
  women, substance abuse 87–91
  workplace substance abuse 97–100
steroids
  adolescent substance use *74*
  defined 555
  drug abuse consequences 312
  minority substance abuse *94*
  overview 119–22
  women *88*
  see also anabolic steroids
stigma, addiction 380
stimulants
  adolescents 80–83
  defined 555
  effects *264–65*
  first-time use statistics *47*, *48*, 50
  pregnancy 58
  prescription drug abuse 285–87
  use statistics *296*
stink weed (slang) 568
stones (slang) 568
strawberries (slang) 568
strawberry fields (slang) 568
street gangs *see* gang activity
"Street Terms: Drugs and the Drug Trade" (Office of National Drug Control Policy) 557n
stress, substance abuse 255–57
"Stress and Substance Abuse" (NIDA) 251n

stroke, withdrawal 402
"Student Drug-Testing Institute -
    Frequently Asked Questions" (US
    Department of Education) 522n
students
    drug tests 522–28
    gang activity 105–6
    health education 528–30
Students Against Destructive
    Decisions, contact information 586
studio fuel (slang) 568
Sublimaze (fentanyl) 161
Suboxone 127–28
substance abuse
    first-time use 45–51, 294–96
    individual rights 451–57
    treatment completion
        statistics 468–75
    treatment statistics
        overview 460–68
    veterans 348–50
    workplace 438–49
    see also addiction; drug abuse
Substance Abuse and Mental
    Health Services Administration
    (SAMHSA)
    contact information 584
    publications
        addictions, recovery 379n
        adolescent drug use
            prevention 510n
        adolescent stimulant use 80n
        cost benefit analysis 11n
        cough medicine 269n
        detoxification 395n
        employee assistance
            programs 447n
        hallucinogens 317n
        individual rights 451n
        inhalants 323n
        methamphetamine 415n
        pain reliever abuse 278n
        religious involvement 543n
        sedative abuse 288n
        state substance abuse
            agencies 571n
        stimulant abuse 285n
        substance abuse 45n
        substance abuse prevalence 3n

Substance Abuse and Mental
    Health Services Administration
    (SAMHSA), continued
    publications, continued
        substance abuse
            treatment 460n, 468n, 471n
        substance dependence, alcohol
            use 294n
        suicide, depression 355n
        support groups 407n
        tranquilizer abuse 282n
        veterans, substance abuse 348n
        workplace substance
            abuse 97n, 444n
        young adult males, substance
            abuse 351n
"Substance Abuse in Brief Fact Sheet,
    Vol. 5, Issue 1: An Introduction to
    Mutual Support Groups for Alcohol
    and Drug Abuse" (SAMHSA) 407n
"Substance Abuse Prevention Dollars
    and Cents: A Cost-Benefit Analysis"
    (SAMHSA) 11n
substance abuse testing 486
Substance Abuse Treatment Locator,
    contact information 538
"Substance Use and Dependence
    Following Initiation of Alcohol or
    Illicit Drug Use" (SAMHSA) 294n
Subutex 127–28
sudden infant death syndrome
    (SIDS), tobacco use 55
sugar (slang) 568
"Suicidal Thoughts, Suicide Attempts,
    Major Depressive Episode, and
    Substance Use among Adults"
    (SAMHSA) 355n
suicide, substance abuse 355–62
"Summary Record of the Ryan Haight
    Online Pharmacy Consumer
    Protection Act of 2008" (Law
    Library of Congress) 33n
"Summary Report CARAVAN Survey
    for SAMHSA on Addiction and
    Recovery" (SAMHSA) 379n
super acid (slang) 185
supergrass (slang) 221
Superman (slang) 568
support groups, overview 407–13

surfer (slang) 568
sweet dreams (slang) 568
"Symptoms and Intervention
Techniques" (DOL) 442n
syringe exchange programs,
overview 337–39
"Syringe Exchange Programs -
United States, 2005" (CDC) 337n

T

"Talking to Your Child about Drugs"
(Nemours Foundation) 497n
tango (slang) 161
tardust (slang) 568
teenagers *see* adolescents
"Teen Marijuana Use Worsens
Depression" (Office of National
Drug Control Policy) 83n
"Teens and Prescriptions Drugs: An
Analysis of Recent Trends on the
Emerging Drug Threat" (Office of
National Drug Control Policy) 75n
"Teen Substance Abuse Continues to
Decline" (NIDA) 74n
temazepam 153–54, *289*
Tennessee, substance abuse
agency contact information 578
tension (slang) 568
Tenuate *286*
testosterone
anabolic steroids 119–20
effects *265*
tetrahydrocannabinol (THC)
defined 555
described 37, 38–39, 201
drugged driving 108–10
effects *265*
medical consequences 329–32
Texas, substance abuse agency
contact information 578
Texas shoe shine (slang) 569
Tex-Mex (slang) 568
thang (slang) 193
THC *see* tetrahydrocannabinol
therapeutic communities
described 420
drug addictions 393–94

thom (slang) 193
3,4-methylenedioxy-
methamphetamine *see* ecstasy
thrust (slang) 569
tic tac (slang) 221, 569
"Timing of Alcohol and Other
Drug Use" (NIAAA) 298n
TNT (slang) 161, 569
tobacco use
addiction treatment 392
adolescent substance use *74*
medical consequences 310
pregnancy 54–55
tohai (slang) 189
tolerance
benzodiazepines 154
defined 556
heroin 172
marijuana 206
toluene 324
Tom and Jerries (slang) 569
tonga (slang) 181
toonies (slang) 569
tootsie roll (slang) 569
top gun (slang) 569
topi (slang) 569
topiramate 392
tops (slang) 569
toxicology screen 486
tox screen 486
toxy (slang) 569
toys (slang) 569
tranquilizers
adolescents *81*
first-time use statistics *47*, *48*, 50, *296*
prescription drug abuse 282–84
use statistics *296*
women *90*
Tranxene *283*
trash (slang) 569
trauma (slang) 569
"Treatment Approaches for Drug
Addiction" (NIDA) 389n
treatment improvement protocols
(TIP) 396–97
"Treatment Outcomes among Clients
Discharged from Residential
Substance Abuse Treatment: 2005"
(SAMHSA) 471n

trenbolone 119
"Trends in Nonmedical Use of
    Prescription Pain Relievers:
    2002 to 2007" (SAMHSA) 278n
triple C (slang) 145
triple crowns (slang) 569
tripstay (slang) 123
truck drivers (slang) 569
tschat (slang) 189
T7 (slang) 123
tuberculosis, substance abuse 336–37
Tuinal *289*
tweety-bird mescaline (slang) 123
tweety birds (slang) 569
twelve-step groups, described 407–9
twinkie (slang) 569
twins studies, adolescent
    substance use 68
2,5-dimethoxy-4-(n)-
    propylthiophenethylamine
    overview 123–25
"2,5-Dimethoxy-4-(n)-
    Propylthiophenethylamine"
    (DEA) 123n
Tylox 217

U

Uncle Milty (slang) 569
"Understanding Drug Abuse and
    Addiction" (NIDA) 245n
"Unintentional Poisoning Deaths -
    United States, 1999-2004" (CDC)
    15n
uppers (slang) 569
uppers, defined 556
US Department of Education,
    student drug testing publication
    522n
US Department of Justice (DOJ),
    publications
    criminal activity 101n
    drug abuse 263n
    drug courts 428n
    drugs of abuse 21n
    drug threat assessment 11n
    khat 189n
    methadone 207n

US Department of Labor (DOL)
    contact information 584
    publications
        glossary 551n
        workplace drug testing 538n
        workplace substance abuse 97n,
            442n, 532n
"Use of Specific Hallucinogens: 2006"
    (SAMHSA) 317n
US Food and Drug Administration (FDA)
    contact information 584
    publications
        drugged driving 107n
        home drug tests 494n
Utah, substance abuse agency
    contact information 578

V

Valium (diazepam) 153–54, *283*
varenicline 392
Ventipulmin Syrup 135
Venus (slang) 569
Vermont, substance abuse agency
    contact information 578
Vetaket 185
Vetamine 185
veterans, substance use
    overview 348–50
Vicodin 78
Violent Crime Control and Law
    Enforcement Act (1994) 429
Virgin Islands, substance abuse
    agency contact information 578
Vistaril *283*
vita-G (slang) 569
vitamin K (slang) 185, 569
vitamin R (slang) 569
vodka acid (slang) 569
Volkow, Nora D. 386, 432
Volpe-Vartanian, Joanna 438n

W

wac (slang) 569
Washington, DC
    see District of Columbia

Washington state, substance abuse
   agency contact information 579
waters (slang) 221
wedding bells (slang) 569
weed (slang) 201
week (slang) 569
weight trainers (slang) 119, 569
West coast (slang) 569
West Virginia, substance abuse
   agency contact information 579
wets (slang) 221
"What Kinds of Things Are
   Paraphernalia?" (DEA) 372n
whippets (slang) 569
white (slang) 569
white ball (slang) 569
white boy (slang) 569
white diamonds (slang) 570
white dragon (slang) 570
white dust (slang) 570
white-haired lady (slang) 570
white lightning (slang) 570
whiteout (slang) 570
white tornado (slang) 570
whiz bang (slang) 570
"Why Drug Tests Are Done"
   (American Association for
   Clinical Chemistry) 488n
wigits (slang) 570
window glass (slang) 570
window pane (slang) 199, 570
wings (slang) 570
Wisconsin, substance abuse
   agency contact information 579
withdrawal
   addiction treatment 391–92
   defined 556
   overview 401–5
   see also detoxification
"Withdrawal" (Melemis) 401n
wolfies (slang) 570
women, substance abuse 87–91
   see also gender factor
"Women and Drugs: Facts and
   Figures" (Office of National
   Drug Control Policy) 87n

Women for Sobriety 409
work (slang) 570
"Worker Substance Abuse,
   by Industry Category"
   (SAMHSA) 97n
Workforce Investment
   Act 451, 454
working man's cocaine
   (slang) 570
"Workplace Resources"
   (NIDA) 532n
workplace substance abuse
   drug screens 490
   drug testing 538–42
   overview 97–100, 438–41
   prevention 532–38
   productivity costs losses *12*
worm (slang) 570
Wyoming, substance abuse
   agency contact information 579

X

Xanax (alprazolam) 153–54, *283*
X-pills (slang) 570
Xyrem 167–69, 313

Y

yangona (slang) 181
yellow (slang) 570
yellow fever (slang) 570
yellow jackets (slang) 570
yellow powder (slang) 570
yellow submarine (slang) 570
"Your Home" (DEA) 501n

Z

zen (slang) 570
zero (slang) 570
zip (slang) 570
zombie weed (slang) 570
zoom (slang) 221, 570

Health Reference Series
Complete Catalog
List price $93 per volume. School and library price $84 per volume.

Adolescent Health Sourcebook, 3rd Edition

Basic Consumer Health Information about Adolescent Growth and Development, Puberty, Sexuality, Reproductive Health, and Physical, Emotional, Social, and Mental Health Concerns of Teens and Their Parents, Including Facts about Nutrition, Physical Activity, Weight Management, Acne, Allergies, Cancer, Diabetes, Growth Disorders, Juvenile Arthritis, Infections, Substance Abuse, and More

Along with Information about Adolescent Safety Concerns, Youth Violence, a Glossary of Related Terms, and a Directory of Resources

Edited by Amy L. Sutton. 600 pages. 2010. 978-0-7808-1140-9.

Adult Health Concerns Sourcebook

Basic Consumer Health Information about Medical and Mental Concerns of Adults, Including Facts about Choosing Healthcare Providers, Navigating Insurance Options, Maintaining Wellness, Preventing Cancer, Heart Disease, Stroke, Diabetes, and Osteoporosis, and Understanding Aging-Related Health Concerns, Including Menopause, Cognitive Changes, and Changes in the Coronary and Vascular Systems

Along with Tips on Caring for Aging Parents and Dealing with Health-Related Work and Travel Issues, a Glossary, and a Directory of Resources for Additional Help and Information

Edited by Sandra J. Judd. 648 pages. 2008. 978-0-7808-0999-4.

"Provides a thorough list of topics that are important to adult health and for caregivers."
—*CHOICE, Nov '08*

"Written in easy-to-understand language... the content is well-organized and is intended to aid adults in making health care-related decisions."
—*AORN Journal, Dec '08*

AIDS Sourcebook, 4th Edition

Basic Consumer Health Information about Human Immunodeficiency Virus (HIV) and Acquired Immunodeficiency Syndrome (AIDS), Featuring Updated Statistics and Facts about Risks, Prevention, Screening, Diagnosis, Treatments, Side Effects, and Complications, and Including a Section about the Impact of HIV/AIDS on the Health of Women, Children, and Adolescents

Along with Tips on Managing Life with AIDS, Reports on Current Research Initiatives and Clinical Trials, a Glossary of Related Terms, and Resource Directories for Further Help and Information

Edited by Ivy L. Alexander. 680 pages. 2008. 978-0-7808-0997-0.

SEE ALSO *Contagious Diseases Sourcebook, 2nd Edition*

Alcoholism Sourcebook, 3rd Edition

Basic Consumer Health Information about Alcohol Use, Abuse, and Dependence, Featuring Facts about the Physical, Mental, and Social Health Effects of Alcohol Addiction, Including Alcoholic Liver Disease, Pancreatic Disease, Cardiovascular Disease, Neurological Disorders, and the Effects of Drinking during Pregnancy

Along with Information about Alcohol Treatment, Medications, and Recovery Programs, in Addition to Tips for Reducing the Prevalence of Underage Drinking, Statistics about Alcohol Use, a Glossary of Related Terms, and Directories of Resources for More Help and Information

Edited by Joyce Brennfleck Shannon. 600 pages. 2010. 978-0-7808-1141-6.

SEE ALSO *Drug Abuse Sourcebook, 3rd Edition*

Allergies Sourcebook, 3rd Edition

Basic Consumer Health Information about Allergic Disorders, Such as Anaphylaxis,

Hives, Eczema, Rhinitis, Sinusitis, and Conjunctivitis, and Their Triggers, Including Pollen, Mold, Dust Mites, Animal Dander, Insects, Chemicals, Food, Food Additives, and Medications

Along with Advice about the Diagnosis and Treatment of Allergy Symptoms, a Glossary of Related Terms, a Directory of Resources for Help and Information, and Suggestions for Additional Reading

Edited by Amy L. Sutton. 588 pages. 2007. 978-0-7808-0950-5.

SEE ALSO Asthma Sourcebook, 2nd Edition

Alzheimer Disease Sourcebook, 4th Edition

Basic Consumer Health Information about Alzheimer Disease, Other Dementias, and Related Disorders, Including Multi-Infarct Dementia, Dementia with Lewy Bodies, Frontotemporal Dementia (Pick Disease), Wernicke-Korsakoff Syndrome (Alcohol-Related Dementia), AIDS Dementia Complex, Huntington Disease, Creutzfeldt-Jacob Disease, and Delirium

Along with Information about Coping with Memory Loss and Forgetfulness, Maintaining Skills, and Long-Term Planning for People with Dementia, and Suggestions Addressing Common Caregiver Concerns, Updated Information about Current Research Efforts, a Glossary of Related Terms, and Directories of Sources for Additional Help and Information

Edited by Karen Bellenir. 603 pages. 2008. 978-0-7808-1001-3.

"An invaluable resource for persons who have received a diagnosis, for caregivers, and for family members dealing with this insidious disease. It is recommended for public, community college, and ready-reference sections in academic libraries."
—American Reference Books Annual, 2009

SEE ALSO Brain Disorders Sourcebook, 3rd Edition

Arthritis Sourcebook, 3rd Edition

Basic Consumer Health Information about the Risk Factors, Symptoms, Diagnosis, and Treatment of Osteoarthritis, Rheumatoid Arthritis, Juvenile Arthritis, Gout, Infectious Arthritis, and Autoimmune Disorders Associated with Arthritis

Along with Facts about Medications, Surgeries, and Self-Care Techniques to Manage Pain and Disability, Tips on Living with Arthritis, a Glossary of Related Terms, and Resources for Additional Help and Information

Edited by Amy L. Sutton. 600 pages. 2010. 978-0-7808-1077-8.

Asthma Sourcebook, 2nd Edition

Basic Consumer Health Information about the Causes, Symptoms, Diagnosis, and Treatment of Asthma in Infants, Children, Teenagers, and Adults, Including Facts about Different Types of Asthma, Common Co-Occurring Conditions, Asthma Management Plans, Triggers, Medications, and Medication Delivery Devices

Along with Asthma Statistics, Research Updates, a Glossary, a Directory of Asthma-Related Resources, and More

Edited by Karen Bellenir. 581 pages. 2006. 978-0-7808-0866-9.

SEE ALSO Lung Disorders Sourcebook; Respiratory Disorders Sourcebook, 2nd Edition

Attention Deficit Disorder Sourcebook

Basic Consumer Health Information about Attention Deficit/Hyperactivity Disorder in Children and Adults, Including Facts about Causes, Symptoms, Diagnostic Criteria, and Treatment Options Such as Medications, Behavior Therapy, Coaching, and Homeopathy

Along with Reports on Current Research Initiatives, Legal Issues, and Government Regulations, and Featuring a Glossary of Related Terms, Internet Resources, and a List of Additional Reading Material

Edited by Dawn D. Matthews. 447 pages. 2002. 978-0-7808-0624-5.

"Recommended reference source."
—Booklist, Jan '03

SEE ALSO Learning Disabilities Sourcebook, 3rd Edition

Autism and Pervasive Developmental Disorders Sourcebook

Basic Consumer Health Information about Autism Spectrum and Pervasive Developmental Disorders, Such as Classical Autism, Asperger Syndrome, Rett Syndrome, and Childhood Disintegrative Disorder, Including Information about Related Genetic Disorders and Medical Problems and Facts about Causes, Screening Methods, Diagnostic Criteria, Treatments and Interventions, and Family and Education Issues

Along with a Glossary of Related Terms, Tips for Evaluating the Validity of Health Claims, and a Directory of Resources for Additional Help and Information

Edited by Sandra J. Judd. 603 pages. 2007. 978-0-7808-0953-6.

"This book provides a current overview of disorders on the autism spectrum and information about various therapies, educational resources, and help for families with practical issues such as workplace adjustments, living arrangements, and estate planning. It is a useful resource for public and consumer health libraries."

—*American Reference Books Annual, 2009*

SEE ALSO *Learning Disabilities Sourcebook, 3rd Edition*

Back and Neck Disorders Sourcebook, 2nd Edition

Basic Consumer Health Information about Spinal Pain, Spinal Cord Injuries, and Related Disorders, Such as Degenerative Disk Disease, Osteoarthritis, Scoliosis, Sciatica, Spina Bifida, and Spinal Stenosis, and Featuring Facts about Maintaining Spinal Health, Self-Care, Pain Management, Rehabilitative Care, Chiropractic Care, Spinal Surgeries, and Complementary Therapies

Along with Suggestions for Preventing Back and Neck Pain, a Glossary of Related Terms, and a Directory of Resources

Edited by Amy L. Sutton. 607 pages. 2004. 978-0-7808-0738-9.

"Recommended... An easy to use, comprehensive medical reference book."

—*E-Streams, Sep '05*

"For anyone who has back or neck problems, this book is ideal. Its easy-to-understand language and variety of topics makes this sourcebook a worthwhile read. The price... is reasonable for the amount of information contained in the book"

—*Occupational Therapy in Health Care, 2007*

Blood & Circulatory Disorders Sourcebook, 3rd Edition

Basic Consumer Health Information about Blood and Circulatory System Disorders, Such as Anemia, Leukemia, Lymphoma, Rh Disease, Hemophilia, Thrombophilia, Other Bleeding and Clotting Deficiencies, and Artery, Vascular, and Venous Diseases, Including Facts about Blood Types, Blood Donation, Bone Marrow and Stem Cell Transplants, Tests and Medications, and Tips for Maintaining Circulatory Health

Along with a Glossary of Related Terms and a List of Resources for Additional Help and Information

Edited by Sandra J. Judd. 600 pages. 2010. 978-0-7808-1081-5.

SEE ALSO *Leukemia Sourcebook*

Brain Disorders Sourcebook, 3rd Edition

Basic Consumer Health Information about Acquired and Traumatic Brain Injuries, Brain Tumors, Cerebral Palsy and Other Genetic and Congenital Brain Disorders, Infections of the Brain, Epilepsy, and Degenerative Neurological Disorders Such as Dementia, Huntington Disease, and Amyotrophic Lateral Sclerosis (ALS)

Along with Information on Brain Structure and Function, Treatment and Rehabilitation Options, a Glossary of Terms Related to Brain Disorders, and a Directory of Resources for More Information

Edited by Joyce Brennfleck Shannon. 600 pages. 2010. 978-0-7808-1083-9.

SEE ALSO *Alzheimer Disease Sourcebook, 4th Edition*

Breast Cancer Sourcebook, 3rd Edition

Basic Consumer Health Information about Breast Health and Breast Cancer, Including Facts about Environmental, Genetic, and Other Risk Factors, Prevention Efforts, Screening and Diagnostic Methods, Surgical Treatment Options and Other Care Choices, Complementary and Alternative Therapies, and Post-Treatment Concerns

Along with Statistical Data, News about Research Advances, a Glossary of Related Terms, and Directories of Resources for Additional Information and Support

Edited by Karen Bellenir. 606 pages. 2009. 978-0-7808-1030-3.

"A very useful reference for people wanting to learn more about breast cancer and how to negotiate their care or the care of a loved one. The third edition is necessary as information/treatment options continue to evolve."
—*Doody's Review Service, 2009*

SEE ALSO *Cancer Sourcebook for Women, 3rd Edition, Women's Health Concerns Sourcebook, 3rd Edition*

■

Breastfeeding Sourcebook

Basic Consumer Health Information about the Benefits of Breastmilk, Preparing to Breastfeed, Breastfeeding as a Baby Grows, Nutrition, and More, Including Information on Special Situations and Concerns Such as Mastitis, Illness, Medications, Allergies, Multiple Births, Prematurity, Special Needs, and Adoption

Along with a Glossary and Resources for Additional Help and Information

Edited by Jenni Lynn Colson. 367 pages. 2002. 978-0-7808-0332-9.

SEE ALSO *Pregnancy and Birth Sourcebook, 3rd Edition*

■

Burns Sourcebook

Basic Consumer Health Information about Various Types of Burns and Scalds, Including Flame, Heat, Cold, Electrical, Chemical, and Sun Burns

Along with Information on Short-Term and Long-Term Treatments, Tissue Reconstruction, Plastic Surgery, Prevention Suggestions, and First Aid

Edited by Allan R. Cook. 604 pages. 1999. 978-0-7808-0204-9.

"This is an exceptional addition to the series and is highly recommended for all consumer health collections, hospital libraries, and academic medical centers."
—*E-Streams, Mar '00*

"This key reference guide is an invaluable addition to all health care and public libraries in confronting this ongoing health issue."
—*American Reference Books Annual, 2000*

SEE ALSO *Dermatological Disorders Sourcebook, 2nd Edition*

■

Cancer Sourcebook, 5th Edition

Basic Consumer Health Information about Major Forms and Stages of Cancer, Featuring Facts about Head and Neck Cancers, Lung Cancers, Gastrointestinal Cancers, Genitourinary Cancers, Lymphomas, Blood Cell Cancers, Endocrine Cancers, Skin Cancers, Bone Cancers, Metastatic Cancers, and More

Along with Facts about Cancer Treatments, Cancer Risks and Prevention, a Glossary of Related Terms, Statistical Data, and a Directory of Resources for Additional Information

Edited by Karen Bellenir. 1105 pages. 2007. 978-0-7808-0947-5.

"The 5th, updated edition of Cancer Sourcebook should be in every public and health lending library collection... An unparalleled discussion essential for any health collections considering an all-in-one basic general reference."
—*California Bookwatch, Aug '07*

SEE ALSO *Breast Cancer Sourcebook, 3rd Edition, Cancer Survivorship Sourcebook, Leukemia Sourcebook*

■

Cancer Sourcebook for Women, 4th Edition

Basic Consumer Health Information about Gynecologic Cancers and Other Cancers of Special Concern to Women, Including Cancers of the Breast, Cervix, Colon, Lung, Ovaries, Thyroid, and Uterus

Along with Facts about Benign Conditions of the Female Reproductive System, Cancer Risk

Factors, Diagnostic and Treatment Procedures, Side Effects of Cancer and Cancer Treatments, Women's Issues in Cancer Survivorship, a Glossary of Related Terms, and a Directory of Resources for Additional Help and Information

Edited by Karen Bellenir. 600 pages. 2010. 978-0-7808-1139-3.

SEE ALSO Breast Cancer Sourcebook, 3rd Edition, Women's Health Concerns Sourcebook, 3rd Edition

Cancer Survivorship Sourcebook

Basic Consumer Health Information about the Physical, Educational, Emotional, Social, and Financial Needs of Cancer Patients from Diagnosis, through Cancer Treatment, and Beyond, Including Facts about Researching Specific Types of Cancer and Learning about Clinical Trials and Treatment Options, and Featuring Tips for Coping with the Side Effects of Cancer Treatments and Adjusting to Life after Cancer Treatment Concludes

Along with Suggestions for Caregivers, Friends, and Family Members of Cancer Patients, a Glossary of Cancer Care Terms, and Directories of Related Resources

Edited by Karen Bellenir. 633 pages. 2007. 978-0-7808-0985-7.

"Well organized and comprehensive in coverage, the book speaks to issues encountered both during and after cancer treatment. Recommended for consumer health and public libraries."
—Library Journal, Aug 1 '07

"Cancer Survivorship Sourcebook will be useful to anyone who has a friend or loved one with a cancer diagnosis."
—American Reference Books Annual, 2008

SEE ALSO Cancer Sourcebook, 5th Edition, Disease Management Sourcebook

Cardiovascular Disorders Sourcebook, 4th Edition

Basic Consumer Health Information about Heart and Blood Vessel Diseases and Disorders, Such as Angina, Heart Attack, Heart Failure, Cardiomyopathy, Arrhythmias, Valve Disease, Atherosclerosis, Aneurysms, and

Congenital Heart Defects, Including Information about Cardiovascular Disease in Women, Men, Children, Adolescents, and Minorities

Along with Facts about Diagnosing, Managing, and Preventing Cardiovascular Disease, a Glossary of Related Medical Terms, and a Directory of Resources for Additional Information

Edited by Amy L. Sutton. 600 pages. 2010. 978-0-7808-1080-8.

Caregiving Sourcebook

Basic Consumer Health Information for Caregivers, Including a Profile of Caregivers, Caregiving Responsibilities and Concerns, Tips for Specific Conditions, Care Environments, and the Effects of Caregiving

Along with Facts about Legal Issues, Financial Information, and Future Planning, a Glossary, and a Listing of Additional Resources

Edited by Joyce Brennfleck Shannon. 583 pages. 2001. 978-0-7808-0331-2.

"Essential for most collections."
—Library Journal, Apr 1 '02

"An ideal addition to the reference collection of any public library. Health sciences information professionals may also want to acquire the Caregiving Sourcebook for their hospital or academic library for use as a ready reference tool by health care workers interested in aging and caregiving."
—E-Streams, Jan '02

Child Abuse Sourcebook, 2nd Edition

Basic Consumer Health Information about the Physical, Sexual, and Emotional Abuse of Children, Neglect, Münchhausen Syndrome by Proxy (MSBP), and Shaken Baby Syndrome, and Featuring Facts about Withholding Medical Care, Corporal Punishment, Child Maltreatment in Youth Sports, and Parental Substance Abuse

Along with Information about Child Protective Services, Foster Care, Adoption, Parenting Challenges, Abuse Prevention Programs, and Intervention, Treatment, and Recovery Guidelines, a Glossary of Related Terms, and Resources for Additional Help and Information

Edited by Joyce Brennfleck Shannon. 600 pages. 2009. 978-0-7808-1037-2.

SEE ALSO Domestic Violence Sourcebook, 3rd Edition

Childhood Diseases and Disorders Sourcebook, 2nd Edition

Basic Consumer Health Information about the Physical, Mental, and Developmental Health of Pre-Adolescent Children, Including Facts about Infectious Diseases, Asthma, Allergies, Diabetes, and Other Acute and Chronic Conditions Affecting the Gastrointestinal Tract, Ears, Nose, Throat, Liver, Kidneys, Heart, Blood, Brain, Muscles, Bones, and Skin

Along with Reports on Recommended Childhood Vaccinations, Wellness Guidelines, a Glossary of Related Medical Terms, and a List of Resources for Parents

Edited by Sandra J. Judd. 694 pages. 2009. 978-0-7808-1031-0.

"The strength of this source is the wide range of information given about childhood health issues... It is most appropriate for public libraries and academic libraries that field medical questions."
—American Reference Books Annual, 2009

SEE ALSO Healthy Children Sourcebook

Colds, Flu and Other Common Ailments Sourcebook

Basic Consumer Health Information about Common Ailments and Injuries, Including Colds, Coughs, the Flu, Sinus Problems, Headaches, Fever, Nausea and Vomiting, Menstrual Cramps, Diarrhea, Constipation, Hemorrhoids, Back Pain, Dandruff, Dry and Itchy Skin, Cuts, Scrapes, Sprains, Bruises, and More

Along with Information about Prevention, Self-Care, Choosing a Doctor, Over-the-Counter Medications, Folk Remedies, and Alternative Therapies, and Including a Glossary of Important Terms and a Directory of Resources for Further Help and Information

Edited by Chad T. Kimball. 622 pages. 2001. 978-0-7808-0435-7.

"A good starting point for research on common illnesses. It will be a useful addition to public and consumer health library collections."
—American Reference Books Annual, 2002

"Will prove valuable to any library seeking to maintain a current, comprehensive reference collection of health resources... Excellent reference."
—The Bookwatch, Aug '01

SEE ALSO Contagious Diseases Sourcebook, 2nd Edition

Communication Disorders Sourcebook

Basic Information about Deafness and Hearing Loss, Speech and Language Disorders, Voice Disorders, Balance and Vestibular Disorders, and Disorders of Smell, Taste, and Touch

Edited by Linda M. Ross. 533 pages. 1996. 978-0-7808-0077-9.

"This is skillfully edited and is a welcome resource for the layperson. It should be found in every public and medical library."
—Booklist Health Sciences Supplement, Oct '97

Complementary & Alternative Medicine Sourcebook, 4th Edition

Basic Consumer Health Information about Ayurveda, Acupuncture, Aromatherapy, Chiropractic Care, Diet-Based Therapies, Guided Imagery, Herbal and Vitamin Supplements, Homeopathy, Hypnosis, Massage, Meditation, Naturopathy, Pilates, Reflexology, Reiki, Shiatsu, Tai Chi, Traditional Chinese Medicine, Yoga, and Other Complementary and Alternative Medical Therapies

Along with Statistics, Tips for Selecting a Practitioner, Treatments for Specific Health Conditions, a Glossary of Related Terms, and a Directory of Resources for Additional Help and Information

Edited by Amy L. Sutton. 600 pages. 2010. 978-0-7808-1082-2.

Congenital Disorders Sourcebook, 2nd Edition

Basic Consumer Health Information about Nonhereditary Birth Defects and Disorders

Related to Prematurity, Gestational Injuries, Congenital Infections, and Birth Complications, Including Heart Defects, Hydrocephalus, Spina Bifida, Cleft Lip and Palate, Cerebral Palsy, and More

Along with Facts about the Prevention of Birth Defects, Fetal Surgery and Other Treatment Options, Research Initiatives, a Glossary of Related Terms, and Resources for Additional Information and Support

Edited by Sandra J. Judd. 619 pages. 2007. 978-0-7808-0945-1.

"Congenital Disorders Sourcebook provides an excellent, non-technical overview of many aspects of pregnancy with the focus on congenital disorders."
—American Reference Books Annual, 2008

"An excellent readable reference aimed at the lay public for difficult to understand medical problems. An excellent starting point for the interested parent or family member who may then be motivated to seek more information."
—Doody's Review Service, 2007

SEE ALSO Pregnancy and Birth Sourcebook, 3rd Edition

Contagious Diseases Sourcebook, 2nd Edition

Basic Consumer Health Information about Diseases Spread from Person to Person through Direct Physical Contact, Airborne Transmissions, Sexual Contact, or Contact with Blood or Other Body Fluids, Including Pneumococcal, Staphylococcal, and Streptococcal Diseases, Colds, Influenza, Lice, Measles, Mumps, Tuberculosis, and Others

Along with Facts about Self-Care and Over-the-Counter Medications, Antibiotics and Drug Resistance, Disease Prevention, Vaccines, and Bioterrorism, a Glossary, and a Directory of Resources for More Information

Edited by Joyce Brennfleck Shannon. 600 pages. 2010. 978-0-7808-1075-4.

SEE ALSO AIDS Sourcebook, 4th Edition, Hepatitis Sourcebook

Cosmetic and Reconstructive Surgery Sourcebook, 2nd Edition

Basic Consumer Information about Plastic Surgery and Non-Surgical Appearance-Enhancing Procedures, Including Facts about Botulinum Toxin, Collagen Replacement, Dermabrasion, Chemical Peels, Eyelid Surgery, Nose Reshaping, Lip Augmentation, Liposuction, Breast Enlargement and Reduction, Tummy Tucking, and Other Skin, Hair, Facial, and Body Shaping Procedures

Along with Information about Reconstructive Procedures for Congenital Disorders, Disfiguring Diseases, Burns, and Traumatic Injuries, a Glossary of Related Terms, and a Directory of Additional Resources

Edited by Karen Bellenir. 483 pages. 2007. 978-0-7808-0951-2.

"A comprehensive source for people considering cosmetic surgery... also recommended for medical students who will perform these procedures later in their careers; and public librarians and academic medical librarians who may assist patrons interested in this information."
—Medical Reference Services Quarterly, Fall '08

"A practical guide for health care consumers and health care workers... This easy-to-read reference guide would be useful for novice and veteran health care consumers, surgical technology students, nursing students, and perioperative nurses new to plastic and reconstructive surgery. It also may be helpful for medical-surgical nurses as a guide for patient teaching in their practices."
—AORN Journal, Aug '08

SEE ALSO Surgery Sourcebook, 2nd Edition

Death and Dying Sourcebook, 2nd Edition

Basic Consumer Health Information about End-of-Life Care and Related Perspectives and Ethical Issues, Including End-of-Life Symptoms and Treatments, Pain Management, Quality-of-Life Concerns, the Use of Life Support, Patients' Rights and Privacy Issues, Advance Directives, Physician-Assisted Suicide, Caregiving, Organ and Tissue Donation, Autopsies, Funeral Arrangements, and Grief

Along with Statistical Data, Information about the Leading Causes of Death, a Glossary, and Directories of Support Groups and Other Resources

Edited by Joyce Brennfleck Shannon. 626 pages. 2006. 978-0-7808-0871-3.

Edited by Sandra J. Judd. 646 pages. 2008. 978-0-7808-1003-7.

"Recommended for public libraries."
—*American Reference Books Annual, 2009*

SEE ALSO Mental Health Disorders Sourcebook, 4th Edition

Dental Care and Oral Health Sourcebook, 3rd Edition

Basic Consumer Health Information about Dental Care and Oral Health Throughout the Lifespan, Including Facts about Cavities, Bad Breath, Cold and Canker Sores, Dry Mouth, Toothaches, Gum Disease, Malocclusion, Temporomandibular Joint and Muscle Disorders, Oral Cancers, and Dental Emergencies

Along with Information about Mouth Hygiene, Crowns, Bridges, Implants, and Fillings, Surgical, Orthodontic, and Cosmetic Dental Procedures, Pain Management, Health Conditions that Impact Oral Care, a Glossary of Related Terms, and a Directory of Additional Resources

Edited by Amy L. Sutton. 619 pages. 2008. 978-0-7808-1032-7.

"Could serve as turning point in the battle to educate consumers in issues concerning oral health. Tightly written in terms the average person can understand, yet comprehensive in scope and authoritative in tone, it is another excellent sourcebook in the Health Reference Series... Should be in the reference department of all public libraries, and in academic libraries that have a public constituency."
—*American Reference Books Annual, 2009*

Depression Sourcebook, 2nd Edition

Basic Consumer Health Information about Unipolar Depression, Bipolar Disorder, Dysthymia, Seasonal Affective Disorder, Postpartum Depression, and Other Depressive Disorders, Including Facts about Populations at Special Risk, Coexisting Medical Conditions, Symptoms, Treatment Options, and Suicide Prevention

Along with Statistical Data, a Glossary of Related Terms, and a Directory of Resources for Additional Help and Information

Dermatological Disorders Sourcebook, 2nd Edition

Basic Consumer Health Information about Conditions and Disorders Affecting the Skin, Hair, and Nails, Such as Acne, Rosacea, Rashes, Dermatitis, Pigmentation Disorders, Birthmarks, Skin Cancer, Skin Injuries, Psoriasis, Scleroderma, and Hair Loss, Including Facts about Medications and Treatments for Dermatological Disorders and Tips for Maintaining Healthy Skin, Hair, and Nails

Along with Information about How Aging Affects the Skin, a Glossary of Related Terms, and a Directory of Resources for Additional Help and Information

Edited by Amy L. Sutton. 617 pages. 2006. 978-0-7808-0795-2.

"Well organized... presents a plethora of information in a manner that is appropriate in style and readability for the intended audience."
—*Physical Therapy, Nov '06*

"Helpfully brings together... sources in one convenient place, saving the user hours of research time."
—*American Reference Books Annual, 2006*

SEE ALSO Burns Sourcebook

Diabetes Sourcebook, 4th Edition

Basic Consumer Health Information about Type 1 and Type 2 Diabetes Mellitus, Gestational Diabetes, Monogenic Forms of Diabetes, and Insulin Resistance, with Guidelines for Lifestyle Modifications and the Medical Management of Diabetes, Including Facts about Insulin, Insulin Delivery Devices, Oral Diabetes Medications, Self-Monitoring of Blood Glucose, Meal Planning, Physical Activity Recommendations, Foot Care, and Treatment Options for People with Kidney Failure

Along with a Section about Diabetes Complications and Co-Occurring Conditions, a Glossary

of Related Terms, and Directories of Resources for Additional Help and Information

Edited by Karen Bellenir. 627 pages. 2008. 978-0-7808-1005-1.

"Completely and comprehensively covering almost everything a student or physician would need to know... well worth the investment."
—*Internet Bookwatch, Dec '08*

SEE ALSO *Endocrine and Metabolic Disorders Sourcebook, 2nd Edition*

Diet and Nutrition Sourcebook, 3rd Edition

Basic Consumer Health Information about Dietary Guidelines and the Food Guidance System, Recommended Daily Nutrient Intakes, Serving Proportions, Weight Control, Vitamins and Supplements, Nutrition Issues for Different Life Stages and Lifestyles, and the Needs of People with Specific Medical Concerns, Including Cancer, Celiac Disease, Diabetes, Eating Disorders, Food Allergies, and Cardiovascular Disease

Along with Facts about Federal Nutrition Support Programs, a Glossary of Nutrition and Dietary Terms, and Directories of Additional Resources for More Information about Nutrition

Edited by Joyce Brennfleck Shannon. 605 pages. 2006. 978-0-7808-0800-3.

"A valuable resource tool for any individual."
—*Journal of Dental Hygiene, Apr '07*

"From different recommended eating habits to reduce disease and common ailments to nutrition advice for those with specific conditions, Diet and Nutrition Sourcebook is especially important because so much is changing in this area, and so rapidly."
—*California Bookwatch, Jun '06*

SEE ALSO *Eating Disorders Sourcebook, 2nd Edition, Vegetarian Sourcebook*

Digestive Diseases and Disorders Sourcebook

Basic Consumer Health Information about Diseases and Disorders that Impact the Upper and Lower Digestive System, Including Celiac Disease, Constipation, Crohn's Disease, Cyclic Vomiting Syndrome, Diarrhea, Diverticulosis and Diverticulitis, Gallstones, Heartburn, Hemorrhoids, Hernias, Indigestion (Dyspepsia), Irritable Bowel Syndrome, Lactose Intolerance, Ulcers, and More

Along with Information about Medications and Other Treatments, Tips for Maintaining a Healthy Digestive Tract, a Glossary, and Directory of Digestive Diseases Organizations

Edited by Karen Bellenir. 323 pages. 2000. 978-0-7808-0327-5.

"An excellent addition to all public or patient-research libraries."
—*American Reference Books Annual, 2001*

"Recommended reference source."
—*Booklist, May '00*

SEE ALSO *Gastrointestinal Diseases and Disorders Sourcebook, 2nd Edition*

Disabilities Sourcebook

Basic Consumer Health Information about Physical and Psychiatric Disabilities, Including Descriptions of Major Causes of Disability, Assistive and Adaptive Aids, Workplace Issues, and Accessibility Concerns

Along with Information about the Americans with Disabilities Act, a Glossary, and Resources for Additional Help and Information

Edited by Dawn D. Matthews. 602 pages. 2000. 978-0-7808-0389-3.

"A must for libraries with a consumer health section."
—*American Reference Books Annual, 2002*

"A much needed addition to the Omnigraphics Health Reference Series. A current reference work to provide people with disabilities, their families, caregivers or those who work with them, a broad range of information in one volume, has not been available until now... It is recommended for all public and academic library reference collections."
—*E-Streams, May '01*

"An excellent source book in easy-to-read format covering many current topics; highly recommended for all libraries."
—*CHOICE, Jan '01*

Disease Management Sourcebook

Basic Consumer Health Information about Coping with Chronic and Serious Illnesses, Navigating the Health Care System, Communicating with Health Care Providers, Assessing Health Care Quality, and Making Informed Health Care Decisions, Including Facts about Second Opinions, Hospitalization, Surgery, and Medications

Along with a Section about Children with Chronic Conditions, Information about Legal, Financial, and Insurance Issues, a Glossary of Related Terms, and Directories of Additional Resources

Edited by Joyce Brennfleck Shannon. 621 pages. 2008. 978-0-7808-1002-0.

"Consumers need to know how to manage their health care the same way they manage anything else in their lives. The text is very readable and is written for the layperson and consumer. The cost is not prohibitive. This book should be in all collections of health care libraries and public libraries."
— American Reference Books Annual, 2009

"The information is very current, and the selection of font and layout make the book easy to read. A hardback that will stand up to much usage, this is an excellent resource for consumers... Recommended. General readers."
—CHOICE, Nov '08

"Intended for lay readers, this resource clarifies the many confusing and overwhelming details associated with chronic disease care. Meticulous and clearly explained, the book even includes diagrams intended to ease comprehension of over-the-counter medication labels. An essential guide to navigating the health-care rapids."
—Library Journal, Aug '08

Domestic Violence Sourcebook, 3rd Edition

Basic Consumer Health Information about Warning Signs, Risk Factors, and Health Consequences of Intimate Partner Violence, Sexual Violence and Rape, Stalking, Human Trafficking, Child Maltreatment, Teen Dating Violence, and Elder Abuse

Along with Facts about Victims and Perpetrators, Strategies for Violence Prevention, and

Emergency Interventions, Safety Plans, and Financial and Legal Tips for Victims, a Glossary of Related Terms, and Directories of Resources for Additional Information and Support

Edited by Joyce Brennfleck Shannon. 634 pages. 2009. 978-0-7808-1038-9.

"A recommended pick for any library interested in consumer health and social issues... A 'must' for any serious health collection."
—California Bookwatch, Jul '09

SEE ALSO *Child Abuse Sourcebook, 2nd Edition*

Drug Abuse Sourcebook, 3rd Edition

Basic Consumer Health Information about the Abuse of Cocaine, Club Drugs, Hallucinogens, Heroin, Inhalants, Marijuana, and Other Illicit Substances, Prescription Medications, and Over-the-Counter Medicines

Along with Facts about Addiction and Related Health Effects, Drug Abuse Treatment and Recovery, Drug Testing, Prevention Programs, Glossaries of Drug-Related Terms, and Directories of Resources for More Information

Edited by Joyce Brennfleck Shannon. 600 pages. 2010. 978-0-7808-1079-2.

SEE ALSO *Alcoholism Sourcebook, 3rd Edition*

Ear, Nose, and Throat Disorders Sourcebook, 2nd Edition

Basic Consumer Health Information about Disorders of the Ears, Hearing Loss, Vestibular Disorders, Nasal and Sinus Problems, Throat and Vocal Cord Disorders, and Otolaryngologic Cancers, Including Facts about Ear Infections and Injuries, Genetic and Congenital Deafness, Sensorineural Hearing Disorders, Tinnitus, Vertigo, Ménière Disease, Rhinitis, Sinusitis, Snoring, Sore Throats, Hoarseness, and More

Along with Reports on Current Research Initiatives, a Glossary of Related Medical Terms, and a Directory of Sources for Further Help and Information

Edited by Sandra J. Judd. 631 pages. 2007. 978-0-7808-0872-0.

"A resource book for the general public that provides comprehensive coverage of basic up-to-date medical information about the causes, symptoms, diagnosis, and treatment of diseases and disorders that affect the ears, nose, sinuses, throat, and voice... The majority of information is presented in question and answer format, much like questions a patient might ask of a health care provider. An extensive index facilitates the reader's ability to easily access information on any specific topic."
—*Journal of Dental Hygiene, Oct '07*

"A handy compilation of information on common and some not so common ailments of the ears, nose, and throat."
—*Doody's Review Service, 2007*

Eating Disorders Sourcebook, 2nd Edition

Basic Consumer Health Information about Anorexia Nervosa, Bulimia, Binge Eating, Compulsive Exercise, Female Athlete Triad, and Other Eating Disorders, Including Facts about Body Image and Other Cultural and Age-Related Risk Factors, Prevention Efforts, Adverse Health Effects, Treatment Options, and the Recovery Process

Along with Guidelines for Healthy Weight Control, a Glossary, and Directories of Additional Resources

Edited by Joyce Brennfleck Shannon. 557 pages. 2007. 978-0-7808-0948-2.

"Recommended for the reference collection of large public libraries."
—*American Reference Books Annual, 2008*

"A basic health reference any health or general library needs."
—*Internet Bookwatch, Jun '07*

SEE ALSO Diet and Nutrition Sourcebook, 3rd Edition, Mental Health Disorders Sourcebook, 4th Edition

---

Emergency Medical Services Sourcebook

Basic Consumer Health Information about Preventing, Preparing for, and Managing Emergency Situations, When and Who to Call for Help, What to Expect in the Emergency Room, the Emergency Medical Team, Patient Issues, and Current Topics in Emergency Medicine

Along with Statistical Data, a Glossary, and Sources of Additional Help and Information

Edited by Jenni Lynn Colson. 472 pages. 2002. 978-0-7808-0420-3.

"Handy and convenient for home, public, school, and college libraries. Recommended."
—*CHOICE, Apr '03*

"This reference can provide the consumer with answers to most questions about emergency care in the United States, or it will direct them to a resource where the answer can be found."
—*American Reference Books Annual, 2003*

SEE ALSO Injury and Trauma Sourcebook

Endocrine and Metabolic Disorders Sourcebook, 2nd Edition

Basic Consumer Health Information about Hormonal and Metabolic Disorders that Affect the Body's Growth, Development, and Functioning, Including Disorders of the Pancreas, Ovaries and Testes, and Pituitary, Thyroid, Parathyroid, and Adrenal Glands, with Facts about Growth Disorders, Addison Disease, Cushing Syndrome, Conn Syndrome, Diabetic Disorders, Multiple Endocrine Neoplasia, Inborn Errors of Metabolism, and More

Along with Information about Endocrine Functioning, Diagnostic and Screening Tests, a Glossary of Related Terms, and Directories of Additional Resources

Edited by Joyce Brennfleck Shannon. 597 pages. 2007. 978-0-7808-0952-9.

SEE ALSO Diabetes Sourcebook, 4th Edition

Environmental Health Sourcebook, 3rd Edition

Basic Consumer Health Information about the Environment and Its Effects on Human Health, Including Facts about Air, Water, and Soil Contamination, Hazardous Chemicals, Foodborne Hazards and Illnesses, Household Hazards Such as Radon, Mold, and Carbon Monoxide, Consumer Hazards from Toxic Products and Imported Goods, and Disorders

Linked to Environmental Causes, Including Chemical Sensitivity, Cancer, Allergies, and Asthma

Along with Information about the Impact of Environmental Hazards on Specific Populations, a Glossary of Related Terms, and Resources for Additional Help and Information.

Edited by Laura Larsen. 600 pages. 2010. 978-0-7808-1078-5

Ethnic Diseases Sourcebook

Basic Consumer Health Information for Ethnic and Racial Minority Groups in the United States, Including General Health Indicators and Behaviors, Ethnic Diseases, Genetic Testing, the Impact of Chronic Diseases, Women's Health, Mental Health Issues, and Preventive Health Care Services

Along with a Glossary and a Listing of Additional Resources

Edited by Joyce Brennfleck Shannon. 648 pages. 2001. 978-0-7808-0336-7.

"Not many books have been written on this topic to date, and the Ethnic Diseases Sourcebook is a strong addition to the list. It will be an important introductory resource for health consumers, students, health care personnel, and social scientists. It is recommended for public, academic, and large hospital libraries."
— American Reference Books Annual, 2002

"Will prove valuable to any library seeking to maintain a current, comprehensive reference collection of health resources... An excellent source of health information about genetic disorders which affect particular ethnic and racial minorities in the U.S."
—The Bookwatch, Aug '01

Eye Care Sourcebook, 3rd Edition

Basic Consumer Health Information about Eye Care and Eye Disorders, Including Facts about the Diagnosis, Prevention, and Treatment of Refractive Disorders, Cataracts, Glaucoma, Macular Degeneration, and Problems Affecting the Cornea, Retina, and Lacrimal Glands

Along with Advice about Preventing Eye Injuries and Tips for Living with Low Vision or Blindness, a Glossary of Related Terms, and Directories of Resources for More Help and Information

Edited by Amy L. Sutton. 646 pages. 2008. 978-0-7808-1000-6.

"A solid reference tool for eye care and a valuable addition to a collection."
—American Reference Books Annual, 2009

Family Planning Sourcebook

Basic Consumer Health Information about Planning for Pregnancy and Contraception, Including Traditional Methods, Barrier Methods, Hormonal Methods, Permanent Methods, Future Methods, Emergency Contraception, and Birth Control Choices for Women at Each Stage of Life

Along with Statistics, a Glossary, and Sources of Additional Information

Edited by Amy Marcaccio Keyzer. 503 pages. 2001. 978-0-7808-0379-4.

"Recommended for public, health, and undergraduate libraries as part of the circulating collection."
—E-Streams, Mar '02

"Will prove valuable to any library seeking to maintain a current, comprehensive reference collection of health resources... Excellent reference."
—The Bookwatch, Aug '01

SEE ALSO Pregnancy and Birth Sourcebook, 3rd Edition

Fitness and Exercise Sourcebook, 3rd Edition

Basic Consumer Health Information about the Physical and Mental Benefits of Fitness, Including Cardiorespiratory Endurance, Muscular Strength, Muscular Endurance, and Flexibility, with Facts about Sports Nutrition and Exercise-Related Injuries and Tips about Physical Activity and Exercises for People of All Ages and for People with Health Concerns

Along with Advice on Selecting and Using Exercise Equipment, Maintaining Exercise Motivation, a Glossary of Related Terms, and a Directory of Resources for More Help and Information

Edited by Amy L. Sutton. 635 pages. 2007. 978-0-7808-0946-8.

"Updates the consumer information on the physical and mental benefits of physical activity throughout the lifespan offered in earlier editions... Recommended. All readers; all levels."
—*CHOICE, Oct '07*

"An exceptionally well-rounded coverage perfect for any concerned about developing and understanding a fitness program."
—*California Bookwatch, Jun '07*

SEE ALSO *Sports Injuries Sourcebook, 3rd Edition*

Food Safety Sourcebook

Basic Consumer Health Information about the Safe Handling of Meat, Poultry, Seafood, Eggs, Fruit Juices, and Other Food Items, and Facts about Pesticides, Drinking Water, Food Safety Overseas, and the Onset, Duration, and Symptoms of Foodborne Illnesses, Including Types of Pathogenic Bacteria, Parasitic Protozoa, Worms, Viruses, and Natural Toxins

Along with the Role of the Consumer, the Food Handler, and the Government in Food Safety, a Glossary, and Resources for Additional Help and Information

Edited by Dawn D. Matthews. 327 pages. 1999. 978-0-7808-0326-8.

"Recommended reference source."
—*Booklist, May '00*

"This book takes the complex issues of food safety and foodborne pathogens and presents them in an easily understood manner. [It does] an excellent job of covering a large and often confusing topic."
— *American Reference Books Annual, 2000*

Forensic Medicine Sourcebook

Basic Consumer Information for the Layperson about Forensic Medicine, Including Crime Scene Investigation, Evidence Collection and Analysis, Expert Testimony, Computer-Aided Criminal Identification, Digital Imaging in the Courtroom, DNA Profiling, Accident Reconstruction, Autopsies, Ballistics, Drugs and Explosives Detection, Latent Fingerprints,

Product Tampering, and Questioned Document Examination

Along with Statistical Data, a Glossary of Forensics Terminology, and Listings of Sources for Further Help and Information

Edited by Annemarie S. Muth. 574 pages. 1999. 978-0-7808-0232-2.

"Given the expected widespread interest in its content and its easy to read style, this book is recommended for most public and all college and university libraries."
—*E-Streams, Feb '01*

"A wealth of information, useful statistics, references are up-to-date and extremely complete. This wonderful collection of data will help students who are interested in a career in any type of forensic field. It is a great resource for attorneys who need information about types of expert witnesses needed in a particular case. It also offers useful information for fiction and nonfiction writers whose work involves a crime. A fascinating compilation. All levels."
—*CHOICE, Jan '00*

"There are several items that make this book attractive to consumers who are seeking certain forensic data... This is a useful current source for those seeking general forensic medical answers."
—*American Reference Books Annual, 2000*

Gastrointestinal Diseases and Disorders Sourcebook, 2nd Edition

Basic Consumer Health Information about the Upper and Lower Gastrointestinal (GI) Tract, Including the Esophagus, Stomach, Intestines, Rectum, Liver, and Pancreas, with Facts about Gastroesophageal Reflux Disease, Gastritis, Hernias, Ulcers, Celiac Disease, Diverticulitis, Irritable Bowel Syndrome, Hemorrhoids, Gastrointestinal Cancers, and Other Diseases and Disorders Related to the Digestive Process

Along with Information about Commonly Used Diagnostic and Surgical Procedures, Statistics, Reports on Current Research Initiatives and Clinical Trials, a Glossary, and Resources for Additional Help and Information

Edited by Sandra J. Judd. 654 pages. 2006. 978-0-7808-0798-3.

"The text is designed for the general reader seeking information on prevention, disease warning signs, diagnostic and therapeutic questions... It is an excellent resource for the general reader to conveniently locate credible, coordinated and indexed information... The sourcebook will prove very helpful for patients, caregivers and should be available in every physician waiting room."
—*Doody's Review Service, 2006*

SEE ALSO Diet and Nutrition Sourcebook, 3rd Edition, Digestive Diseases and Disorders Sourcebook

■

Genetic Disorders Sourcebook, 4th Edition

Basic Consumer Health Information about Hereditary Diseases and Disorders, Including Facts about the Human Genome, Genetic Inheritance Patterns, Disorders Associated with Specific Genes, Such as Sickle Cell Disease, Hemophilia, and Cystic Fibrosis, Chromosome Disorders, Such as Down Syndrome, Fragile X Syndrome, and Turner Syndrome, and Complex Diseases and Disorders Resulting from the Interaction of Environmental and Genetic Factors, Such as Allergies, Cancer, and Obesity

Along with Facts about Genetic Testing, Suggestions for Parents of Children with Special Needs, Reports on Current Research Initiatives, a Glossary of Genetic Terminology, and Resources for Additional Help and Information

Edited by Sandra J. Judd. 600 pages. 2010. 978-0-7808-1076-1.

■

Head Trauma Sourcebook

Basic Information for the Layperson about Open-Head and Closed-Head Injuries, Treatment Advances, Recovery, and Rehabilitation

Along with Reports on Current Research Initiatives

Edited by Karen Bellenir. 414 pages. 1997. 978-0-7808-0208-7.

■

Headache Sourcebook

Basic Consumer Health Information about Migraine, Tension, Cluster, Rebound and Other Types of Headaches, with Facts about the Cause and Prevention of Headaches, the Effects of Stress and the Environment, Headaches during Pregnancy and Menopause, and Childhood Headaches

Along with a Glossary and Other Resources for Additional Help and Information

Edited by Dawn D. Matthews. 342 pages. 2002. 978-0-7808-0337-4.

"Highly recommended for academic and medical reference collections."
—*Library Bookwatch, Sep '02*

SEE ALSO Pain Sourcebook, 3rd Edition

■

Healthy Aging Sourcebook

Basic Consumer Health Information about Maintaining Health through the Aging Process, Including Advice on Nutrition, Exercise, and Sleep, Help in Making Decisions about Midlife Issues and Retirement, and Guidance Concerning Practical and Informed Choices in Health Consumerism

Along with Data Concerning the Theories of Aging, Different Experiences in Aging by Minority Groups, and Facts about Aging Now and Aging in the Future; and Featuring a Glossary, a Guide to Consumer Help, Additional Suggested Reading, and Practical Resource Directory

Edited by Jenifer Swanson. 537 pages. 1999. 978-0-7808-0390-9.

"Recommended reference source."
—*Booklist, Feb '00*

SEE ALSO Adult Health Sourcebook, Physical and Mental Issues in Aging Sourcebook

■

Healthy Children Sourcebook

Basic Consumer Health Information about the Physical and Mental Development of Children between the Ages of 3 and 12, Including Routine Health Care, Preventative Health Services, Safety and First Aid, Healthy Sleep, Dental Care, Nutrition, and Fitness, and Featuring Parenting Tips on Such Topics as Bedwetting, Choosing Day Care, Monitoring TV and Other Media, and Establishing a Foundation for Substance Abuse Prevention

Along with a Glossary of Commonly Used Pediatric Terms and Resources for Additional Help and Information.

Edited by Chad T. Kimball. 624 pages. 2003. 978-0-7808-0247-6.

"Should be required reading for parents and teachers."
—*E-Streams, Jun '04*

"It is hard to imagine that any other single resource exists that would provide such a comprehensive guide of timely information on health promotion and disease prevention for children aged 3 to 12."
—*American Reference Books Annual, 2004*

"This easy-to-read volume is a tremendous resource."
—*AORN Journal, May '05*

SEE ALSO *Childhood Diseases and Disorders Sourcebook, 2nd Edition*

Healthy Heart Sourcebook for Women

Basic Consumer Health Information about Cardiac Issues Specific to Women, Including Facts about Major Risk Factors and Prevention, Treatment and Control Strategies, and Important Dietary Issues

Along with a Special Section Regarding the Pros and Cons of Hormone Replacement Therapy and Its Impact on Heart Health, and Additional Help, Including Recipes, a Glossary, and a Directory of Resources

Edited by Dawn D. Matthews. 321 pages. 2000. 978-0-7808-0329-9.

"A good reference source and recommended for all public, academic, medical, and hospital libraries."
—*Medical Reference Services Quarterly, Summer '01*

"Contains very important information about coronary artery disease that all women should know. The information is current and presented in an easy-to-read format. The book will make a good addition to any library."
—*American Medical Writers Association Journal, Summer '00*

SEE ALSO *Cardiovascular Diseases and Disorders Sourcebook, 4th Edition, Women's Health Concerns Sourcebook, 3rd Edition*

Hepatitis Sourcebook

Basic Consumer Health Information about Hepatitis A, Hepatitis B, Hepatitis C, and Other Forms of Hepatitis, Including Autoimmune Hepatitis, Alcoholic Hepatitis, Nonalcoholic Steatohepatitis, and Toxic Hepatitis, with Facts about Risk Factors, Screening Methods, Diagnostic Tests, and Treatment Options

Along with Information on Liver Health, Tips for People Living with Chronic Hepatitis, Reports on Current Research Initiatives, a Glossary of Terms Related to Hepatitis, and a Directory of Sources for Further Help and Information

Edited by Sandra J. Judd. 570 pages. 2006. 978-0-7808-0749-5.

"The breadth of information found in this one book would not be readily found in another source. Highly recommended."
—*American Reference Books Annual, 2006*

SEE ALSO *Contagious Diseases Sourcebook, 2nd Edition*

Household Safety Sourcebook

Basic Consumer Health Information about Household Safety, Including Information about Poisons, Chemicals, Fire, and Water Hazards in the Home

Along with Advice about the Safe Use of Home Maintenance Equipment, Choosing Toys and Nursery Furniture, Holiday and Recreation Safety, a Glossary, and Resources for Further Help and Information

Edited by Dawn D. Matthews. 587 pages. 2002. 978-0-7808-0338-1.

"As a sourcebook on household safety this book meets its mark. It is encyclopedic in scope and covers a wide range of safety issues that are commonly seen in the home."
—*E-Streams, Jul '02*

Hypertension Sourcebook

Basic Consumer Health Information about the Causes, Diagnosis, and Treatment of High Blood Pressure, with Facts about Consequences, Complications, and Co-Occurring Disorders, Such as Coronary Heart Disease, Diabetes, Stroke, Kidney Disease, and Hypertensive Retinopathy, and Issues in Blood Pressure

Control, Including Dietary Choices, Stress Management, and Medications

Along with Reports on Current Research Initiatives and Clinical Trials, a Glossary, and Resources for Additional Help and Information

Edited by Dawn D. Matthews and Karen Bellenir. 588 pages. 2004. 978-0-7808-0674-0.

"Academic, public, and medical libraries will want to add the Hypertension Sourcebook to their collections."
—E-Streams, Aug '05

"The strength of this source is the wide range of information given about hypertension."
—American Reference Books Annual, 2005

SEE ALSO Stroke Sourcebook, 2nd Edition

Immune System Disorders Sourcebook, 2nd Edition

Basic Consumer Health Information about Disorders of the Immune System, Including Immune System Function and Response, Diagnosis of Immune Disorders, Information about Inherited Immune Disease, Acquired Immune Disease, and Autoimmune Diseases, Including Primary Immune Deficiency, Acquired Immunodeficiency Syndrome (AIDS), Lupus, Multiple Sclerosis, Type 1 Diabetes, Rheumatoid Arthritis, and Graves' Disease

Along with Treatments, Tips for Coping with Immune Disorders, a Glossary, and a Directory of Additional Resources

Edited by Joyce Brennfleck Shannon. 643 pages. 2005. 978-0-7808-0748-8.

"Highly recommended for academic and public libraries."
—American Reference Books Annual, 2006

"The updated second edition is a 'must' for any consumer health library seeking a solid resource covering the treatments, symptoms, and options for immune disorder sufferers... An excellent guide."
—MBR Bookwatch, Jan '06

SEE ALSO AIDS Sourcebook, 4th Edition, Arthritis Sourcebook, 3rd Edition

Infant and Toddler Health Sourcebook

Basic Consumer Health Information about the Physical and Mental Development of Newborns, Infants, and Toddlers, Including Neonatal Concerns, Nutrition Recommendations, Immunization Schedules, Common Pediatric Disorders, Assessments and Milestones, Safety Tips, and Advice for Parents and Other Caregivers

Along with a Glossary of Terms and Resource Listings for Additional Help

Edited by Jenifer Swanson. 570 pages. 2000. 978-0-7808-0246-9.

"As a reference for the general public, this would be useful in any library."
—E-Streams, May '01

"Recommended reference source."
—Booklist, Feb '01

Infectious Diseases Sourcebook

Basic Consumer Health Information about Non-Contagious Bacterial, Viral, Prion, Fungal, and Parasitic Diseases Spread by Food and Water, Insects and Animals, or Environmental Contact, Including Botulism, E. Coli, Encephalitis, Legionnaires' Disease, Lyme Disease, Malaria, Plague, Rabies, Salmonella, Tetanus, and Others, and Facts about Newly Emerging Diseases, Such as Hantavirus, Mad Cow Disease, Monkeypox, and West Nile Virus

Along with Information about Preventing Disease Transmission, the Threat of Bioterrorism, and Current Research Initiatives, with a Glossary and Directory of Resources for More Information

Edited by Karen Bellenir. 610 pages. 2004. 978-0-7808-0675-7.

"This reference continues the excellent tradition of the Health Reference Series in consolidating a wealth of information on a selected topic into a format that is easy to use and accessible to the general public."
—American Reference Books Annual, 2005

"Recommended for public and academic libraries."
—E-Streams, Jan '05

SEE ALSO Environmental Health Sourcebook, 3rd Edition

Injury and Trauma Sourcebook

Basic Consumer Health Information about the Impact of Injury, the Diagnosis and Treatment of Common and Traumatic Injuries, Emergency Care, and Specific Injuries Related to Home, Community, Workplace, Transportation, and Recreation

Along with Guidelines for Injury Prevention, a Glossary, and a Directory of Additional Resources

Edited by Joyce Brennfleck Shannon. 675 pages. 2002. 978-0-7808-0421-0.

"Practitioners should be aware of guides such as this in order to facilitate their use by patients and their families."
—*Doody's Health Sciences Book Review Journal, Sep-Oct '02*

"Recommended reference source."
—*Booklist, Sep '02*

"Highly recommended for academic and medical reference collections."
—*Library Bookwatch, Sep '02*

SEE ALSO *Emergency Medical Services Sourcebook, Sports Injuries Sourcebook, 3rd Edition*

Learning Disabilities Sourcebook, 3rd Edition

Basic Consumer Health Information about Dyslexia, Auditory and Visual Processing Disorders, Communication Disorders, Dyscalculia, Dysgraphia, and Other Conditions That Impede Learning, Including Attention Deficit/ Hyperactivity Disorder, Autism Spectrum Disorders, Hearing and Visual Impairments, Chromosome-Based Disorders, and Brain Injury

Along with Facts about Brain Function, Assessment, Therapy and Remediation, Accommodations, Assistive Technology, Legal Protections, and Tips about Family Life, School Transitions, and Employment Strategies, a Glossary of Related Terms, and Directories of Additional Resources

Edited by Joyce Brennfleck Shannon. 613 pages. 2009. 978-0-7808-1039-6.

"Intended to be a starting point for people who need to know about learning disabilities. Each chapter on a specific disability includes read-

able, well-organized descriptions... The book is well indexed and a glossary is included. Chapters on organizations and helpful websites will aid the reader who needs more information."
—*American Reference Books Annual, 2009*

"This book provides the necessary information to better understand learning disabilities and work with children who have them... It would be difficult to find another book that so comprehensively explains learning disabilities without becoming incomprehensible to the average parent who needs this information."
—*Doody's Review Service, 2009*

SEE ALSO *Attention Deficit Disorder Sourcebook, Autism and Pervasive Developmental Disorders Sourcebook*

Leukemia Sourcebook

Basic Consumer Health Information about Adult and Childhood Leukemias, Including Acute Lymphocytic Leukemia (ALL), Chronic Lymphocytic Leukemia (CLL), Acute Myelogenous Leukemia (AML), Chronic Myelogenous Leukemia (CML), and Hairy Cell Leukemia, and Treatments Such as Chemotherapy, Radiation Therapy, Peripheral Blood Stem Cell and Marrow Transplantation, and Immunotherapy

Along with Tips for Life During and After Treatment, a Glossary, and Directories of Additional Resources

Edited by Joyce Brennfleck Shannon. 564 pages. 2003. 978-0-7808-0627-6.

"Unlike other medical books for the layperson... the language does not talk down to the reader... This volume is highly recommended for all libraries."
—*American Reference Books Annual, 2004*

"A fine title which ranges from diagnosis to alternative treatments, staging, and tips for life during and after diagnosis."
—*The Bookwatch, Dec '03*

SEE ALSO *Blood & Circulatory Disorders Sourcebook, 3rd Edition, Cancer Sourcebook, 5th Edition*

Liver Disorders Sourcebook

Basic Consumer Health Information about the Liver and How It Works; Liver Diseases, Including Cancer, Cirrhosis, Hepatitis, and

Toxic and Drug Related Diseases; Tips for Maintaining a Healthy Liver; Laboratory Tests, Radiology Tests, and Facts about Liver Transplantation

Along with a Section on Support Groups, a Glossary, and Resource Listings

Edited by Joyce Brennfleck Shannon. 580 pages. 2000. 978-0-7808-0383-1.

"This title is recommended for health sciences and public libraries with consumer health collections."
—E-Streams, Oct '00

"Recommended reference source."
—Booklist, Jun '00

SEE ALSO Gastrointestinal Diseases and Disorders Sourcebook, 2nd Edition, Hepatitis Sourcebook

Lung Disorders Sourcebook

Basic Consumer Health Information about Emphysema, Pneumonia, Tuberculosis, Asthma, Cystic Fibrosis, and Other Lung Disorders, Including Facts about Diagnostic Procedures, Treatment Strategies, Disease Prevention Efforts, and Such Risk Factors as Smoking, Air Pollution, and Exposure to Asbestos, Radon, and Other Agents

Along with a Glossary and Resources for Additional Help and Information

Edited by Dawn D. Matthews. 657 pages. 2002. 978-0-7808-0339-8.

"Highly recommended for academic and medical reference collections."
—Library Bookwatch, Sep '02

SEE ALSO Asthma Sourcebook, 2nd Edition, Respiratory Disorders Sourcebook, 2nd Edition

Medical Tests Sourcebook, 3rd Edition

Basic Consumer Health Information about X-Rays, Blood Tests, Stool and Urine Tests, Biopsies, Mammography, Endoscopic Procedures, Ultrasound Exams, Computed Tomography, Magnetic Resonance Imaging (MRI), Nuclear Medicine, Genetic Testing, Home-Use Tests, and More

Along with Facts about Preventive Care and Screening Test Guidelines, Screening and

Assessment Tests Associated with Such Specific Concerns as Cancer, Heart Disease, Allergies, Diabetes, Thyroid Disfunction, and Infertility, a Glossary of Related Terms, and a Directory of Resources for Additional Help and Information

Edited by Karen Bellenir. 627 pages. 2008. 978-0-7808-1040-2

"This volume has a wide scope that makes it useful... Can be a valuable reference guide."
—American Reference Books Annual, 2009

"Would be a valuable contribution to any consumer health or public library."
—Doody's Book Review Service, 2009

Men's Health Concerns Sourcebook, 3rd Edition

Basic Consumer Health Information about Wellness in Men and Gender-Related Differences in Health, With Facts about Heart Disease, Cancer, Traumatic Injury, and Other Leading Causes of Death in Men, Reproductive Concerns, Sexual Dysfunction, Disorders of the Prostate, Penis, and Testes, Sex-Linked Genetic Disorders, and Other Medical and Mental Concerns of Men

Along with Statistical Data, a Glossary of Related Terms, and a Directory of Resources for Additional Information

Edited by Sandra J. Judd. 632 pages. 2009. 978-0-7808-1033-4.

"A good addition to any reference shelf in academic, consumer health, or hospital libraries."
—ARBAOnline, Oct '09

SEE ALSO Prostate and Urological Disorders Sourcebook

Mental Health Disorders Sourcebook, 4th Edition

Basic Consumer Health Information about the Causes and Symptoms of Mental Health Problems, Including Depression, Bipolar Disorder, Anxiety Disorders, Posttraumatic Stress Disorder, Obsessive-Compulsive Disorder, Eating Disorders, Addictions, and Personality and Psychotic Disorders

Along with Information about Medications and Treatments, Mental Health Concerns in

Children, Adolescents, and Adults, Tips on Living with Mental Health Disorders, a Glossary of Related Terms, and a Directory of Resources for Additional Help and Information

Edited by Amy L. Sutton. 680 pages. 2009. 978-0-7808-1041-9.

"Mental health concerns are presented in everyday language and intended for patients and their families as well as the general public... This resource is comprehensive and up to date... The easy-to-understand writing style helps to facilitate assimilation of needed facts and specifics on often challenging topics."
—ARBAOnline, Oct '09

"No health collection should be without this resource, which will reach into many a general lending library as well."
—Internet Bookwatch, Oct '09

SEE ALSO Depression Sourcebook, 2nd Edition, Stress-Related Disorders Sourcebook, 2nd Edition

Mental Retardation Sourcebook

Basic Consumer Health Information about Mental Retardation and Its Causes, Including Down Syndrome, Fetal Alcohol Syndrome, Fragile X Syndrome, Genetic Conditions, Injury, and Environmental Sources

Along with Preventive Strategies, Parenting Issues, Educational Implications, Health Care Needs, Employment and Economic Matters, Legal Issues, a Glossary, and a Resource Listing for Additional Help and Information

Edited by Joyce Brennfleck Shannon. 627 pages. 2000. 978-0-7808-0377-0.

"Public libraries will find the book useful for reference and as a beginning research point for students, parents, and caregivers."
—American Reference Books Annual, 2001

"The strength of this work is that it compiles many basic fact sheets and addresses for further information in one volume. It is intended and suitable for the general public."
—E-Streams, Nov '00

"An invaluable overview."
—Reviewer's Bookwatch, Jul '00

Movement Disorders Sourcebook, 2nd Edition

Basic Consumer Health Information about the Symptoms and Causes of Movement Disorders, Including Parkinson Disease, Amyotrophic Lateral Sclerosis, Cerebral Palsy, Muscular Dystrophy, Multiple Sclerosis, Myasthenia, Myoclonus, Spina Bifida, Dystonia, Essential Tremor, Choreatic Disorders, Huntington Disease, Tourette Syndrome, and Other Disorders That Cause Slowed, Absent, or Excessive Movements

Along with Information about Surgical and Nonsurgical Interventions, Physical Therapies, Strategies for Independent Living, a Glossary of Related Terms, and a Directory of Resources for Additional Help and Information

Edited by Amy L. Sutton. 618 pages. 2009. 978-0-7808-1034-1.

"The second updated edition of Movement Disorders Sourcebook is a winner, providing the latest research and health findings on all kinds of movement disorders in children and adults... a top pick for any health or general lending library's health reference collection."
—California Bookwatch, Aug '09

SEE ALSO Muscular Dystrophy Sourcebook

Multiple Sclerosis Sourcebook

Basic Consumer Health Information about Multiple Sclerosis (MS) and Its Effects on Mobility, Vision, Bladder Function, Speech, Swallowing, and Cognition, Including Facts about Risk Factors, Causes, Diagnostic Procedures, Pain Management, Drug Treatments, and Physical and Occupational Therapies

Along with Guidelines for Nutrition and Exercise, Tips on Choosing Assistive Equipment, Information about Disability, Work, Financial, and Legal Issues, a Glossary of Related Terms, and a Directory of Additional Resources

Edited by Joyce Brennfleck Shannon. 553 pages. 2007. 978-0-7808-0998-7.

Muscular Dystrophy Sourcebook

Basic Consumer Health Information about Congenital, Childhood-Onset, and Adult-Onset

633

Forms of Muscular Dystrophy, Such as Duchenne, Becker, Emery-Dreifuss, Distal, Limb-Girdle, Facioscapulohumeral (FSHD), Myotonic, and Ophthalmoplegic Muscular Dystrophies, Including Facts about Diagnostic Tests, Medical and Physical Therapies, Management of Co-Occurring Conditions, and Parenting Guidelines

Along with Practical Tips for Home Care, a Glossary, and Directories of Additional Resources

Edited by Joyce Brennfleck Shannon. 552 pages. 2004. 978-0-7808-0676-4.

"This book is highly recommended for public and academic libraries as well as health care offices that support the information needs of patients and their families."
—E-Streams, Apr '05

"Excellent reference."
—The Bookwatch, Jan '05

SEE ALSO Movement Disorders Sourcebook, 2nd Edition

Obesity Sourcebook

Basic Consumer Health Information about Diseases and Other Problems Associated with Obesity, and Including Facts about Risk Factors, Prevention Issues, and Management Approaches

Along with Statistical and Demographic Data, Information about Special Populations, Research Updates, a Glossary, and Source Listings for Further Help and Information

Edited by Wilma Caldwell and Chad T. Kimball. 360 pages. 2001. 978-0-7808-0333-6.

"The book synthesizes the reliable medical literature on obesity into one easy-to-read and useful resource for the general public."
—American Reference Books Annual, 2002

"Well suited for the health reference collection of a public library or an academic health science library that serves the general population."
—E-Streams, Sep '01

Osteoporosis Sourcebook

Basic Consumer Health Information about Primary and Secondary Osteoporosis and Juvenile Osteoporosis and Related Conditions, Including Fibrous Dysplasia, Gaucher Disease, Hyperthyroidism, Hypophosphatasia,

Myeloma, Osteopetrosis, Osteogenesis Imperfecta, and Paget's Disease

Along with Information about Risk Factors, Treatments, Traditional and Non-Traditional Pain Management, a Glossary of Related Terms, and a Directory of Resources

Edited by Allan R. Cook. 568 pages. 2001. 978-0-7808-0239-1.

"This resource is recommended as a great reference source for public, health, and academic libraries, and is another triumph for the editors of Omnigraphics."
—American Reference Books Annual, 2002

"Will prove valuable to any library seeking to maintain a current, comprehensive reference collection of health resources... From prevention to treatment and associated conditions, this provides an excellent survey."
—The Bookwatch, Aug '01

SEE ALSO Healthy Aging Sourcebook, Women's Health Concerns Sourcebook, 3rd Edition

---

Pain Sourcebook, 3rd Edition

Basic Consumer Health Information about Acute and Chronic Pain, Including Nerve Pain, Bone Pain, Muscle Pain, Cancer Pain, and Disorders Characterized by Pain, Such as Arthritis, Temporomandibular Muscle and Joint (TMJ) Disorder, Carpal Tunnel Syndrome, Headaches, Heartburn, Sciatica, and Shingles, and Facts about Diagnostic Tests and Treatment Options for Pain, Including Over-the-Counter and Prescription Drugs, Physical Rehabilitation, Injection and Infusion Therapies, Implantable Technologies, and Complementary Medicine

Along with Tips for Living with Pain, a Glossary of Related Terms, and a Directory of Additional Resources

Edited by Joyce Brennfleck Shannon. 644 pages. 2008. 978-0-7808-1006-8.

"Excellent for ready-reference users and can be used for beginning students in health fields... appropriate for the consumer health collection in both public and academic libraries."
—American Reference Books Annual, 2009

SEE ALSO Arthritis Sourcebook, 3rd Edition; Back and Neck Sourcebook, 2nd Edition;

Headache Sourcebook; Sports Injuries Sourcebook, 3rd Edition

Pediatric Cancer Sourcebook

Basic Consumer Health Information about Leukemias, Brain Tumors, Sarcomas, Lymphomas, and Other Cancers in Infants, Children, and Adolescents, Including Descriptions of Cancers, Treatments, and Coping Strategies

Along with Suggestions for Parents, Caregivers, and Concerned Relatives, a Glossary of Cancer Terms, and Resource Listings

Edited by Edward J. Prucha. 575 pages. 1999. 978-0-7808-0245-2.

"An excellent source of information. Recommended for public, hospital, and health science libraries with consumer health collections."
—*E-Streams, Jun '00*

"A valuable addition to all libraries specializing in health services and many public libraries."
—*American Reference Books Annual, 2000*

SEE ALSO *Childhood Diseases and Disorders Sourcebook, 2nd Edition, Healthy Children Sourcebook*

Physical and Mental Issues in Aging Sourcebook

Basic Consumer Health Information on Physical and Mental Disorders Associated with the Aging Process, Including Concerns about Cardiovascular Disease, Pulmonary Disease, Oral Health, Digestive Disorders, Musculoskeletal and Skin Disorders, Metabolic Changes, Sexual and Reproductive Issues, and Changes in Vision, Hearing, and Other Senses

Along with Data about Longevity and Causes of Death, Information on Acute and Chronic Pain, Descriptions of Mental Concerns, a Glossary of Terms, and Resource Listings for Additional Help

Edited by Jenifer Swanson. 660 pages. 1999. 978-0-7808-0233-9.

"This is a treasure of health information for the layperson."
—*CHOICE Health Sciences Supplement, May '00*

"Recommended for public libraries."
—*American Reference Books Annual, 2000*

SEE ALSO *Healthy Aging Sourcebook*

Podiatry Sourcebook, 2nd Edition

Basic Consumer Health Information about Disorders, Diseases, and Deformities that Affect the Foot and Ankle, Including Sprains, Corns, Calluses, Bunions, Plantar Warts, Plantar Fasciitis, Neuromas, Clubfoot, Flat Feet, Achilles Tendonitis, and Much More

Along with Information about Selecting a Foot Care Specialist, Foot Fitness, Shoes and Socks, Diagnostic Tests and Corrective Procedures, Financial Assistance for Corrective Devices, a Glossary of Related Terms, and a Directory of Resources for Additional Help and Information

Edited by Ivy L. Alexander. 516 pages. 2007. 978-0-7808-0944-4.

"An excellent resource... Although there have been various types of 'foot books' published in the past, none are as comprehensive as this one. 5 Stars (out of 5)!"
—*Doody's Review Service, 2007*

"Perfect for both health libraries and general-interest lending collections."
—*Internet Bookwatch, Jul '07*

Pregnancy and Birth Sourcebook, 3rd Edition

Basic Consumer Health Information about Pregnancy and Fetal Development, Including Facts about Fertility and Conception, Physical and Emotional Changes during Pregnancy, Prenatal Care and Diagnostic Tests, High-Risk Pregnancies and Complications, Labor, Delivery, and the Postpartum Period

Along with Tips on Maintaining Health and Wellness during Pregnancy and Caring for Newborn Infants, a Glossary of Related Terms, and Directories of Resources for Additional Help and Information

Edited by Amy L. Sutton. 645 pages. 2009. 978-0-7808-1074-7.

SEE ALSO *Breastfeeding Sourcebook, Congenital Disorders Sourcebook, 2nd Edition, Family Planning Sourcebook, Women's Health Concerns Sourcebook, 3rd Edition*

Prostate and Urological Disorders Sourcebook

Basic Consumer Health Information about Urogenital and Sexual Disorders in Men, Including Prostate and Other Andrological Cancers, Prostatitis, Benign Prostatic Hyperplasia, Testicular and Penile Trauma, Cryptorchidism, Peyronie Disease, Erectile Dysfunction, and Male Factor Infertility, and Facts about Commonly Used Tests and Procedures, Such as Prostatectomy, Vasectomy, Vasectomy Reversal, Penile Implants, and Semen Analysis

Along with a Glossary of Andrological Terms and a Directory of Resources for Additional Information

Edited by Karen Bellenir. 604 pages. 2006. 978-0-7808-0797-6.

"Certain to be a popular pick among library reference holdings... No prior knowledge is assumed for any of the conditions or terms herein, making it a most accessible general-interest reference."
—*California Bookwatch, Apr '06*

SEE ALSO *Men's Health Concerns Sourcebook, 3rd Edition, Urinary Tract and Kidney Diseases and Disorders Sourcebook, 2nd Edition*

Prostate Cancer Sourcebook

Basic Consumer Health Information about Prostate Cancer, Including Information about the Associated Risk Factors, Detection, Diagnosis, and Treatment of Prostate Cancer

Along with Information on Non-Malignant Prostate Conditions, and Featuring a Section Listing Support and Treatment Centers and a Glossary of Related Terms

Edited by Dawn D. Matthews. 340 pages. 2001. 978-0-7808-0324-4.

"Recommended reference source."
—*Booklist, Jan '02*

"A valuable resource for health care consumers seeking information on the subject... All text is written in a clear, easy-to-understand language that avoids technical jargon. Any library that collects consumer health resources would strengthen their collection with the addition of the Prostate Cancer Sourcebook."
—*American Reference Books Annual, 2002*

SEE ALSO *Cancer Sourcebook, 5th Edition, Men's Health Concerns Sourcebook, 3rd Edition*

Rehabilitation Sourcebook

Basic Consumer Health Information about Rehabilitation for People Recovering from Heart Surgery, Spinal Cord Injury, Stroke, Orthopedic Impairments, Amputation, Pulmonary Impairments, Traumatic Injury, and More, Including Physical Therapy, Occupational Therapy, Speech/Language Therapy, Massage Therapy, Dance Therapy, Art Therapy, and Recreational Therapy

Along with Information on Assistive and Adaptive Devices, a Glossary, and Resources for Additional Help and Information

Edited by Dawn D. Matthews. 519 pages. 2000. 978-0-7808-0236-0.

"This is an excellent resource for public library reference and health collections."
—*American Reference Books Annual, 2001*

"Recommended reference source."
—*Booklist, May '00*

Respiratory Disorders Sourcebook, 2nd Edition

Basic Consumer Health Information about Infectious, Inflammatory, and Chronic Conditions Affecting the Lungs and Respiratory System, Including Pneumonia, Bronchitis, Influenza, Tuberculosis, Sarcoidosis, Asthma, Cystic Fibrosis, Chronic Obstructive Pulmonary Disease, Lung Abscesses, Pulmonary Embolism, Occupational Lung Diseases, and Other Bacterial, Viral, and Fungal Infections

Along with Facts about the Structure and Function of the Lungs and Airways, Methods of Diagnosing Respiratory Disorders, and Treatment and Rehabilitation Options, a Glossary of Related Terms, and a Directory of Resources for Additional Help and Information

Edited by Sandra L. Judd. 638 pages. 2008. 978-0-7808-1007-5.

"An excellent book for patients, their families, or for those who are just curious about respiratory disease. Public libraries and physician offices would find this a valuable resource as well. 4 Stars! (out of 5)"
—*Doody's Review Service, 2009*

"A great addition for public and school libraries because it provides concise health information... readers can start with this reference source and get satisfactory answers before proceeding to other medical reference tools for

more in depth information... A good guide for health education on lung disorders."
—*American Reference Books Annual, 2009*

SEE ALSO *Asthma Sourcebook, 2nd Edition, Lung Disorders Sourcebook*

Sexually Transmitted Diseases Sourcebook, 4th Edition

Basic Consumer Health Information about Chlamydial Infections, Gonorrhea, Hepatitis, Herpes, HIV/AIDS, Human Papillomavirus, Pubic Lice, Scabies, Syphilis, Trichomoniasis, Vaginal Infections, and Other Sexually Transmitted Diseases, Including Facts about Risk Factors, Symptoms, Diagnosis, Treatment, and the Prevention of Sexually Transmitted Infections

Along with Updates on Current Research Initiatives, a Glossary of Related Terms, and Resources for Additional Help and Information

Edited by Laura Larsen. 623 pages. 2009. 978-0-7808-1073-0.

"**Extremely beneficial... The question-and-answer format along with the index and table of contents make this well-organized resource extremely easy to reference, read, and comprehend... an invaluable medical reference source for lay readers, and a highly appropriate addition for public library collections, health clinics, and any library with a consumer health collection**"
—*ARBAOnline, Oct '09*

SEE ALSO *AIDS Sourcebook, 4th Edition, Contagious Diseases Sourcebook, 2nd Edition, Men's Health Concerns Sourcebook, 3rd Edition, Women's Health Concerns Sourcebook, 3rd Edition*

Sleep Disorders Sourcebook, 3rd Edition

Basic Consumer Health Information about Sleep Disorders, Including Insomnia, Sleep Apnea and Snoring, Jet Lag and Other Circadian Rhythm Disorders, Narcolepsy, and Parasomnias, Such as Sleep Walking and Sleep Talking, and Featuring Facts about Other Health Problems that Affect Sleep, Why Sleep Is Necessary, How Much Sleep Is Needed, the Physical and Mental Effects of Sleep Deprivation, and Pediatric Sleep Issues

Along with Tips for Diagnosing and Treating Sleep Disorders, a Glossary of Related Terms, and a List of Resources for Additional Help and Information

Edited by Sandra J. Judd. 600 pages. 2010. 978-0-7808-1084-6.

Smoking Concerns Sourcebook

Basic Consumer Health Information about Nicotine Addiction and Smoking Cessation, Featuring Facts about the Health Effects of Tobacco Use, Including Lung and Other Cancers, Heart Disease, Stroke, and Respiratory Disorders, Such as Emphysema and Chronic Bronchitis

Along with Information about Smoking Prevention Programs, Suggestions for Achieving and Maintaining a Smoke-Free Lifestyle, Statistics about Tobacco Use, Reports on Current Research Initiatives, a Glossary of Related Terms, and Directories of Resources for Additional Help and Information

Edited by Karen Bellenir. 595 pages. 2004. 978-0-7808-0323-7.

"**Provides everything needed for the student or general reader seeking practical details on the effects of tobacco use.**"
—*The Bookwatch, Mar '05*

"**Public libraries and consumer health care libraries will find this work useful.**"
—*American Reference Books Annual, 2005*

SEE ALSO *Respiratory Disorders Sourcebook, 2nd Edition*

Sports Injuries Sourcebook, 3rd Edition

Basic Consumer Health Information about Sprains and Strains, Fractures, Growth Plate Injuries, Overtraining Injuries, and Injuries to the Head, Face, Shoulders, Elbows, Hands, Spinal Column, Knees, Ankles, and Feet, and with Facts about Heat-Related Illness, Steroids and Sport Supplements, Protective Equipment, Diagnostic Procedures, Treatment Options, and Rehabilitation

Along with a Glossary of Related Terms and a Directory of Resources for Additional Help and Information

Edited by Sandra J. Judd. 623 pages. 2007. 978-0-7808-0949-9.

SEE ALSO Fitness and Exercise Sourcebook, 3rd Edition, Podiatry Sourcebook, 2nd Edition

Stress-Related Disorders Sourcebook, 2nd Edition

Basic Consumer Health Information about Stress and Stress-Related Disorders, Including Types of Stress, Sources of Acute and Chronic Stress, the Impact of Stress on the Body's Systems, and Mental and Emotional Health Problems Associated with Stress, Such as Depression, Anxiety Disorders, Substance Abuse, Posttraumatic Stress Disorder, and Suicide

Along with Advice about Getting Help for Stress-Related Disorders, Information about Stress Management Techniques, a Glossary of Stress-Related Terms, and a Directory of Resources for Additional Help and Information

Edited by Amy L. Sutton. 608 pages. 2007. 978-0-7808-0996-3.

"Accessible to the lay reader. Highly recommended for medical and psychiatric collections."
—*Library Journal, Mar '08*

"Well-written for a general readership, the 2nd Edition of Stress-Related Disorders Sourcebook is a useful addition to the health reference literature."
—*American Reference Books Annual, 2008*

SEE ALSO Mental Health Disorders Sourcebook, 4th Edition

Stroke Sourcebook, 2nd Edition

Basic Consumer Health Information about Stroke, Including Ischemic, Hemorrhagic, and Mini Strokes, as Well as Risk Factors, Prevention Guidelines, Diagnostic Tests, Medications and Surgical Treatments, and Complications of Stroke

Along with Rehabilitation Techniques and Innovations, Tips on Staying Healthy and Maintaining Independence after Stroke, a Glossary of Related Terms, and a Directory of Resources for Stroke Survivors and Their Families

Edited by Amy L. Sutton. 626 pages. 2008. 978-0-7808-1035-8.

"An encyclopedic handbook on stroke that is written in a language the layperson can understand... This is one of the most helpful, readable books on stroke. This volume is highly recommended and should be in every medical, hospital and public library; in addition, every family practitioner should have a copy in his or her office."
—*American Reference Books Annual, 2009*

SEE ALSO Brain Disorders Sourcebook, 3rd Edition, Hypertension Sourcebook

Surgery Sourcebook, 2nd Edition

Basic Consumer Health Information about Common Inpatient and Outpatient Surgeries, Including Critical Care and Trauma, Gastrointestinal, Gynecologic and Obstetric, Cardiac and Vascular, Neurologic, Ophthalmologic, Orthopedic, Reconstructive and Cosmetic, and Other Major and Minor Surgeries

Along with Information about Anesthesia and Pain Relief Options, Risks and Complications, Postoperative Recovery Concerns, and Innovative Surgical Techniques and Tools, a Glossary of Related Terms, and a Directory of Additional Resources

Edited by Amy L. Sutton. 645 pages. 2008. 978-0-7808-1004-4.

"Large public libraries and medical libraries would benefit from this material in their reference collections."
—*American Reference Books Annual, 2009*

SEE ALSO Cosmetic and Reconstructive Surgery Sourcebook, 2nd Edition

Thyroid Disorders Sourcebook

Basic Consumer Health Information about Disorders of the Thyroid and Parathyroid Glands, Including Hypothyroidism, Hyperthyroidism, Graves Disease, Hashimoto Thyroiditis, Thyroid Cancer, and Parathyroid Disorders, Featuring Facts about Symptoms, Risk Factors, Tests, and Treatments

Along with Information about the Effects of Thyroid Imbalance on Other Body Systems, Environmental Factors That Affect the Thyroid Gland, a Glossary, and a Directory of Additional Resources

Edited by Joyce Brennfleck Shannon. 573 pages. 2005. 978-0-7808-0745-7.

"Recommended for consumer health collections."
—*American Reference Books Annual, 2006*

"Highly recommended pick for Basic Consumer health reference holdings at all levels."
—*The Bookwatch, Aug '05*

SEE ALSO Endocrine and Metabolic Disorders Sourcebook, 2nd Edition

Transplantation Sourcebook

Basic Consumer Health Information about Organ and Tissue Transplantation, Including Physical and Financial Preparations, Procedures and Issues Relating to Specific Solid Organ and Tissue Transplants, Rehabilitation, Pediatric Transplant Information, the Future of Transplantation, and Organ and Tissue Donation

Along with a Glossary and Listings of Additional Resources

Edited by Joyce Brennfleck Shannon. 610 pages. 2002. 978-0-7808-0322-0.

"Recommended for libraries with an interest in offering consumer health information."
—*E-Streams, Jul '02*

"This is a unique and valuable resource for patients facing transplantation and their families."
—*Doody's Review Service, Jun '02*

Traveler's Health Sourcebook

Basic Consumer Health Information for Travelers, Including Physical and Medical Preparations, Transportation Health and Safety, Essential Information about Food and Water, Sun Exposure, Insect and Snake Bites, Camping and Wilderness Medicine, and Travel with Physical or Medical Disabilities

Along with International Travel Tips, Vaccination Recommendations, Geographical Health Issues, Disease Risks, a Glossary, and a Listing of Additional Resources

Edited by Joyce Brennfleck Shannon. 619 pages. 2000. 978-0-7808-0384-8.

"Recommended reference source."
—*Booklist, Feb '01*

"This book is recommended for any public library, any travel collection, and especially any collection for the physically disabled."
—*American Reference Books Annual, 2001*

SEE ALSO Worldwide Health Sourcebook

Urinary Tract and Kidney Diseases and Disorders Sourcebook, 2nd Edition

Basic Consumer Health Information about the Urinary System, Including the Bladder, Urethra, Ureters, and Kidneys, with Facts about Urinary Tract Infections, Incontinence, Congenital Disorders, Kidney Stones, Cancers of the Urinary Tract and Kidneys, Kidney Failure, Dialysis, and Kidney Transplantation

Along with Statistical and Demographic Information, Reports on Current Research in Kidney and Urologic Health, a Summary of Commonly Used Diagnostic Tests, a Glossary of Related Terms, and a Directory of Resources for Additional Help and Information

Edited by Ivy L. Alexander. 621 pages. 2005. 978-0-7808-0750-1.

"A good choice for a consumer health information library or for a medical library needing information to refer to their patients."
—*American Reference Books Annual, 2006*

SEE ALSO Prostate and Urological Disorders Sourcebook

Vegetarian Sourcebook

Basic Consumer Health Information about Vegetarian Diets, Lifestyle, and Philosophy, Including Definitions of Vegetarianism and Veganism, Tips about Adopting Vegetarianism, Creating a Vegetarian Pantry, and Meeting Nutritional Needs of Vegetarians, with Facts Regarding Vegetarianism's Effect on Pregnant and Lactating Women, Children, Athletes, and Senior Citizens

Along with a Glossary of Commonly Used Vegetarian Terms and Resources for Additional Help and Information

Edited by Chad T. Kimball. 337 pages. 2002. 978-0-7808-0439-5.

"Organizes into one concise volume the answers to the most common questions concerning vegetarian diets and lifestyles. This title is recommended for public and secondary school libraries."

—*E-Streams, Apr '03*

"Invaluable reference for public and school library collections alike."
—*Library Bookwatch, Apr '03*

"The articles in this volume are easy to read and come from authoritative sources. The book does not necessarily support the vegetarian diet but instead provides the pros and cons of this important decision... Recommended for public libraries and consumer health libraries."
—*American Reference Books Annual, 2003*

SEE ALSO *Diet and Nutrition Sourcebook, 3rd Edition*

Women's Health Concerns Sourcebook, 3rd Edition

Basic Consumer Health Information about Issues and Trends in Women's Health and Health Conditions of Special Concern to Women, Including Endometriosis, Uterine Fibroids, Menstrual Irregularities, Menopause, Sexual Dysfunction, Infertility, Cancer in Women, and Other Such Chronic Disorders as Lupus, Fibromyalgia, and Thyroid Disease

Along with Statistical Data, Tips for Maintaining Wellness, a Glossary, and a Directory of Resources for Further Help and Information

Edited by Sandra J. Judd. 679 pages. 2009. 978-0-7808-1036-5.

"This useful resource provides information about a wide range of topics that will help women understand their bodies, prevent or treat disease, and maintain health... A detailed index helps readers locate information. This is a useful addition to public and consumer health library collections"
—*ARBAOnline, Jun '09*

SEE ALSO *Breast Cancer Sourcebook, 3rd Edition, Cancer Sourcebook for Women, 4th Edition, Healthy Heart Sourcebook for Women*

Workplace Health and Safety Sourcebook

Basic Consumer Health Information about Workplace Health and Safety, Including the Effect of Workplace Hazards on the Lungs,

Skin, Heart, Ears, Eyes, Brain, Reproductive Organs, Musculoskeletal System, and Other Organs and Body Parts

Along with Information about Occupational Cancer, Personal Protective Equipment, Toxic and Hazardous Chemicals, Child Labor, Stress, and Workplace Violence

Edited by Chad T. Kimball. 610 pages. 2000. 978-0-7808-0231-5.

"As a reference for the general public, this would be useful in any library."
—*E-Streams, Jun '01*

"Provides helpful information for primary care physicians and other caregivers interested in occupational medicine... General readers; professionals."
—*CHOICE, May '01*

Worldwide Health Sourcebook

Basic Information about Global Health Issues, Including Malnutrition, Reproductive Health, Disease Dispersion and Prevention, Emerging Diseases, Risky Health Behaviors, and the Leading Causes of Death

Along with Global Health Concerns for Children, Women, and the Elderly, Mental Health Issues, Research and Technology Advancements, and Economic, Environmental, and Political Health Implications, a Glossary, and a Resource Listing for Additional Help and Information

Edited by Joyce Brennfleck Shannon. 597 pages. 2001. 978-0-7808-0330-5.

"Named an Outstanding Academic Title."
—*CHOICE, Jan '02*

"Yet another handy but also unique compilation in the extensive Health Reference Series, this is a useful work because many of the international publications reprinted or excerpted are not readily available. Highly recommended."
—*CHOICE, Nov '01*

SEE ALSO *Traveler's Health Sourcebook*

Teen Health Series
Complete Catalog
List price $69 per volume. School and library price $62 per volume.

Abuse and Violence Information for Teens

Health Tips about the Causes and Consequences of Abusive and Violent Behavior

Including Facts about the Types of Abuse and Violence, the Warning Signs of Abusive and Violent Behavior, Health Concerns of Victims, and Getting Help and Staying Safe

Edited by Sandra Augustyn Lawton. 411 pages. 2008. 978-0-7808-1008-2.

"A useful resource for schools and organizations providing services to teens and may also be a starting point in research projects."
—*Reference and Research Book News, Aug '08*

"Violence is a serious problem for teens... This resource gives teens the information they need to face potential threats and get help—either for themselves or for their friends."
—*American Reference Books Annual, 2009*

Accident and Safety Information for Teens

Health Tips about Medical Emergencies, Traumatic Injuries, and Disaster Preparedness

Including Facts about Motor Vehicle Accidents, Burns, Poisoning, Firearms, Natural Disasters, National Security Threats, and More

Edited by Karen Bellenir. 420 pages. 2008. 978-0-7808-1046-4.

"Aimed at teenage audiences, this guide provides practical information for handling a comprehensive list of emergencies, from sport injuries and auto accidents to alcohol poisoning and natural disasters."
—*Library Journal, Apr 1, '09*

"Useful in the young adult collections of public libraries as well as high school libraries."
—*American Reference Books Annual, 2009*

SEE ALSO *Sports Injuries Information for Teens, 2nd Edition*

Alcohol Information for Teens, 2nd Edition

Health Tips about Alcohol and Alcoholism

Including Facts about Alcohol's Effects on the Body, Brain, and Behavior, the Consequences of Underage Drinking, Alcohol Abuse Prevention and Treatment, and Coping with Alcoholic Parents

Edited by Lisa Bakewell. 410 pages. 2009. 978-0-7808-1043-3.

"This handbook, written for a teenage audience, provides information on the causes, effects, and preventive measures related to alcohol abuse among teens... The chapters are quick to make a connection to their teenage reading audience. The prose is straightforward and the book lends itself to spot reading. It should be useful both for practical information and for research, and it is suitable for public and school libraries."
—*ARBAOnline, Jun '09*

SEE ALSO *Drug Information for Teens, 2nd Edition*

Allergy Information for Teens

Health Tips about Allergic Reactions Such as Anaphylaxis, Respiratory Problems, and Rashes

Including Facts about Identifying and Managing Allergies to Food, Pollen, Mold, Animals, Chemicals, Drugs, and Other Substances

Edited by Karen Bellenir. 410 pages. 2006. 978-0-7808-0799-0.

"This is a comprehensive, readable text on the subject of allergic diseases in teenagers. 5 Stars (out of 5)!"
—*Doody's Review Service, Jun '06*

"This authoritative and useful self-help title is a solid addition to YA collections, whether for personal interest or reports."
—*School Library Journal, Jul '06*

Asthma Information for Teens, 2nd Ed.

Health Tips about Managing Asthma and Related Concerns

641

Including Facts about Asthma Causes, Triggers and Symptoms, Diagnosis, and Treatment

Edited by Kim Wohlenhaus. 400 pages. 2010. 978-0-7808-1086-0.

Body Information for Teens
Health Tips about Maintaining Well-Being for a Lifetime
Including Facts about the Development and Functioning of the Body's Systems, Organs, and Structures and the Health Impact of Lifestyle Choices

Edited by Sandra Augustyn Lawton. 458 pages. 2007. 978-0-7808-0443-2.

Cancer Information for Teens, 2nd Edition
Health Tips about Cancer Awareness, Symptoms, Prevention, Diagnosis, and Treatment
Including Facts about Common Cancers Affecting Teens, Causes, Detection, Coping Strategies, Clinical Trials, Nutrition and Exercise, Cancer in Friends or Family, and More

Edited by Karen Bellenir and Lisa Bakewell. 445 pages. 2010. 978-0-7808-1085-3.

Complementary and Alternative Medicine Information for Teens
Health Tips about Non-Traditional and Non-Western Medical Practices
Including Information about Acupuncture, Chiropractic Medicine, Dietary and Herbal Supplements, Hypnosis, Massage Therapy, Prayer and Spirituality, Reflexology, Yoga, and More

Edited by Sandra Augustyn Lawton. 407 pages. 2007. 978-0-7808-0966-6.

"This volume covers CAM specifically for teenagers but of general use also. It should be a welcome addition to both public and academic libraries."
—American Reference Books Annual, 2008

"This volume provides a solid foundation for further investigation of the subject, making it useful for both public and high school libraries."
—VOYA: Voice of Youth Advocates, Jun '07

Diabetes Information for Teens
Health Tips about Managing Diabetes and Preventing Related Complications
Including Information about Insulin, Glucose Control, Healthy Eating, Physical Activity, and Learning to Live with Diabetes

Edited by Sandra Augustyn Lawton. 410 pages. 2006. 978-0-7808-0811-9.

"A comprehensive instructional guide for teens... some of the material may also be directed towards parents or teachers. 5 stars (out of 5)!"
—Doody's Review Service, 2006

"Students dealing with their own diabetes or that of a friend or family member or those writing reports on the topic will find this a valuable resource."
—School Library Journal, Aug '06

"This text is directed to the teen population and would be an excellent library resource for a health class or for the teacher as a reference for class preparation. It can, however, serve a much wider audience. The clinical educator on diabetes may find it valuable to educate the newly diagnosed client regardless of age. It also would be an excellent reference and education tool for a preventive medicine seminar on diabetes."
—Physical Therapy, Mar '07

Diet Information for Teens, 2nd Edition
Health Tips about Diet and Nutrition
Including Facts about Dietary Guidelines, Food Groups, Nutrients, Healthy Meals, Snacks, Weight Control, Medical Concerns Related to Diet, and More

Edited by Karen Bellenir. 432 pages. 2006. 978-0-7808-0820-1.

"A very quick and pleasant read in spite of the fact that it is very detailed in the information it gives... A book for anyone concerned about diet and nutrition."
—American Reference Books Annual, 2007

SEE ALSO Eating Disorders Information for Teens, 2nd Edition

Drug Information for Teens, 2nd Edition

Health Tips about the Physical and Mental Effects of Substance Abuse

Including Information about Marijuana, Inhalants, Club Drugs, Stimulants, Hallucinogens, Opiates, Prescription and Over-the-Counter Drugs, Herbal Products, Tobacco, Alcohol, and More

Edited by Sandra Augustyn Lawton. 468 pages. 2006. 978-0-7808-0862-1.

"As with earlier installments in Omnigraphics' Teen Health Series, Drug Information for Teens is designed specifically to meet the needs and interests of middle and high school students... Strongly recommended for both academic and public libraries."
—*American Reference Books Annual, 2007*

"Solid thoughtful advice is given about how to handle peer pressure, drug-related health concerns, and treatment strategies."
—*School Library Journal, Dec '06*

SEE ALSO *Alcohol Information for Teens, 2nd Edition, Tobacco Information for Teens, 2nd Edition*

Eating Disorders Information for Teens, 2nd Edition

Health Tips about Anorexia, Bulimia, Binge Eating, And Other Eating Disorders

Including Information about Risk Factors, Diagnosis and Treatment, Prevention, Related Health Concerns, and Other Issues

Edited by Sandra Augustyn Lawton. 377 pages. 2009. 978-0-7808-1044-0.

"This handy reference offers basic information and addresses specific disorders, consequences, prevention, diagnosis and treatment, healthy eating, and more. It is written in a conversational style that is easy to understand... Will provide plenty of facts for reports as well as browsing potential for students with an interest in the topic."
—*School Library Journal, Jun '09*

"Written in a straightforward style that will appeal to its teenage audience. The author does not play down the danger of living with an eating disorder and urges those struggling with this problem to seek professional help.

This work, as well as others in this series, will be a welcome addition to high school and undergraduate libraries."
—*American Reference Books Annual, 2009*

SEE ALSO *Diet Information for Teens, 2nd Edition*

Fitness Information for Teens, 2nd Edition

Health Tips about Exercise, Physical Well-Being, and Health Maintenance

Including Facts about Conditioning, Stretching, Strength Training, Body Shape and Body Image, Sports Nutrition, and Specific Activities for Athletes and Non-Athletes

Edited by Lisa Bakewell. 432 pages. 2009. 978-0-7808-1045-7.

"This no-nonsense guide packs a great deal into its pages... This is a helpful reference for basic diet and exercise information for health reports or personal use."
—*School Library Journal, April 2009*

"An excellent source for general information on why teens should be active, making time to exercise, the equipment people might need, various types of activities to try, how to maintain health and wellness, and how to avoid barriers to becoming healthier... This would still be an excellent addition to a public library ready-reference collection or a high school health library collection."
—*American Reference Books Annual, 2009*

"This easy to read, well-written, up-to-date overview of fitness for teenagers provides excellent wellness and exercise tips, information, and directions... It is a useful tool for them to obtain a base knowledge in fitness topics and different sports."
—*Doody's Review Service, 2009*

SEE ALSO *Diet Information for Teens, 2nd Edition, Sports Injuries Information for Teens, 2nd Edition*

Learning Disabilities Information for Teens

Health Tips about Academic Skills Disorders and Other Disabilities That Affect Learning

Including Information about Common Signs of Learning Disabilities, School Issues, Learning to Live with a Learning Disability, and Other Related Issues

Edited by Sandra Augustyn Lawton. 400 pages. 2006. 978-0-7808-0796-9.

"This book provides a wealth of information for any reader interested in the signs, causes, and consequences of learning disabilities, as well as related legal rights and educational interventions... Public and academic libraries should want this title for both students and general readers."

—*American Reference Books Annual, 2006*

Mental Health Information for Teens, 3rd Edition
Health Tips about Mental Wellness and Mental Illness
Including Facts about Mental and Emotional Health, Depression and Other Mood Disorders, Anxiety Disorders, Behavior Disorders, Self-Injury, Psychosis, Schizophrenia, and More

Edited by Karen Bellenir. 400 pages. 2010. 978-0-7808-1087-7.

SEE ALSO Stress Information for Teens, Suicide Information for Teens, 2nd Edition

---

Pregnancy Information for Teens
Health Tips about Teen Pregnancy and Teen Parenting
Including Facts about Prenatal Care, Pregnancy Complications, Labor and Delivery, Postpartum Care, Pregnancy-Related Lifestyle Concerns, and More

Edited by Sandra Augustyn Lawton. 434 pages. 2007. 978-0-7808-0984-0.

Sexual Health Information for Teens, 2nd Edition
Health Tips about Sexual Development, Reproduction, Contraception, and Sexually Transmitted Infections
Including Facts about Puberty, Sexuality, Birth Control, Chlamydia, Gonorrhea, Herpes, Human Papillomavirus, Syphilis, and More

Edited by Sandra Augustyn Lawton. 430 pages. 2008. 978-0-7808-1010-5.

"This offering represents the most up-to-date information available on an array of topics including abstinence-only sexual education and pregnancy-prevention methods... The range of coverage—from puberty and anatomy to sexually transmitted diseases—is thorough and extensive. Each chapter includes a bibliographic citation, and the three back sections containing additional resources, further reading, and the index are all first-rate... This volume will be well used by students in need of the facts, whether for educational or personal reasons."

—*School Library Journal, Nov '08*

"Presents information related to the emotional, physical, and biological development of both males and females that occurs during puberty. It also strives to address some of the issues and questions that may arise... The text is easy to read and understand for young readers, with satisfactory definitions within the text to explain new terms."

—*American Reference Books Annual, 2009*

Skin Health Information for Teens, 2nd Edition
Health Tips about Dermatological Concerns and Skin Cancer Risks
Including Facts about Acne, Warts, Hives, and Other Conditions and Lifestyle Choices, Such as Tanning, Tattooing, and Piercing, That Affect the Skin, Nails, Scalp, and Hair

Edited by Edited by Kim Wohlenhaus. 418 pages. 2009. 978-0-7808-1042-6.

"The material in this work will be easily understood by teenagers and young adults. The publisher has liberally used bulleted lists and sidebars to keep the reader's attention... A useful addition to school and public library collections."

—*ARBAOnline, Oct '09*

Sleep Information for Teens
Health Tips about Adolescent Sleep Requirements, Sleep Disorders, and the Effects of Sleep Deprivation
Including Facts about Why People Need Sleep, Sleep Patterns, Circadian Rhythms, Dreaming, Insomnia, Sleep Apnea, Narcolepsy, and More

Edited by Karen Bellenir. 355 pages. 2008. 978-0-7808-1009-9.

"Clear, concise, and very readable and would be a good source of sleep information for anyone—not just teenagers. This work is highly recommended for medical libraries, public school libraries, and public libraries."
—*American Reference Books Annual, 2009*

SEE ALSO *Body Information for Teens*

▪

Sports Injuries Information for Teens, 2nd Edition
Health Tips about Acute, Traumatic, and Chronic Injuries in Adolescent Athletes
Including Facts about Sprains, Fractures, and Overuse Injuries, Treatment, Rehabilitation, Sport-Specific Safety Guidelines, Fitness Suggestions, and More

Edited by Karen Bellenir. 429 pages. 2008. 978-0-7808-1011-2.

"An engaging selection of informative articles about the prevention and treatment of sports injuries... The value of this book is that the articles have been vetted and are often augmented with inserts of useful facts, definitions of technical terms, and quick tips. Sensitive topics like injuries to genitalia are discussed openly and responsibly. This revised edition contains updated articles and defines sport more broadly than the first edition."
—*School Library Journal, Nov '08*

"This work will be useful in the young adult collections of public libraries as well as high school libraries... A useful resource for student research."
—*American Reference Books Annual, 2009*

SEE ALSO *Accident and Safety Information for Teens*

▪

Stress Information for Teens
Health Tips about the Mental and Physical Consequences of Stress
Including Information about the Different Kinds of Stress, Symptoms of Stress, Frequent Causes of Stress, Stress Management Techniques, and More

Edited by Sandra Augustyn Lawton. 392 pages. 2008. 978-0-7808-1012-9.

"Understanding what stress is, what causes it, how the body and the mind are impacted by it, and what teens can do are the general categories addressed here... The chapters are brief but informative, and the list of community-help organizations is exhaustive. Report writers will find information quickly and easily, as will those who have personal concerns. The print is clear and the format is readable, making this an accessible resource for struggling readers and researchers."
—*School Library Journal, Dec '08*

"The articles selected will specifically appeal to young adults and are designed to answer their most common questions."
— *American Reference Books Annual, 2009*

SEE ALSO *Mental Health Information for Teens, 3rd Edition*

▪

Suicide Information for Teens, 2nd Edition
Health Tips about Suicide Causes and Prevention
Including Facts about Depression, Risk Factors, Getting Help, Survivor Support, and More

Edited by Kim Wohlenhaus. 400 pages. 2010. 978-0-7808-1088-4.

SEE ALSO *Mental Health Information for Teens, 3rd Edition*

▪

Tobacco Information for Teens, 2nd Edition
Health Tips about the Hazards of Using Cigarettes, Smokeless Tobacco, and Other Nicotine Products
Including Facts about Nicotine Addiction, Nicotine Delivery Systems, Secondhand Smoke, Health Consequences of Tobacco Use, Related Cancers, Smoking Cessation, and Tobacco Use Statistics

Edited by Karen Bellenir. 400 pages. 2010. 978-0-7808-1153-9.

SEE ALSO *Drug Information for Teens, 2nd Edition*

Health Reference Series

Adolescent Health Sourcebook, 3rd Edition

Adult Health Concerns Sourcebook

AIDS Sourcebook, 4th Edition

Alcoholism Sourcebook, 3rd Edition

Allergies Sourcebook, 3rd Edition

Alzheimer Disease Sourcebook, 4th Edition

Arthritis Sourcebook, 3rd Edition

Asthma Sourcebook, 2nd Edition

Attention Deficit Disorder Sourcebook

Autism & Pervasive Developmental Disorders
Sourcebook

Back & Neck Sourcebook, 2nd Edition

Blood & Circulatory Disorders Sourcebook,
3rd Edition

Brain Disorders Sourcebook, 3rd Edition

Breast Cancer Sourcebook, 3rd Edition

Breastfeeding Sourcebook

Burns Sourcebook

Cancer Sourcebook for Women, 4th Edition

Cancer Sourcebook, 5th Edition

Cancer Survivorship Sourcebook

Cardiovascular Disorders Sourcebook,
4th Edition

Caregiving Sourcebook

Child Abuse Sourcebook

Childhood Diseases & Disorders Sourcebook,
2nd Edition

Colds, Flu & Other Common Ailments
Sourcebook

Communication Disorders Sourcebook

Complementary & Alternative Medicine
Sourcebook, 4th Edition

Congenital Disorders Sourcebook, 2nd Edition

Contagious Diseases Sourcebook

Cosmetic & Reconstructive Surgery
Sourcebook, 2nd Edition

Death & Dying Sourcebook, 2nd Edition

Dental Care & Oral Health Sourcebook,
3rd Edition

Depression Sourcebook, 2nd Edition

Dermatological Disorders Sourcebook,
2nd Edition

Diabetes Sourcebook, 4th Edition

Diet & Nutrition Sourcebook, 3rd Edition

Digestive Diseases & Disorder Sourcebook

Disabilities Sourcebook

Disease Management Sourcebook

Domestic Violence Sourcebook, 3rd Edition

Drug Abuse Sourcebook, 3rd Edition

Ear, Nose & Throat Disorders Sourcebook,
2nd Edition

Eating Disorders Sourcebook, 3rd Edition

Emergency Medical Services Sourcebook

Endocrine & Metabolic Disorders Sourcebook,
2nd Edition

Environmental Health Sourcebook, 3rd Edition

Ethnic Diseases Sourcebook

Eye Care Sourcebook, 3rd Edition

Family Planning Sourcebook

Fitness & Exercise Sourcebook, 4th Edition

Food Safety Sourcebook

Forensic Medicine Sourcebook

Gastrointestinal Diseases & Disorders
Sourcebook, 2nd Edition

Genetic Disorders Sourcebook, 3rd Edition

Head Trauma Sourcebook

Headache Sourcebook

Health Insurance Sourcebook

Healthy Aging Sourcebook

Healthy Children Sourcebook

Healthy Heart Sourcebook for Women

Hepatitis Sourcebook

Household Safety Sourcebook

Hypertension Sourcebook

Immune System Disorders Sourcebook,
2nd Edition

Infant & Toddler Health Sourcebook

Infectious Diseases Sourcebook

Injury & Trauma Sourcebook